Here are your

1995 WORLD BOOK HEALTH & MEDICAL ANNUAL Cross-Reference Tabs

For insertion in your WORLD BOOK set

The Cross-Reference Tab System is designed to help link THE WORLD BOOK HEALTH & MEDICAL ANNUAL's major articles to related WORLD BOOK articles. When you later look up some topic in your WORLD BOOK and find a Tab by the article, you will know that one of your HEALTH & MEDICAL ANNUALS has newer or more detailed information.

How to use these Tabs

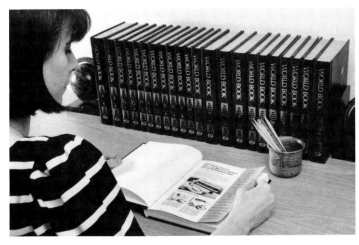

First, remove this page from THE HEALTH & MEDICAL ANNUAL.

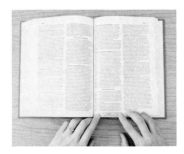

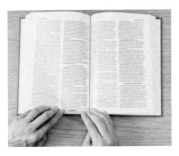

Begin with the first Tab, **ALZHEIMER'S DISEASE.** Take the *A* volume of your WORLD BOOK set and find the **ALZ-HEIMER'S DISEASE** article. Moisten the **ALZHEIMER'S DISEASE** tab and affix it to that page by the article.

Glue all the other Tabs in the appropriate WORLD BOOK volumes.

Special Report
ALZHEIMER'S DISEASE
1995 Health & Medical Annual, p. 202

Health Matters
BURN
1995 Health & Medical Annual, p. 36

Health Matters
CATARACT
1995 Health & Medical Annual, p. 32

Special Report
CHILD
1995 Health & Medical Annual, p. 74

Special Report
DIABETES
1995 Health & Medical Annual, p. 160

Special Report
DISEASE
1995 Health & Medical Annual, p. 44

Special Report
DIZZINESS
1995 Health & Medical Annual, p. 188

Health Matters
FAT
1995 Health & Medical Annual, p. 16

Health Studies
GENETICS
1995 Health & Medical Annual, p. 218

Health Matters
HEALTH CARE PLANS
1995 Health & Medical Annual, p. 20

Special Report
MENTAL ILLNESS
1995 Health & Medical Annual, p. 174

Special Report
NERVOUS SYSTEM
1995 Health & Medical Annual, p. 132

Health Matters
PET
1995 Health & Medical Annual, p. 12

Health Matters
POSTURE
1995 Health & Medical Annual, p. 24

Special Report
PHYSICAL FITNESS
1995 Health & Medical Annual, p. 102

Special Report
SAFETY
1995 Health & Medical Annual, p. 146

Health Matters
SKIN
1995 Health & Medical Annual, p. 28

Special Report
SLEEP
1995 Health & Medical Annual, p. 118

Special Report
ULCER
1995 Health & Medical Annual, p. 88

Special Report
VITAMIN
1995 Health & Medical Annual, p. 60

The Year's Major Health Stories

From the announcement of a cure for most peptic ulcers to various proposals for health care reform, it was an eventful year in medicine. On these two pages are stories that *Health & Medical Annual* editors selected as among the year's most important, memorable, or promising, along with information about where to find them in the book.

The Editors

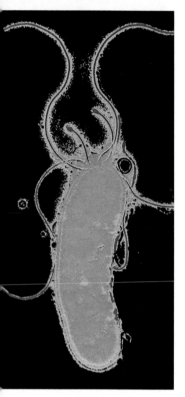

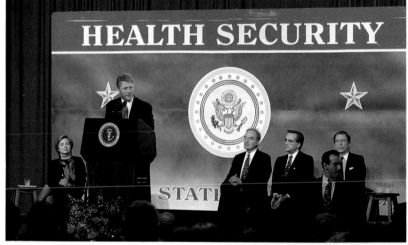

Debate over health care reform
President Bill Clinton urges support for his health care reform plan in a speech in late 1993. Debate on reform continues during 1994. In the Health & Medical News Update section, see HEALTH CARE ISSUES.

The ulcer bug
Most cases of peptic ulcers are caused by bacteria and respond to antibiotics, a panel of experts concludes in February 1994. In the Special Reports section, see BAGGING THE ULCER BUG.

Fraud in breast cancer study
Scientific misconduct is revealed in 1994 in tests of the effectiveness of a breast cancer therapy that saves the patient's breast. In the Health & Medical News Update section, see CANCER.

A genetic cause?
Researchers came closer to understanding the genetic basis of Alzheimer's disease in late 1993 and 1994. In the Special Reports section, see COPING WITH ALZHEIMER'S DISEASE. In the Health & Medical News Update section, see BRAIN AND NERVOUS SYSTEM.

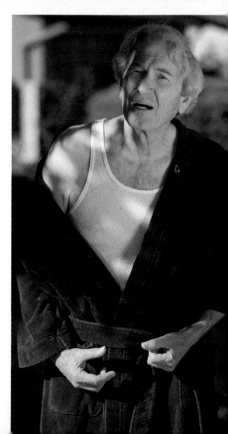

World Book, Inc.
525 W. Monroe
Chicago, IL 60661

ISBN 0-7166-1195-3
ISSN 0890-4480
Library of Congress Catalog Card Number: 87-648075
Printed in the United States of America

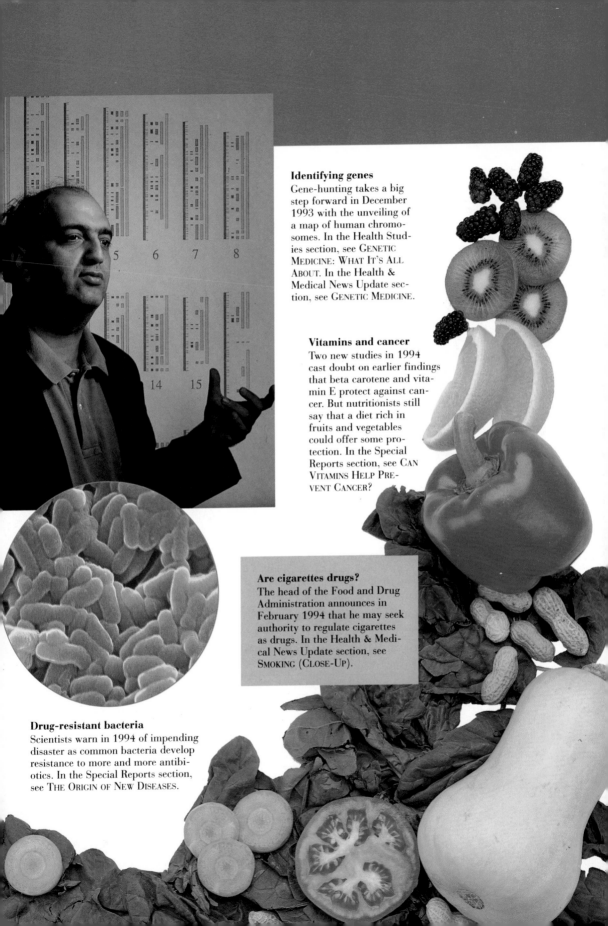

Identifying genes
Gene-hunting takes a big step forward in December 1993 with the unveiling of a map of human chromosomes. In the Health Studies section, see GENETIC MEDICINE: WHAT IT'S ALL ABOUT. In the Health & Medical News Update section, see GENETIC MEDICINE.

Vitamins and cancer
Two new studies in 1994 cast doubt on earlier findings that beta carotene and vitamin E protect against cancer. But nutritionists still say that a diet rich in fruits and vegetables could offer some protection. In the Special Reports section, see CAN VITAMINS HELP PREVENT CANCER?

Are cigarettes drugs?
The head of the Food and Drug Administration announces in February 1994 that he may seek authority to regulate cigarettes as drugs. In the Health & Medical News Update section, see SMOKING (CLOSE-UP).

Drug-resistant bacteria
Scientists warn in 1994 of impending disaster as common bacteria develop resistance to more and more antibiotics. In the Special Reports section, see THE ORIGIN OF NEW DISEASES.

Contents

The Year's Major Health Stories   2

A review of the top health stories in the news and where
to find information about them in this edition of *The World
Book Health & Medical Annual.*

Health Matters   10

Eight articles provide practical, up-to-date information on
a variety of health matters of concern to families.

Friends Indeed: Pets and Your Health	12
Which Fats Are Worse Than Others?	16
The Managed Care Prescription	20
Standing Tall: Why Posture Matters	24
A Guide to Dry Skin and Moisturizers	28
What You Should Know About Cataracts	32
Treating Burns	36
Health Information by Phone	40

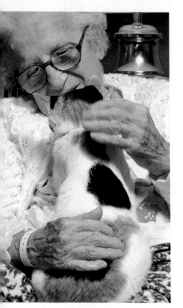

See page 12.

Special Reports   42

Feature articles present in-depth information about topics
of current interest in the fields of health and medicine.

The Origin of New Diseases by Robin Marantz Henig	44
Can Vitamins Help Prevent Cancer? by John Grossmann	60
Dr. Spock Talks About Raising Children Today A conversation with the editors	74
Bagging the Ulcer Bug by Robin Netherton	88
Exercise: The Gain Made Plain by Richard Saltus	102
Getting a Good Night's Sleep by Dianne Hales	118
New Hope for Spinal Cord Injuries by Richard Saltus	132
Home, Safe Home by Michael Woods	146

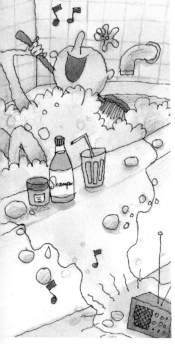

See page 153.

Understanding Type II Diabetes   160
by Mark Stolar

Medicines for the Mind   174
by Bernard Salzman

When the World Turns: Dizziness and Its Causes   188
by Bruce H. Dobkin

Coping with Alzheimer's Disease   202
by Donna Cohen

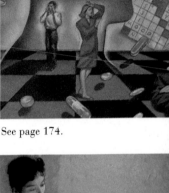

Health Studies   216

In five separate, short articles, *The World Book Health & Medical Annual* takes a look at recent advances in our understanding of genes and the diseases genes cause and at efforts to develop genetic therapies for those diseases.

Genetic Medicine: What It's All About   218
by Yvonne Baskin

See page 174.

Health & Medical News Update   238

Forty alphabetically arranged articles report on the year's major developments in health and medicine, from "Aging" and "AIDS" to "Veterinary Medicine" and "Weight Control." In addition, five Close-Up articles focus on noteworthy developments.

Defeating Prostate Cancer Through Better Detection   266

Estrogen Mimics in the Environment   288

After the Quake: Post-Traumatic Stress Disorder   318

A Genetically Engineered Cow Hormone Sparks Consumer Ire   322

A Commissioner's Crusade: Regulating Cigarettes   338

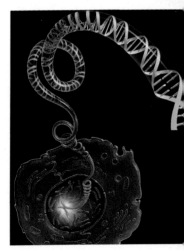

See page 210.

Index   353

A cumulative index of topics covered in the 1995, 1994, and 1993 issues of *The World Book Health & Medical Annual.*

Cross-Reference Tabs

A tear-out page of cross-reference tabs for insertion in *The World Book Encyclopedia* appears before page 1.

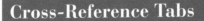

See page 219.

Staff

Editorial

Executive Editor
Darlene R. Stille

Managing Editor
Karin C. Rosenberg

Senior Editors
Meira Ben-Gad
Mary Carvlin
David L. Dreier
Mark Dunbar
Carol L. Hanson
Patricia Ohlenroth

Contributing Editors
Jinger Hoop
Rod Such

Editorial Assistant
Ethel Matthews

Cartographic Services
H. George Stoll, Head
Wayne K. Pichler

Index Services
David Pofelski

Art

Executive Director
Roberta Dimmer

**Senior Designer,
Health & Medical Annual**
Melanie J. Lawson

Senior Designers
Cari L. Biamonte
Brenda Tropinski

Contributing Artist
Isaiah Sheppard

Art Production Assistant
Stephanie Tunney

Senior Photographs Editor
Sandra M. Dyrlund

Photographs Editor
Julie Laffin

Research Services
Mary Norton, Director

Library Services
Mary Ann Urbashich, Head

Product Production
Daniel N. Bach, Vice President of
Production and Technology

Manufacturing/Pre-Press
Sandra Van den Broucke, Director
Barbara Podczerwinski
Joann Seastrom

Proofreaders
Anne Dillon
Daniel Marotta

Text Processing
Curley Hunter
Gwendolyn Johnson

Permissions Editor
Janet Peterson

Editor in Chief
W. Richard Dell

President
John E. Frere

Editorial Advisory Board

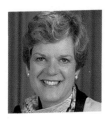

Linda H. Clever, M.D., is Chairman of the Department of Occupational Health at California Pacific Medical Center and Clinical Professor of Medicine at the University of California at San Francisco. She received the A.B. degree in 1962 and the M.D. degree in 1965, both from Stanford University. Dr. Clever served on the Board of Governors of the American College of Physicians from 1984 to 1989 and currently serves as Vice Chairman of its Board of Regents. Since 1990, she has been Editor of the *Western Journal of Medicine.* She is a member of the Institute of Medicine of the National Academy of Sciences.

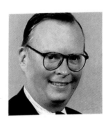

C. Anderson Hedberg, M.D., is Associate Professor of Medicine, Rush Medical College, and Senior Attending Physician at Rush-Presbyterian-St. Luke's Medical Center. Dr. Hedberg received the B.A. degree from Harvard College in 1957 and the M.D. degree from Cornell University Medical College in 1961. He is a fellow of the American College of Physicians and is a member of the American Gastroenterology Association and the Chicago Society of Internal Medicine.

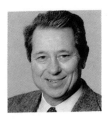

Jerome Kagan, Ph.D., is the Daniel and Amy Starch Professor of Psychology at Harvard University. He received the B.S. degree from Rutgers University in 1950 and the Ph.D. from Yale University in 1954. He received Distinguished Scientist awards from the American Psychological Association in 1987 and the Society for Research in Child Development in 1989 and was awarded the Hofheimer Prize for Research from the American Psychiatric Association in 1962. He is a fellow of the American Academy of Arts and Sciences and a member of the Institute of Medicine of the National Academy of Sciences.

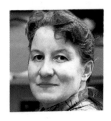

June E. Osborn, M.D., is on the faculty of the University of Michigan, where she is Professor of Epidemiology in the School of Public Health and Professor of Pediatrics and Communicable Diseases in the Medical School. Dr. Osborn received the B.A. degree from Oberlin College in 1957 and the M.D. degree from Case Western Reserve University in 1961. She was Chairman of the National Commission on AIDS from 1989 to 1993 and a member of the World Health Organization's Global Commission on AIDS from 1988 to 1992. She is a fellow of the American Academy of Pediatrics and a member of the Institute of Medicine of the National Academy of Sciences.

Contributors

Balk, Robert A., M.D.
Director of Pulmonary Medicine,
Rush-Presbyterian-St. Luke's
Medical Center.
[*Respiratory System*]

Barlough, Jeffrey E.,
D.V.M., Ph.D.
Postdoctoral Fellow,
School of Veterinary Medicine,
University of California at Davis.
[*Veterinary Medicine*]

Barone, Jeanine, M.S.
Writer and Editor,
*University of California at
Berkeley Wellness Letter.*
[Health Matters: *Which Fats Are
Worse Than Others; Nutrition and
Food*]

Baskin, Yvonne, B.A.
Free-lance Science Writer.
[Health Studies: *Genetic Medicine:
What It's All About*]

Birnbaum, Gary, M.D.
Professor of Neurology,
University of Minnesota.
[*Brain and Nervous System*]

Bowers, Kathryn E., M.D.
Clinical Instructor,
Dermatology,
Harvard Medical School.
[Health Matters: *A Guide to Dry
Skin and Moisturizers; Skin*]

Cohen, Donna, Ph.D.
Professor and Chairman, Department of Aging and Mental Health,
University of South Florida.
[Special Report: *Coping with
Alzheimer's Disease*]

Crawford, Michael H., M.D.
Chief, Division of Cardiology,
University of New Mexico
School of Medicine.
[*Heart and Blood Vessels*]

Dobkin, Bruce H., M.D.
Professor of Neurology,
University of California at
Los Angeles School of Medicine.
[Special Report: *When the World
Turns: Dizziness and Its Causes*]

Foreman, Julie, M.S.
Program Administrator,
American Medical Association.
[*Ear and Hearing; Eye and Vision;
Stroke; Surgery;* Health Matters:
*What You Should Know About
Cataracts*]

Franklin, James L., M.D.
Associate Professor of Medicine,
Rush-Presbyterian-St. Luke's
Medical Center.
[*Digestive System*]

Friedman, Emily, B.A.
Health Policy Columnist,
*Journal of the American Medical
Association.*
[*Health Care Issues*]

Gartland, John J., M.D.
Medical Editor and
Emeritus Professor of
Orthopedic Surgery,
Thomas Jefferson University.
[*Bone Disorders*]

Gerber, Glenn S., M.D.
Assistant Professor,
Division of Urology,
University of Chicago.
[Close-Up: *Cancer; Urology*]

Gourley, Mark F., M.D.
Senior Staff Fellow, National
Institute of Arthritis and Musculoskeletal and Skin Diseases.
[*Arthritis and Connective
Tissue Disorders*]

Grossmann, John, M.S.J.
Free-lance Writer.
[Special Report: *Can Vitamins Help
Prevent Cancer?*]

Hales, Dianne, M.A.
Free-lance Writer.
[Special Report: *Getting a Good
Night's Sleep;* Close-Up: *Mental
Health*]

Hamilton, Gayle R., Ph.D.
Associate Research Professor,
Center for Health Promotion,
George Mason University.
[*Alcohol and Drug Abuse;
Smoking;* Close-Up: *Smoking*]

Hart, Lynette A., Ph.D.
Director, Center for
Animals in Society,
School of Veterinary Medicine,
University of California at Davis.
[Health Matters: *Friends Indeed:
Pets and Your Health*]

Henig, Robin Marantz, B.A., B.S.
Free-lance Writer.
[Special Report: *The Origin
of New Diseases*]

Hussar, Daniel A., Ph.D.
Remington Professor of Pharmacy,
Philadelphia College of
Pharmacy and Science.
[*Drugs*]

Klippel, John, M.D.
Clinical Director, National
Institute of Arthritis and Musculoskeletal and Skin Diseases.
[*Arthritis and Connective
Tissue Disorders*]

Levine, Carol, M.A.
Executive Director,
The Orphan Project,
Fund for the City of New York.
[*Medical Ethics*]

Lewis, Ricki, Ph.D.
Adjunct Assistant Professor of
Biology, State University of
New York at Albany.
[*Weight Control*]

Maugh, Thomas H., II, Ph.D.
Science Writer,
Los Angeles Times.
[*Environmental Health*]

McInerney, Joseph D.,
M.A., M.S.
Director, Biological Sciences
Curriculum Study,
Colorado College.
[*Genetic Medicine*]

Minotti, Dominick A.,
M.D., M.P.H.
Clinical Associate
Professor of Medicine,
University of Washington
Medical Center.
[*Allergies and Asthma*]

Moore, Margaret E.,
A.M.L.S., M.P.H.
Head, Education Services,
Health Sciences Library,
University of North Carolina
at Chapel Hill.
[*Books of Health and Medicine*]

Netherton, Robin, A.B., B.J.
Free-lance Writer and Editor.
[Special Report: *Bagging the
Ulcer Bug*]

Raloff, Janet, M.S.J.
Senior Editor,
Science News magazine.
[Close-Up: *Environmental Health*]

Rinehart, Rebecca D.,
Associate Director, Publications,
American College of Obstetricians
and Gynecologists.
[*Pregnancy and Childbirth*]

Roodman, G. David,
M.D., Ph.D.
Professor of Medicine,
University of Texas
Health Science Center.
[*Blood*]

Saltus, Richard, B.A.
Science Writer,
The Boston Globe.
[Special Reports: *Exercise: The
Gain Made Plain; New Hope for
Spinal Cord Injuries*]

Salzman, Bernard, M.D.
Unit Chief, Adult Psychiatry,
Bellevue Hospital Center.
[Special Report: *Medicines
for the Mind*]

Siscovick, David S.,
M.D., M.P.H.
Associate Professor of Medicine
and Epidemiology,
University of Washington.
[*Exercise and Fitness*]

Stephenson, Joan, Ph.D.
Chief, Chicago Bureau,
International Medical News Group.
[Health Matters: *The Managed
Care Prescription*]

Stolar, Mark, B.A., M.D.
Associate Professor of
Clinical Medicine,
Northwestern University.
[Special Report: *Understanding
Type II Diabetes*]

Stone, Katherine, M.D.
Medical Epidemiologist,
Centers for Disease Control.
[*Sexually Transmitted Diseases*]

Terr, Lenore, M.D.
Clinical Professor of Psychiatry,
University of California at
San Francisco.
[*Child Development; Mental
Health*]

Thomas, Scott, B.A.
Free-lance Writer.
[Health Matters: *Standing Tall:
Why Posture Matters*]

Thompson, Jeffrey R., M.D.
Dallas Kidney Specialists;
Clinical Assistant Professor of
Medicine, University of Texas
Southwestern Medical School.
[*Kidney*]

Tideiksaar, Rein, Ph.D.
Assistant Professor,
Department of Geriatrics,
Mount Sinai Medical Center.
[*Aging*]

Trubo, Richard, M.A.
Free-lance Medical Writer.
[*AIDS; Diabetes*]

Van Herle, Andre J., M.D.
Professor of Medicine,
University of California at
Los Angeles School of Medicine.
[*Glands and Hormones*]

Voelker, Rebecca, M.S.J.
Senior Editor,
American Medical News.
[Health Matters: *Treating Burns*]

Waalen, Jill, M.S.
Free-lance Science Writer.
[*Cancer*]

Woods, Michael, B.S.
Science Editor,
The Toledo Blade.
[Special Report: *Home, Safe Home;
Dentistry; Infectious Diseases;
Safety;* Close-Up: *Nutrition*]

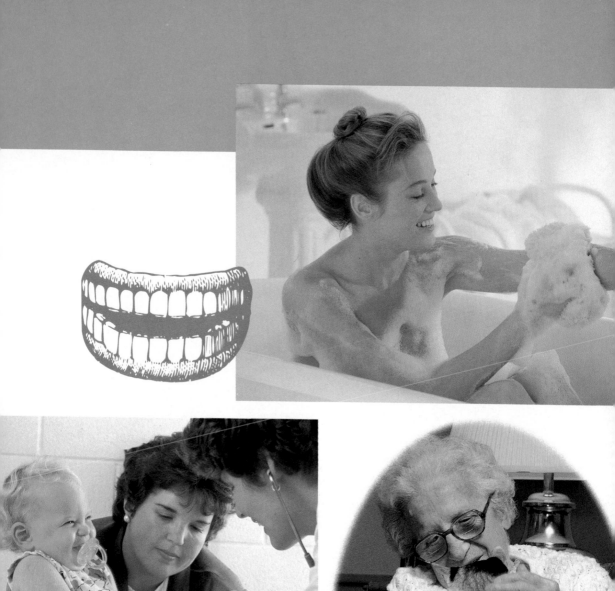
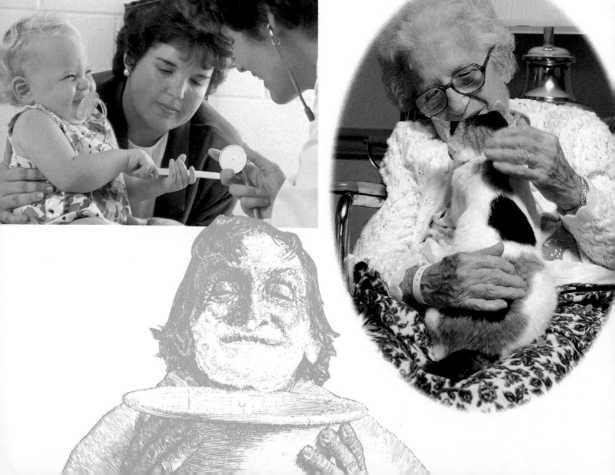

Health Matters

Eight articles present practical, up-to-date information on health topics of concern to families.

Friends Indeed: Pets and Your Health   12

Which Fats Are Worse Than Others?   16

The Managed Care Prescription   20

Standing Tall: Why Posture Matters   24

A Guide to Dry Skin and Moisturizers   28

What You Should Know About Cataracts   32

Treating Burns   36

Health Information by Phone   40

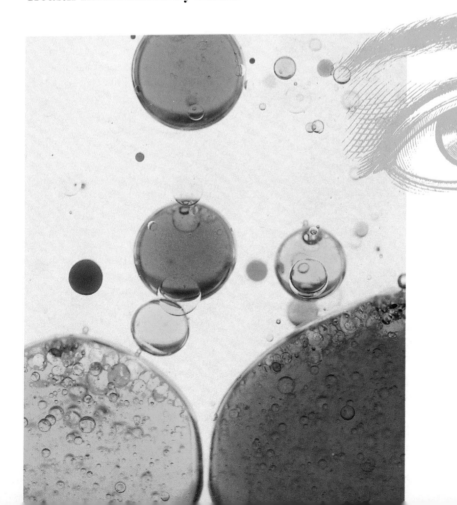

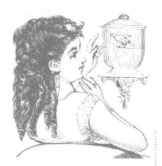

Friends Indeed: Pets and Your Health

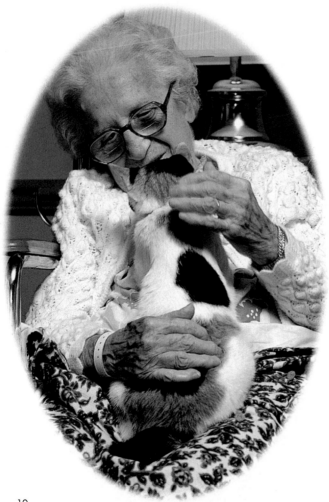

We tend to think of dogs and cats as enriching the lives of children. But many adults without children also own pets. In fact, the majority of American households have at least one dog or cat, and most people say that the love and companionship their animals provide more than offsets the cost of food and other expenses involved in maintaining the health of a furry or feathery friend. Now, scientists have found a surprise bonus in possessing a Rover or a Tabby: improved health, including a reduced risk of heart disease.

Three studies in the 1990's have investigated whether pets provide their owners with health benefits. The first study, reported in 1992, looked at blood pressure levels and levels of cholesterol and triglyceride fats in the blood of pet owners and nonowners. The researchers, Warwick Anderson and colleagues at the Baker Medical Research Institute in Australia, questioned 5,741 men and women attending a heart disease risk clinic on their lifestyle and whether they had a pet. Then, they compared screening-test results of the pet owners with the test results of the nonowners. High blood pressure and high blood levels of cholesterol and triglycerides put people at a greater-than-average risk of a heart attack.

The 784 people who owned pets, particularly the men, had significantly lower blood pressure and lower levels of triglycerides and cholesterol than the men and women without pets. On average, men who owned pets had triglyceride levels that were 13 percent lower than those of men without pets. If these low levels had been found only among dog owners, it could be as-

Potential health rewards of owning a pet

Recent studies have turned up some surprising health benefits for people who own pets, including:

- Reduced risk for heart attacks, because of lower blood pressure and lower blood levels of artery-clogging fats and cholesterol.
- Fewer headaches.
- Less difficulty sleeping.
- Fewer bouts of indigestion.
- Protection against loneliness and depression.
- Fewer physician visits following stress-producing events, such as the death of a loved one.
- A sense of optimism about the future.

sumed that exercise in the form of walking the dog had influenced the results. But the dog owners and the owners of other pets had similar test results. Owning a pet, the researchers said, was as effective in lowering blood pressure as switching to a low-salt diet or reducing alcohol consumption.

A second 1992 study evaluated the effect of owning a dog or cat on its owner's health over a period of months. James Serpell at Cambridge University in the United Kingdom recruited three groups of people who did not own a pet. They all completed questionnaires on the frequency of minor health problems, such as headaches, difficulty sleeping, and indigestion. One group then received dogs, the second group received cats, and the third group had no pets.

The three groups began the study with no significant differences in their scores on the health questionnaire. Differences began to appear after one month and continued throughout the 10-month study. The two groups with pets reported that

their general health had greatly improved, though the group with dogs fared slightly better than the group with cats. And dog ownership also meant that people got more exercise than they previously had.

Serpell's research continued in 1994 in an effort to find out if the results would hold up over a longer period of time—18 months—and among larger groups. Early results confirmed his original findings.

The third study of the health benefits of pet ownership concentrated on older people. It involved the number of medical visits made by almost 1,000 people covered by Medicare, the federal health insurance program for people receiving social security benefits. The research was reported in 1991 by epidemiologist Judith Siegel of the University of California at Los Angeles.

Siegel interviewed the participants by telephone every two months for one year. At the end of that time, she found that pet owners had reported fewer visits to the doctor than nonowners. While participants in general saw a doctor more often during stressful times—for example, after the death of a relative or friend—dog owners reported fewer such visits.

Like Serpell, Siegel found increased recreational walking among dog owners. She reported that dog owners spent an average of 1.4 hours each day outdoors with their dogs. Even cats appeared to motivate some owners to be more active than people without an animal companion.

Increased physical activity can translate into improved health in several ways: by strengthening the heart muscle and improving blood circulation and by slowing the loss of bone tissue that commonly accompanies aging. Thus, the capacity of a dog to motivate a person to increase outdoor activity may be one of the most important contributions dogs make to human health.

In addition to improving an owner's physical health, animals contribute to a sense of psychological and social well-being. And this sense of well-being may account for some of the improvements in physical health reported by various researchers throughout the 1980's. These included drops in pet owners' blood pressure when the pet was present, presumably because the pet had a soothing effect.

Other research in the 1990's has investigated the power of pets to relieve stress. For example, in 1991, Karen Allen and her colleagues at the State University of New York at Buffalo monitored women who were attempting to solve arithmetic problems. She then had friends of the participants sit in on the problem-solving sessions. This increased stress and resulted in fewer correct answers than when the women worked alone. Finally, Allen brought in the participants' dogs. The women's stress levels dropped, even though they continued to work on challenging arithmetic problems.

Other studies have shown that animals are buffers against ongoing problems, such as loneliness. An older person who lives alone, for example, may be vulnerable to loneliness or depression. Peter Peretti at Richard J. Daley College in Chicago found in 1990 that a majority of 128 older dog owners living alone reported that their dog was their only friend. And a 1986 study by John Goldmeier at the University of Maryland in Baltimore found that among 116 older women living alone, those who had pets showed a greater sense of well-being as measured by four criteria: absence of agitation, degree of optimism, absence of loneliness, and ability to think of the future.

Older people become especially vulnerable to isolation and depression after the death of a spouse. In 1989, a research group headed by Thomas Garrity at the University of Kentucky College of Medicine in Lexington found that bereaved people who had a strong attachment to a pet rarely suffered from depression, even when they lacked close friends.

Since 1988, I and my colleagues at the Center for Animals in Society at the University of California at Davis have concentrated on the socializing role of pets. In one study of older pet owners, we found that all the dog owners talked to their pets during regular walks. They often spoke to other people during these walks, focusing primarily on their dogs but also conversing on current, rather

Getting off to a good start with a new companion

Pets can trigger allergies and spread infections, and some may bite. But you can guard against such risks by taking a few precautions:

- Purchase a pet from a reliable dealer to ensure its good health or, if you prefer, choose a healthy-looking animal from a shelter. Find out what immunizations a dog or cat has had, and have a veterinarian give the animal a thorough checkup.

- Establish and follow a preventive-care program for a dog or cat that includes annual checkups for parasites, such as worms, and immunizations against disease.

- Provide a nutritious diet, fresh water, clean housing, adequate ventilation, and regular exercise to keep your pet in peak health.

- Teach children in the household how to approach and handle the pet and how to recognize the animal's warning signs.

Adapted with permission from the December 1993 *Harvard Health Letter*.

than on past, events. And neighbors stopped to talk about the dog whether the dog was present or not.

Another of our studies of older pet owners revealed that even a pet rabbit or turtle attracted adults and children who initiated conversations, though they had never met the owner. These socializing effects also applied to pet owners with disabilities. Many people feel awkward about striking up a conversation with someone in a wheelchair. But we found that people often spoke to children and adults in wheelchairs who also had dogs.

Animal companions also present some risks to the owner. Some animals bite, and pets can also transmit disease-causing viruses, bacteria, parasites, and fungi to people.

Bites are most commonly inflicted by dogs, but cats also bite. Bites pose a double threat. First, the wound itself can be painful and may require stitches. Second, infectious microbes can enter the wound from the animal's saliva and cause illness.

Dog bites can be prevented by selecting a breed known to be nonaggressive. However, if a dog behaves in an aggressive manner, immediate steps should be taken to thwart the behavior, such as giving the animal obedience training.

Pets can also transmit diseases to people without biting them. One way is through their waste. Gastrointestinal diseases caused by bacteria can be transmitted to people in the feces of infected dogs, birds, and aquarium pets such as frogs and reptiles. Cats can carry protozoa that cause toxoplasmosis. This flulike disease is very serious in a pregnant woman, because it can lead to mental retardation, blindness, and other birth defects. People may be infected if they do not wash their hands after cleaning an infected cat's litter box.

People can contract other diseases by touching an infected animal. Tularemia, a bacterial infection also known as rabbit fever, is transmitted directly through the skin by handling an infected animal or being bitten by it. Ringworm, a common fungal infection of dogs and cats, is easily acquired by touching the characteristic red, scaly rings on the animal's skin. By inhaling dust or bird excrement from the cage of an infected bird, people can develop psittacosis, a lung infection spread by parakeets, parrots, and canaries.

In some areas of the United States, people can get diseases carried by ticks that pets pick up from wild animals. Lyme disease and Rocky Mountain spotted fever are both transmitted through tick bites. And fleas are more than an itchy nuisance to Rover and Tabby: They can spread tapeworm or even bubonic plague in some areas of the country.

People also can become hosts to common parasites of dogs. Mites can burrow into human skin and bring on a rash, hair loss, and itching. Hookworms and roundworms from puppies can invade the human digestive tract.

In general, getting a disease from a pet poses a health risk primarily to children, pregnant women, the elderly, and people who have weakened immune systems. But the risks can be made negligible by observing reasonable hygiene, avoiding situations that provoke an animal to bite or scratch, and keeping the animals' veterinary care and vaccinations current. Such good friends deserve good care indeed.

☐ Lynette A. Hart

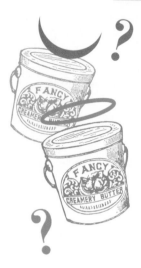

Which Fats Are Worse Than Others?

Fat has traditionally been seen as a nutritional villain. A high-fat diet has been linked with many chronic diseases, including heart disease and some forms of cancer. And because fat is packed with calories, it increases the risk of obesity.

The issue of dietary fat would seem to be quite straightforward: Eat less fat and you will be healthier. But it's not quite as simple as that, and consumers may occasionally find themselves in a quandary.

One problem is that food labels have often been misleading. Many labels boasted, for example, that a food product contained no cholesterol, which many people confuse with fat, while failing to mention that the product had a high fat content. But new federal labeling regulations, which took effect on Aug. 8, 1994, should make it easier for shoppers to compare the fat content of various products.

Another complication, however, is that not all fats are bad for us. Scientists have found that some fats serve a beneficial—indeed, an essential—role in the body and that others might actually have a protective effect against heart disease. So what are the right fats to eat?

Fats are found in both animals and plants. Most plant fats are liquid at room temperature and are called oils. These edible oils are generally more healthful than most animal fats.

Fats make up one of three primary classes of nutrients. The other two classes are carbohydrates, the nutrients we obtain from such foods as grains and beans; and proteins, which are a major constituent of meat, fish, and dairy products.

We need a certain amount of fat in our diet because it helps with the absorption of fat-soluble vitamins such as vitamins A, D, and E. Fats also contain substances called fatty acids, long strings of carbon atoms with hydrogen molecules attached to them. Some of these, known as essential fatty acids, are necessary

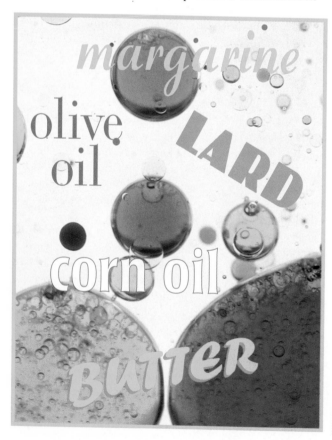

The facts on fats

Fats and oils differ widely in their nutritional content. Only animal fats, such as butter and lard, contain cholesterol. But some vegetable oils, such as coconut oil, are loaded with saturated fat, which can contribute to the development of heart disease by raising cholesterol levels in the blood. Other oils are higher in more healthful unsaturated fat. There are two kinds of unsaturated fat—monounsaturated, found in abundance in canola and olive oils, and polyunsaturated, the main constituent of corn, safflower, and soybean oils. Recent research indicates that monounsaturated fat may be better for us than polyunsaturated fat.

Fat or oil*	Calories	Cholesterol (milligrams)	Saturated fat (grams)	Polyunsaturated fat (grams)	Monounsaturated fat (grams)
Butter	100	33	7	0.4	3
Canola oil	120	0	0.8	4	9
Coconut oil	120	0	11	0.3	0.8
Corn oil	120	0	2	8	4
Lard	115	12	5	2	6
Margarine (spread)	90	0	1	5	4
Margarine (stick)	100	0	2	4	5
Olive oil	120	0	2	1	11
Palm oil	120	0	7	1	5
Peanut oil	120	0	2	5	7
Safflower oil	120	0	1	11	2
Soybean oil	120	0	2	8	3
Vegetable shortening	115	0	3	3	6

*Figures given are for one tablespoon of fat or oil. Amounts of cholesterol over one milligram per tablespoon or of saturated, polyunsaturated, or monounsaturated fat over one gram per tablespoon are rounded to the nearest whole number.

Source: United States Department of Agriculture and other sources.

for the growth and maintenance of the body.

Fatty acids vary chemically by their length and by how saturated they are. A fatty acid molecule is said to be saturated if its carbon atoms are linked to as many hydrogen atoms as possible.

A fat containing saturated fatty acid molecules is known as a saturated fat. Most saturated fats are solid at room temperature. Saturated fats are found mainly in animal-derived foods such as dairy products and meat. But palm and coconut oils are also loaded with saturated fats.

Some fatty acids, because of the way their carbon atoms bond together, have fewer bonding sites available for hydrogen atoms. Such fatty acids, and the fats containing them, are called unsaturated.

The most highly unsaturated fats—those that exclude the largest number of hydrogen atoms—are called polyunsaturated. Those fats are found in safflower, sesame, sunflower, soybean, and corn oils.

A monounsaturated fat has just one point in its carbon chain where hydrogen atoms cannot join. Canola, olive, and peanut oils are high in monounsaturated fats, as are avocados and many kinds of nuts.

A polyunsaturated oil can be made monounsaturated or saturated by artificially adding hydrogen atoms to it. This process, known as hydrogenation, is used to produce margarine and shortening from oils. Shortening (which may also be made from animal fat) is used in many commercial cookies and snack foods.

The fatty acids in hydrogenated fats have a different structure than fatty acids that formed naturally. The artificially altered molecules are known as trans fatty acids.

As if the different kinds of fats weren't enough for consumers to keep straight, there is also the matter of cholesterol to consider. Although many people think of fat and cholesterol as essentially the same, cholesterol is a different nutrient. It is a waxy, fatlike substance the body uses to insulate nerve fibers and manufacture hormones and cell walls.

Most of the cholesterol in the body is formed in the liver. But cholesterol is also present in many foods, though only in animal products, mainly eggs, meats—particularly organ meats—and dairy items.

Cholesterol comes in two main forms, one of which is good for you, the other bad. Actually, it isn't cholesterol itself that varies, but rather the molecules, called lipoproteins,

that ferry it in the bloodstream. The two molecules are called high-density lipoproteins (HDL's) and low-density lipoproteins (LDL's).

LDL's deposit cholesterol molecules in cells, and elevated levels of LDL's in the blood can promote the development of deposits in the arteries. For that reason, LDL cholesterol is known as "bad cholesterol."

HDL's, on the other hand, clear cholesterol from the bloodstream and carry it to the liver, where it is broken down into harmless compounds. Cholesterol attached to HDL molecules is thus referred to as "good cholesterol," and high levels of it in the blood are thought to be protective.

Cholesterol and fat are intimately linked in the body. That is because the fats we eat can raise the amount of LDL cholesterol in the blood and contribute to the development of heart disease. Research indicates, in fact, that fat intake plays a much greater role in raising blood cholesterol than does the consumption of cholesterol itself.

In this process, saturated fat appears to be the biggest culprit. Saturated fat apparently increases LDL cholesterol levels by suppressing the liver's ability to remove cholesterol from the bloodstream.

But even this seemingly clear-cut issue has been complicated by a study reported in 1991 by a team of scientists at the University of Texas Southwestern Medical Center in Dallas. They found that stearic acid, one of the main saturated fatty acids in beef, actually lowers LDL cholesterol levels. That doesn't mean, however, that fatty steaks should be a regular part of one's diet. Beef also contains a variety of saturated fats that can raise the levels of bad cholesterol.

Fortunately, some fats—the un-

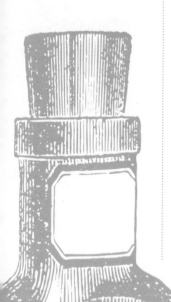

Watching for saturated fat

A number of ingredients commonly listed on food labels contain significant amounts of saturated fat:

Beef fat

Butterfat

Chicken fat

Coconut oil

Cream

Hydrogenated oil

Lard

Palm oil

Shortening

Whole-milk solids

Source: Hope Health Institute.

saturated ones—lower LDL cholesterol levels. So doctors thought that the more unsaturated a fat was, the better. Accordingly, they urged patients to use polyunsaturated oils, and margarines made from them, for all their dietary needs. That seemed like sound advice, but once again things weren't quite as simple as they seemed.

A study reported in 1993 by researchers at the Harvard School of Public Health in Boston indicated that trans fatty acids might not be good for us. The scientists analyzed data on the dietary habits of 85,000 women and compared the information with the women's medical histories. They found that the consumption of foods containing large amounts of hydrogenated oils—margarine, cookies, cake, and white bread—was associated with up to a 50 percent greater risk of suffering from heart disease. The highest association was for women who had eaten margarine daily for at least 10 years.

But even polyunsaturated fats that haven't been hydrogenated may not be as beneficial as once thought. Although these fats do lower blood levels of LDL cholesterol, they also seem to reduce levels of HDL cholesterol.

Furthermore, heart disease isn't the only risk associated with polyunsaturated fats. Animal studies have indicated that a diet high in polyunsaturated fats, like one rich in saturated fats, may increase the risk of some types of cancer. Polyunsaturated fats may also depress the body's disease-fighting immune system.

So what's the solution to this dilemma? Aren't there any fats we can eat without doing ourselves at least some harm? Of course, no fat should be eaten to excess, because too much of any fat can lead to obesity. But there is one class of fats—monounsaturated fats—that, used in moderation, may be genuinely good for us.

Scientists are taking an especially close look at olive oil, which has been used for thousands of years in countries around the Mediterranean Sea. The incidence of heart disease is relatively low in Mediterranean societies, and the prevalence of olive oil in their cuisines may be a major reason why.

Many experimental studies in both human subjects and animals have shown that when olive oil is substituted for saturated fat in the diet, the amount of LDL cholesterol in the blood drops. Moreover, that reduction occurs without a lowering of HDL cholesterol levels.

People in Mediterranean countries also eat a lot of fish, which seems to be good for the heart. Scientists have found that certain fish oils, called omega-3 fatty acids, may reduce the risk of heart disease by helping prevent the formation of blood clots in the arteries.

In sorting through the sometimes confusing and contradictory information on fats, the best policy, many doctors say, is to exercise moderation together with a bit of caution. A soft margarine, which has much less saturated fat than butter and half that of stick margarine, is a sensible choice for regular use. In selecting an oil for cooking and salad dressings, olive oil or another oil high in monounsaturated fats is probably best. And for dinner, a broiled fish filet is a more healthful choice than a steak.

□ Jeanine Barone

19

The Managed Care Prescription

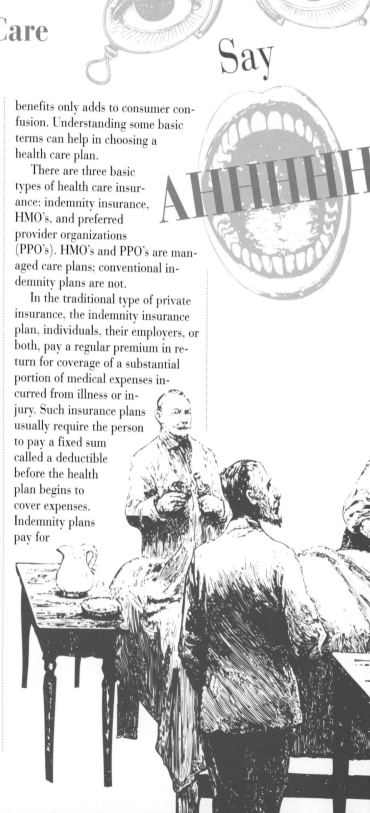

Say AHHHHHH

Even as politicians in 1994 debate proposals to reform a health care system plagued by runaway costs and inadequate medical coverage, the previous several years have already brought sweeping changes in the ways medical care is financed and delivered in the United States. Central to these changes is the concept of managed care, which most Americans are familiar with in the form of plans known as health maintenance organizations (HMO's).

The managed care approach has two major aims: to control health care costs, including doctors' fees, and to reduce the volume of unnecessary medical services. Managed care plans rely on a variety of strategies to accomplish these goals.

One strategy common to all managed care plans is that they finance and deliver health care through an organized network of providers—doctors, hospitals, and other medical professionals or organizations. Such arrangements reduce costs because the providers agree to deliver services at fixed or discounted rates.

In addition, managed care plans rely heavily on primary care physicians—medical generalists, such as family practitioners, internists, and pediatricians—who act as "gatekeepers." Gatekeepers approve a visit to a medical specialist only when they believe the patient needs such care.

The array of available options in health care coverage can be confusing, and a mixing and matching of benefits only adds to consumer confusion. Understanding some basic terms can help in choosing a health care plan.

There are three basic types of health care insurance: indemnity insurance, HMO's, and preferred provider organizations (PPO's). HMO's and PPO's are managed care plans; conventional indemnity plans are not.

In the traditional type of private insurance, the indemnity insurance plan, individuals, their employers, or both, pay a regular premium in return for coverage of a substantial portion of medical expenses incurred from illness or injury. Such insurance plans usually require the person to pay a fixed sum called a deductible before the health plan begins to cover expenses. Indemnity plans pay for

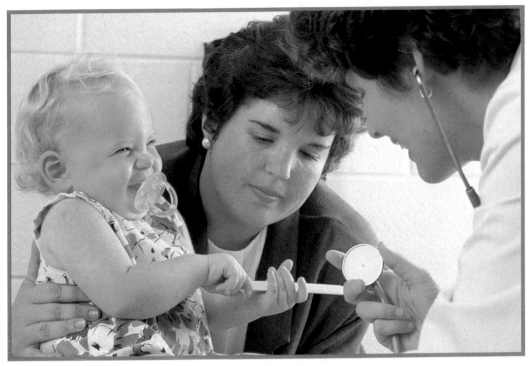

Many managed care plans emphasize such preventive medical services as well-baby care.

services related to serious illnesses up to a fixed amount, and the individual pays any expenses after that fixed amount.

Indemnity insurance plans generally pay providers a fee for each service performed, as long as the type of care is included in the plan's stated benefits. This is called fee-for-service.

Indemnity insurance plans have several drawbacks. The plans generally exclude routine physical examinations and screening tests, such as Pap smears and vision tests. In addition, they often do not cover medical conditions that existed before the person joined the plan. Patients also typically have greater out-of-pocket costs with indemnity insurance plans.

At the same time, indemnity plans have some advantages. Patients in these plans have freedom to choose physicians and hospitals. And

physicians paid under these plans generally enjoy greater independence in medical decision making than they do under managed care plans.

Indemnity plans, however, have provided little incentive for doctors to limit the services they recommend or deliver to patients, or for patients to consider the cost of their care. For many years, insurance companies also had little incentive to control rising medical costs, because they could pass the expense along to consumers by raising premium rates or by reducing benefits.

The continued escalation of medical costs as well as competition from other types of insurance plans has prompted some indemnity insurers to implement managed care strategies. Some of these insurers now require that patients obtain approval for certain procedures, either from the insurance company itself or from a utilization review firm that assesses a patient's case

21

and decides whether a recommended course of action—such as a diagnostic test, surgery, or a hospital stay—is medically necessary.

In an HMO, members or their employers pay a regular, set fee and receive coverage not only for illnesses but also for certain diagnostic tests, routine physical exams, and vaccinations. In general, people who choose HMO's believe they receive better benefits for their premiums than if they had indemnity plans, and they are spared the bother of insurance claim forms.

HMO patients generally have more modest out-of-pocket expenses because HMO's usually do not require a deductible and because they require only a small copayment from the patient for office visits and drugs. Preventive measures, such as well-baby care, mammograms, Pap smears, and cholesterol screenings, may also be covered.

Standard HMO's have a significant drawback, however. Members of these HMO's are usually covered only if they use doctors or medical facilities designated by the plan.

But not all HMO's are alike. Some plans, called open-ended HMO's or point-of-service (POS) plans, offer members the option of using providers outside the plan, though the plans cover a reduced portion of the cost. Some plans provide service in HMO-staffed health centers, whereas others contract with independent doctors who also can see patients outside the plan.

HMO's generally pay doctors a fixed amount for each patient they serve, regardless of the type and number of services actually provided to the patient. This system of payment is called capitation.

PPO's combine features of indemnity insurance and of HMO's. A PPO is a network of doctors and hospitals that provides services to an insurance company or an employer at a discounted rate. People who join a basic PPO can see any doctor in the plan, including specialists, whenever they need to. They may choose to see a doctor outside the network, but they will incur greater out-of-pocket expenses if they do so. PPO's also may require approval from the plan's ad-

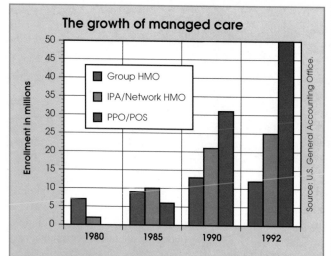

The growth of managed care

Enrollment in millions

- Group HMO
- IPA/Network HMO
- PPO/POS

1980   1985   1990   1992

Source: U.S. General Accounting Office.

The most common managed care plans today are the health maintenance organization (HMO) and the preferred provider organization (PPO). HMO's and PPO's also offer various plans.

HMO: A plan that covers physical examinations, screening tests, and medical treatment for a fixed monthly or yearly fee. Patients use only doctors and hospitals affiliated with the HMO. An HMO may be organized as a group practice, known as a group-model HMO, or as an individual practice association (IPA).

Group-model HMO: An HMO in which physicians have offices at a clinic run by the HMO.

Individual practice association (IPA) or **network HMO:** An HMO in which independent doctors provide services in their own offices.

PPO: A network of doctors and hospitals that offers a discount to the organization that contracts for their services, usually an employer or an insurance company. A patient may choose any doctor within the network.

Point-of-service (POS) plan: A PPO that permits a patient to use physicians outside the network, though the patient pays the difference between the "preferred provider's" discounted fee and the outside physician's fee. Some HMO's also offer this plan.

ministrators for expensive tests or major procedures.

Not all PPO's are alike. For example, a gatekeeper PPO requires members to choose a primary-care physician, just as an HMO does. An exclusive-provider organization (EPO) pays no benefits for health care that a member obtains outside the network.

Another type of managed care consists of specialized networks that provide services only for specific types of medical problems, such as substance abuse or mental illness. Employers purchase services from these networks at discounted rates. Employees can seek treatment outside the network, but the program will cover less of their costs.

There are other potential drawbacks to managed care plans besides the restricted choice of physicians. For example, a patient needing emergency care might be allowed to go to a hospital or physician outside the network, but plan administrators could disagree with the patient as to what constitutes an emergency and pay only part or none of the bill. To avoid such situations, patients and their family members need to know their plan's rules and, if required, get approval before heading to a hospital or other provider.

Critics of managed care plans also charge that measures aimed at pressuring physicians to be cost-efficient create an incentive to undertreat patients. For example, some plans give doctors bonuses for holding down costs. And in plans that pay by the patient, a doctor can lose money if the cost of caring for the patient exceeds the fixed payment. Doctors can be penalized financially if they send too many patients to hospitals or specialists.

Some HMO patients complain

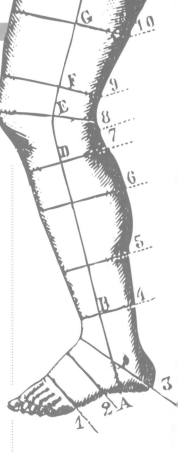

that instead of enjoying a traditional, long-term relationship with a family doctor, they are forced to switch physicians if their doctor leaves the plan. Other patients contend that they have to wait weeks for nonemergency appointments, though one nationwide survey of HMO members suggests that they wait only slightly longer for a doctor's appointment than people with traditional insurance do.

Physicians working for managed care plans have their own trade-offs. Many doctors, particularly specialists, do not mind charging less money than they otherwise would to ensure a steady stream of patients. Others, notably family physicians, can earn more because of the demand for their services as primary caregivers.

A major drawback to managed care for doctors is the erosion of their independence in making medical decisions. Many physicians in managed care systems find themselves burdened by negotiations with insurance companies and utilization review firms to justify diagnostic tests or treatment that they believe their patients need.

Managed care has generally been an important feature in the health care proposals put forth in the national political arena. Although the individual proposals continue to be the subject of endless debate, most health policy experts agree that managed care is a feature that is here to stay.

The managed care approach to meeting our nation's health needs is still in the developmental stage. Whether it will ultimately achieve one of its major goals, which is to control our soaring health care costs, remains to be seen.

☐ Joan Stephenson

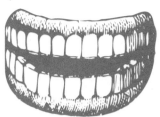

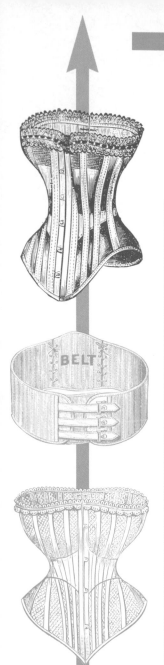

Standing Tall: Why Posture Matters

Parents have probably always admonished children, especially adolescents, to stand up straight. This parental anxiety over posture is usually less a concern about good health than about body language. A slouching adolescent, after all, is not exactly putting his or her best foot forward. A person with slumping shoulders appears downhearted and insecure, whereas someone who stands tall conveys an air of assurance and self-confidence. And children who develop poor posture habits tend to carry these habits—along with the image they express—into adulthood.

But doctors have long recognized a connection between a person's posture and his or her health. Poor posture can improperly distribute weight on the muscles and joints, which may contribute to chronic back pain. In 1741, a French physician suggested that lifelong suffering could be avoided if poor posture were corrected in childhood. But even correcting the habit of bad posture in adulthood can bring relief from disabling aches and pains.

Posture simply means the body's position while sitting, standing, or moving. An individual's posture depends on the degree to which muscles—especially those in the legs, abdomen, and back—succeed in holding the body upright against the force of gravity, which constantly pulls the body downward. Essentially, a person has good posture when body weight is evenly balanced around the body's center of gravity, located in the lower back and pelvis.

In someone with well-balanced posture while standing, the earlobes, shoulders, center of the hips, back of the kneecaps, and ankle joints form a straight, vertical line. Behind the neck and lower back, there should be slight inward curves, and the chin should be parallel to the ground. In good sitting posture, body weight should be supported by the hips and the backs of the thighs, so that the earlobes, shoulders, and hips form a straight line.

Slouching is the most common form of poor posture. When a person slouches, the shoulders roll forward and the head slumps, straining the upper back and neck. Slouching shortens the chest muscles, thereby reducing their flexibility. Slouching also compresses the *diaphragm* (the chief muscle used in breathing), and it leaves less room for the lungs to expand.

Some people who slouch, especially those with weak abdominal muscles, also thrust the stomach forward, creating a swayback—an exaggerated curve in the backbone

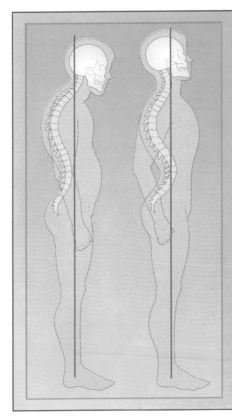

Evaluating your posture

People who feel too tall or who have insufficient muscle strength in the back and abdomen may slouch, rolling the shoulders forward and, sometimes, thrusting the lower back inward and the stomach out, *far left*. In the so-called military posture, the knees lock and the head and shoulders are pulled back, creating an unnatural sway in the spine, *near left*. You may be following one of these poor posture habits if you answer no to the following questions.

Standing sideways in front of a mirror:

- Draw an imaginary line through the earlobe, the front of the shoulder, the center of the hip, the kneecap, and the front of the ankle. Is the line straight and vertical?
- Are there slight inward curves behind the neck and lower back and a slight outward curve behind the upper back?
- Is the bottom of the chin parallel to the floor?

Ask the same questions when sitting in a straight, armless chair, checking for an imaginary vertical line from the earlobe to the hip.

Adapted with permission from the *University of California at Berkeley Wellness Letter*, March 1992.

between the pelvis and ribs. In an extreme example of swayback posture, a condition called lordosis, the chest and upper back appear to lean backward. The swayback stance exerts tremendous pressure on the lower back and can result in serious back problems.

Another form of poor posture is the so-called military stance, which many people mistakenly regard as an example of very good posture. In the military stance, the head and shoulders are thrust stiffly back and the knees are locked, creating an exaggerated curve in the lower back. Like the swayback posture, the military stance puts significant strain on the muscles of the spine.

You can check the curves in your upper and lower spine by standing against a door or wall with your heels about 3 inches (8 centimeters) from the base. Place your right hand, palm out, behind your waist, and your left hand, palm in, behind your neck. If you are standing properly, your hands should nearly fill the hollows.

To evaluate your posture from the front, stand or sit while facing a full-length mirror. Your shoulders should rest at an equal height, your knees should face forward, and your ankles should be straight. For additional ways to check your posture, see the box above.

If you do have poor posture, one reason may be a physical disorder. For instance, injury to the ligaments that support the bones of the spine can curve the back unnaturally and reduce flexibility. Bone disorders that affect older people, such as *osteoporosis* (a thinning of bone tissue), can sometimes give rise to a "hunchback," known in medical terms as kyphosis. Arthritis also can cause posture problems in older adults.

In children over the age of 9, poor posture can be a sign of scoliosis, a bone disorder marked by a side-to-side curve in the spine. Although mild scoliosis usually does not require treatment, more severe cases can lead to deformity if not treated before the child's skeleton has stopped developing during adolescence. Doctors usually prescribe a back brace to treat moderate scoliosis, though surgery may be needed to straighten the spine in severe cases. A physician should examine any child with habitual poor posture to rule out scoliosis or other physical abnormalities.

While physical conditions cause some cases of poor posture, experts agree that most posture problems result from bad habits or poor physical fitness. According to physical therapists, weak, unsupple muscles in the abdomen and the upper body are the leading cause of poor posture. Sagging abdominal muscles, for example, push the pelvis down and back. The resulting pelvic rotation can throw the spine out of line, causing swayback. Overweight people and pregnant women who lack muscle tone in the back and abdomen are also likely to develop swayback.

In many cases, poor posture is simply the result of years of positioning the body incorrectly, by habitually slumping down in deep chairs, for instance, or by leaning over a desk. People whose work requires them to sit for long periods, bend over frequently, or carry abnormally heavy loads may slouch as they try to relieve back strain incurred on the job. And for women,

regularly wearing high-heeled shoes can throw the body out of balance, forcing the back to arch unnaturally and the heel (Achilles) tendon to shorten, making it uncomfortable to wear flat-heeled shoes.

The good news, according to physicians and physical education experts, is that most common posture problems can be reversed by a combination of simple exercises and practice. To strengthen weak abdominal muscles, for instance, experts recommend this easy-to-do exercise: Simply tighten your stomach muscles for as long as 30 seconds, then release. Repeat the procedure three or four times, several times a day.

Experts also recommend a number of other simple strategies for improving posture. The most important one is: Think tall. Stretch to your full height by imagining a string attached to the top of your head, pulling it upward. Do this throughout the day, whether you are standing, sitting, or walking.

If you must stand in one place for long periods, you can reduce the strain on your lower back by shifting your weight from one foot to the other. Placing one foot on a low stool or other object about 8 inches (20 centimeters) off the floor helps reduce strain on the lower back.

When sitting, choose a straight chair and press your shoulders firmly against the chair back, keeping your upper back straight. Rest both feet on the floor or on a footstool, preferably with the knees slightly higher than the hips. If you cross your legs, cross them at the ankles, not at the knees. Try to get up and move about every 30 to 40 minutes. Place work at a comfortable height to minimize stress on

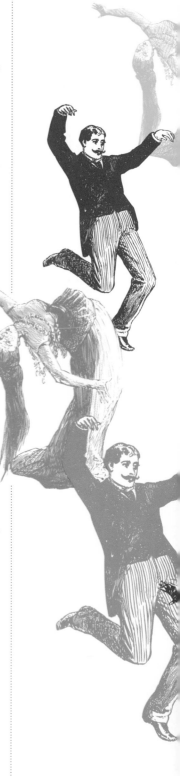

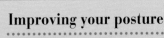

Improving your posture

When the body is properly aligned, the earlobe, shoulder, center of the hip, kneecap, and ankle should form a straight line, *right*. The following tips can help correct poor posture.

- Imagine a string attached to the top of the head, pulling it upward. Relax the shoulders and let them drop.
- To practice correct posture, stand against a wall with the head straight, chin tucked in, and feet slightly apart, then tilt the hips so the lower back moves closer to the wall.
- Strengthen the abdominal muscles by slowly tightening them, then holding the position for several seconds before relaxing. Repeat three or four times.
- When sitting, use a straight-backed chair. Keep the upper back straight and the knees slightly higher than the hips. A rolled-up towel or small, firm pillow can provide extra lower-back support. Get up every half-hour to stretch and change position.
- Sleep on a firm mattress. If possible, sleep on your side, keeping the knees bent. Choose a pillow that supports the neck and keeps it straight.

Adapted with permission from the *University of California at Berkeley Wellness Letter*, March 1992.

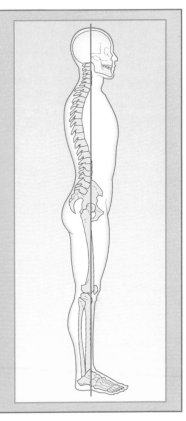

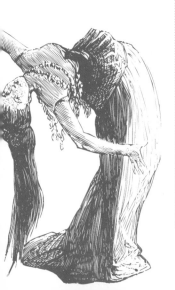

your neck, shoulders, upper back, elbows, and wrists.

To maintain good posture while walking, let the heel of the leading leg touch the ground first, then shift the body's weight forward to the toes. Swing the legs easily from the hips, and keep the torso relaxed to decrease jarring. Let the arms swing gently from the shoulders.

You can also help reduce back strain by watching your posture when bending down or lifting heavy loads. Start by bending from the knees, never the waist. When lifting something, stand up slowly, keeping the object close to you. Turn from the feet, not the waist, if you have to turn while holding the object.

If you experience chronic back or neck pain that your own efforts fail to correct, see your doctor or an *orthopedist* (specialist in disorders of the bones and joints). The doctor

may recommend a physical therapy program to help you realign misplaced bones, muscles, and joints.

Maintaining correct posture is a simple way to encourage good health and to project a positive image. Moreover, psychologists suggest that good posture not only suggests self-confidence but instills it as well. People who stand up straight look better to others and feel better about themselves.

The best news about good posture, however, is that it may be the world's easiest diet and cheapest face-lift. According to beauty experts, standing tall lends a more youthful appearance and can give the impression of a 5-to-7 pound (2-to-3 kilogram) weight loss. With health, youth, and beauty at stake, parents' perennial advice to teenagers is well worth following.

☐ Scott Thomas

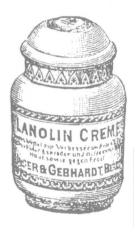

A Guide to Dry Skin and Moisturizers

Dry skin, known medically as xerosis, is one of the most common skin disorders and one that I and my colleagues in the field of dermatology often see. Although dry skin becomes more likely in a cold climate or with old age, it can afflict almost anybody. Despite being a frequent source of distress and discomfort, the condition can be treated easily and inexpensively.

Extremely dry skin consists of rough, flaky scales that send out annoying sensations of burning or itching. The reasons for itching are only partially understood, but it occurs when something stimulates nerve endings beneath the skin's surface. Scratching provides temporary relief because it disturbs the nerve endings even more, momentarily drowning out the initial irritation. Scratching is never a good idea, however, because it can open the skin to infection.

When your skin is in this sensitive state, many things can make it feel worse. The clothes you wear, for example, may either irritate or soothe it. Wool and polyester often intensify itching. Some people who notice this assume they are allergic

Although a steaming bath may relieve the itching of dry skin temporarily, hot water dries the skin further by stripping surface oils. Applying moisturizer to skin that's still damp helps seal in water absorbed during a bath.

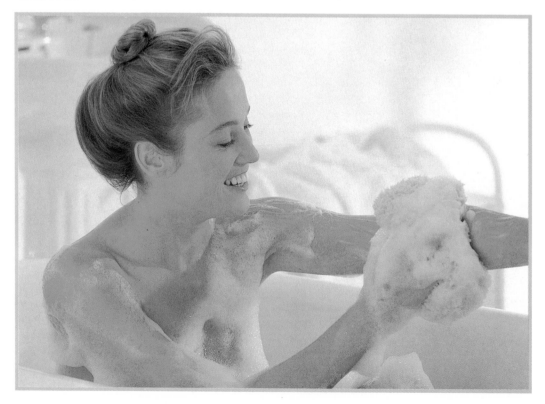

to wool, when the wool is merely irritating their already-sensitive skin.
Cotton and silk, on the other hand,
usually feel good against the skin.

Stress can aggravate dry, itchy
skin, in part by lowering the thresh-
old at which irritation sets in. Even
undressing and hopping into bed
can make matters worse, probably
because air currents stimulate the
skin's nerve endings and because
warm bedclothes are an irritant.

Whether your skin feels dry or
moist depends on the condition of its
outermost cells, which make up the
stratum corneum, or horny layer.
Cells of the stratum corneum are
dead, yet they prevent dryness by
trapping water. For your skin to appear and feel normal, these cells
must consist of at least 10 percent
water. Water enters these cells from
both inside and outside the body.
Blood vessels provide water that
spreads through the skin's three layers, reaches the surface, and evaporates. The skin secretes oils that help
seal in moisture. How quickly water
travels through your skin, and how
quickly it evaporates, determines
your skin's degree of moistness. Dry
skin is much less common during
humid weather than during cold, because less water escapes and evaporates when humidity is high.

As skin ages, it is less able to retain moisture. The skin's top layer,
or epidermis, thins with age, leaving
fewer cells to capture water. Older
skin also produces less oil. For
these reasons, dry skin is common among older people. Some
studies have found that
100 percent of people over
the age of 80 have dry skin.
Certain medicines can dry out
skin. They include H$_2$-
blockers (used to
treat stomach ul-
cers), lithi-

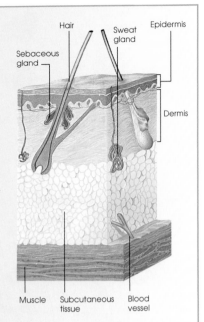

Inside the skin
Your skin's three layers
of tissue—the epider-
mis, dermis, and subcu-
taneous tissue—each
help keep it moist. The
epidermis absorbs wa-
ter from outside the
body and prevents wa-
ter from escaping.
Sebaceous glands
within the dermis se-
crete an oil that limits
water evaporation
from the skin. The sub-
cutaneous layer con-
tains blood vessels that
bring water to the skin.

um (used for manic-depressive illness), and phenothiazines (used for
nausea or psychiatric disorders).
Dry skin occasionally is caused by
an underlying illness or condition,
including malnutrition, vitamin A
deficiency, diabetes, an underactive
thyroid gland, and certain liver and
kidney diseases.

Dry skin can be accompanied by
dermatitis, an inflammation that
makes the skin red and itchy and
sometimes swollen and crusted.
Dermatitis can develop in response
to harsh detergents or other chemical agents. New parents—who dip
their hands into soapy water frequently—often develop painful
dermatitis on their hands. Dermatitis also can result from an allergic reaction. It's a good idea to
consult a dermatologist if you
see signs of dermatitis.

To treat dry skin, you must
increase the amount of water in
the stratum corneum. Your
skin soaks up water
during a bath or
shower, though

How to avoid dry skin

- During cold weather, drink lots of water and use a humidifier.
- Use a sunscreen with a protective factor of between 15 and 30 when going out in the sun, even during winter.
- Avoid hot water. Apply moisturizer over the entire skin after a bath or shower.
  - Choose a moisturizing soap or nonsoap skin cleanser. Rinse well after use.
  - Use an oil-in-water moisturizer during warm weather or if you have oily skin. Use a water-in-oil moisturizer during cold weather or if you have dry skin.
  - Check moisturizers for ingredients that can irritate the skin, such as fragrance or preservatives.
  - To minimize the itching that accompanies dry skin, wear clothes made from nonirritating fibers such as cotton and silk. Common irritants include wool and polyester.

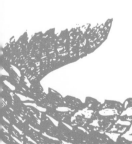

removes oils from the skin. Deodorant soap tends to be the most irritating; mild moisturizing bars less so; and nonsoap cleansers the least irritating. Make sure to rinse all soap and shampoo from your skin, as residue can dry it.

During winter cold, a combination of low humidity and blasting radiators or heat vents can suck even more water than usual from your skin. You can fight these drying conditions by drinking lots of water and using a humidifier.

Sun exposure prematurely ages and dries skin. Sun exposure, in fact, is the main cause of wrinkling. Even during the winter, outdoor activities can expose your skin to significant amounts of sunlight reflected off snow and ice. Regular, year-round use of a sunscreen with a sun protective factor (SPF) of between 15 and 30 will help reduce sun-related aging and dryness. One way to protect your skin is to use a moisturizer that contains a sunscreen. If the label does not reveal the SPF factor, assume it is inadequate.

All skin-care products work on the basic principle of adding moisture to the stratum corneum. Moisturizers follow one of two formulas: oil-in-water or water-in-oil. Which formula is best for you depends on several factors, including your skin condition and the weather. Oil-in-water moisturizers have water as their main ingredient. These moisturizers are ideal for the face, especially if your skin is prone to acne,

it's a good idea to avoid very hot water. Although hot water temporarily relieves itchy skin by stunning the nerve endings, it also strips oils from the skin's surface. This in turn allows water to escape more quickly from the skin. While your skin is still moist after a bath or shower, apply moisturizer to your body to help seal in the water. You can also rub your skin with a mixture of baby oil and water and rinse off the excess while you are still in the shower. Be careful: The oil may make the tub slippery.

The soap you use also can make a difference. Soap can cause discomfort because it and for use as a lighter body moisturizer during warm months. Water-in-oil moisturizers, which consist mainly of lanolin (an oil found on wool fibers) or mineral oil, are best applied to drier skin, worn as a night cream, or used during harsh winter months.

Moisturizers cater to specific skin types—dry, oily, or combination—by varying the ratio of water to oil. People with acne-prone complexions can avoid worsening the condition by using oil-free products that contain substances such as talc, clay, or starch.

Moisturizers contain substances that keep the skin moist in different ways. Oils—such as animal fats, lanolin, and the petroleum products petrolatum and propylene glycol—slow water loss. Substances called humectants draw water from the air or deeper layers of the skin. The terms glycerin, urea, gelatin, sorbitol, and hyaluronic acid on moisturizer labels indicate the presence of humectants. Other substances, including colloidal oatmeal baths, act as a barrier that seals the skin.

Almost any moisturizer will relieve slightly dry skin. When dryness is more severe, a combination of humectants and oil will keep the skin moist for a longer time. A moisturizer high in oils helps dry skin that is extremely itchy. People with genetic forms of dry skin or with very thickened skin will gain more relief from products containing alphahydroxy acid or lactic acid. Over-the-counter preparations contain 5 percent lactic acid, while prescription products contain 12 percent. Alphahydroxy acid and lactic acid also have become popular as possible antiaging therapies that reduce fine wrinkles and rejuvenate the skin.

A moisturizing cream or lotion consists of the moisturizing substance itself suspended in other ingredients, known as the vehicle or medium. Substances that make up this vehicle—such as fragrance, preservatives, emulsifiers, and solvents—can be irritating to your skin or cause an allergic reaction. If a product makes your skin uncomfortable, the most likely culprit is fragrance, followed by preservatives such as Germall 115 (imidazolidinyl urea) and Dowicil 200 (quaternium 15). Emulsifiers keep water and oil from separating and thereby help the skin retain moisture. But a common emulsifier, PEG-4 dilaurate, can irritate skin when highly concentrated. Propylene glycol, a solvent that also acts as a humectant, also may bother your skin.

Whatever moisturizer you select, you must apply it regularly to banish dry skin. Your local drugstore or supermarket carries a large variety of products that can moisturize your skin. You don't need to spend top dollar—more expensive moisturizers may smell or feel better, but that doesn't make them more effective.

☐ Kathryn E. Bowers

Why fingers wrinkle

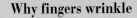

Fingers and toes wrinkle after soaking in water because the outer layer of the skin becomes bloated with water but the layer underneath does not. This difference in water content makes the skin shrivel. The water is absorbed by keratin, a protein in the body's outermost cells, which traps water and holds it inside the body or soaks it up from outside. Cells containing keratin make up the stratum corneum, or horny layer, of the epidermis, the skin's outer layer. The stratum corneum is especially thick on the hands and feet, which is why they pucker more than other parts of the body. The loose skin of fingers and toes also makes them prone to puckering.

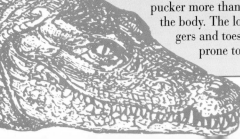

What You Should Know About Cataracts

The most common surgical procedure performed in the United States in 1994 was the removal of cataracts—the nation's leading cause of vision loss. Approximately 1.5 million cataract operations are performed annually to restore sight.

A cataract is a painless clouding of the normally transparent lens of the eye. The lens focuses light rays that pass through it so that a clear image forms on the *retina*—the light-sensitive area at the back of the eyeball. By clouding the lens, a cataract hampers the passage of light rays. As a result, images that form on the retina are less clear.

The most common reason for the lens's loss of transparency is the natural process of aging. For reasons not fully understood, aging causes a progressive hardening of the center of the lens. The lens normally bends to focus light. As the lens loses flexibility, it loses its ability to focus light, and in many cases loses its transparency as well.

The frequency and predictability of cataracts in the older population has led *ophthalmologists* (physicians who specialize in eye diseases) to conclude that cataracts may be an inevitable part of aging. By age 65, most people have developed some clouding, usually around the edge of the lens, which does not greatly interfere with vision. By age 75, most people have experienced at least minor vision loss due to a cataract. A cataract associated with aging can develop as early as age 40, however. More than 700,000 new cases are diagnosed annually, according to the American Academy of Ophthalmology.

Most cataracts develop slowly

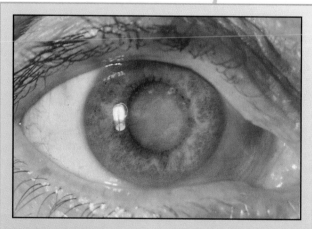

What is a cataract?
A cataract is a clouding of the normally clear lens of the eye, *above*. As light passes through a transparent lens, *top right*, it is focused on the retina at the back of the eye. But when the lens becomes opaque—usually as a result of aging—it blocks the transmission of light, *bottom right*.

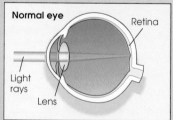

Normal eye
Retina
Light rays
Lens

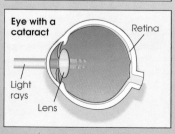

Eye with a cataract
Retina
Light rays
Lens

over many years. The rate of development varies from individual to individual and can vary even in a single pair of eyes. It is generally impossible for a physician to predict how fast an individual's cataract will progress.

How much vision is lost depends on the location and extent of the cataract. If it is small and located on the outer edge of the lens, a person can usually see around it. If the cataract is large, in the center of the lens, or both, vision loss can be profound. Cataracts, however, do not lead to total blindness. Even a severely clouded lens allows some transmission of light.

Besides loss of vision, the main symptom of a cataract is sensitivity to glare. In many cases, this sensitivity makes it difficult to drive at night. Night vision also becomes poor as cataracts progress, because so little light can reach the retina.

People with cataracts may also experience other vision problems, such as distorted depth perception. In many cases, they find that they need to change eyeglass prescriptions frequently and need a brighter than usual light for reading.

Other factors than age can cause a cataract. For example, a baby may be born with cataracts as the result of certain rare genetic disorders. Cataracts also can develop as a result of eye injury, eye surgery, or a particle entering the lens. Certain medications, such as steroids, appear to trigger development as well. Physicians also believe that unprotected, long-term exposure to radiation, including X rays and the sun's ultraviolet radiation, can lead to cataract development.

Diabetes mellitus, a disease in which blood sugar levels are high, can result in cataracts, especially in

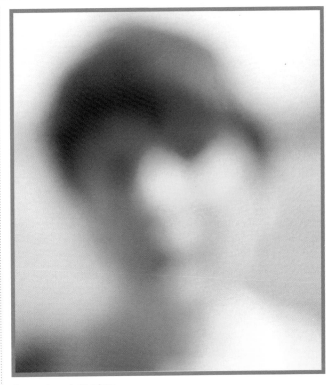

As a cataract develops, vision may become hazy or blurred. A cataract in the center of the lens impairs vision more than one that forms to the side.

young people. In many cases, these cataracts progress rapidly over a few months.

A cataract may require no treatment if it blurs vision only slightly. And a change in eyeglasses can sometimes improve vision temporarily. But surgery is the only permanent treatment for cataracts.

Cataract surgery involves removing the clouded lens from the eye. In most cases, the focusing power of the natural lens is restored by implanting a permanent, plastic lens slightly larger than Lincoln's head on a penny. After measuring the eye to calculate the shape of the implant needed to restore vision, the examining ophthalmologist prescribes the replacement lens.

Cataract surgery may be performed using general or local anesthesia. In either case, the procedure is painless. A patient is given eyedrops to widen the pupil, ex-

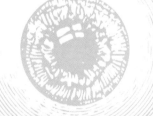

posing most of the front surface of the lens. The physician uses an instrument with a diamond tip to make an incision around the upper edge of the cornea. The cornea consists of transparent tissue that lies like a watch crystal over the colored part of the eye.

The surgeon then removes much of the front of the capsule enclosing the lens and carefully squeezes out the hard core of the lens, removing it from the eye. The remaining soft parts of the lens are cleared away, and the artificial lens is slipped into place. The incision on the cornea is sewn closed with nylon thread half the diameter of a human hair.

When the operation is finished, the surgeon usually places a shield over the eye to be worn temporarily as protection against infection and injury. Patients generally go home after a short stay in the outpatient recovery area. Although lens transplants can correct distance vision, people may need reading glasses for close vision. New eyeglasses are prescribed after the curvature of the cornea has stabilized.

Approximately 1 cataract patient in 4 develops blurred vision after surgery, when the back of the lens capsule becomes cloudy. This problem can occur months or years after surgery and can be treated with laser surgery. In this procedure, the laser's concentrated beam of light cuts a small hole in the center of the capsule, allowing light to again reach the retina. Laser sur-

A cataract is treated by surgically removing the clouded lens. If vision becomes blurred after surgery, a physician can use a laser's concentrated beam of light to open a small hole in the lens capsule, letting light through, *below*.

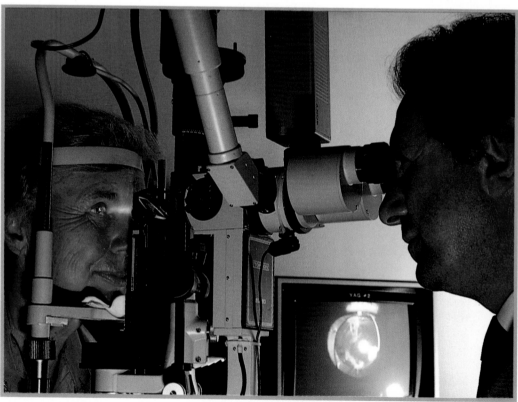

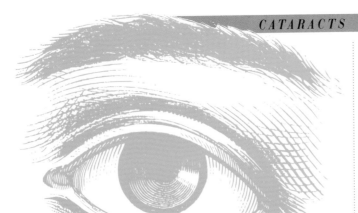

gery is never part of the original cataract operation.

More than 90 per cent of all cataract surgeries successfully improve vision. However, eye disorders unrelated to cataracts can affect the success of the surgery. These conditions include a deterioration of the retina called macular degeneration and vision loss due to glaucoma.

A nationwide study conducted in 1993 by Johns Hopkins School of Hygiene and Public Health in Baltimore found that the benefits of cataract surgery far outweighed the disadvantages of living with limited vision. People who chose to live with limited sight from a cataract, the study found, experienced a measurable decline in quality of life. Cataract-related vision problems were linked to increased hip fractures, a higher rate of automobile accidents, earlier admission to nursing homes, premature retirement, and higher mortality rates.

Ophthalmologists generally recommend cataract surgery when loss of sight affects a person's work or life style. But a more conservative approach to surgery was advocated by a panel of experts convened in 1993 by the United States Public Health Service.

Because delaying cataract surgery does not lower the chances of surgical success, the panel advised trying other remedies before turning to surgery and issued guidelines for alternate treatments. These included changing eyeglasses, using magnifying lenses, and improving home lighting. In contrast to the Johns Hopkins findings, the panel suggested that quality of life, in many cases, is not reduced enough by the cataract to warrant surgery.

The U.S. government requested the Public Health Service guidelines in part because it pays for the majority of the 1.5 million cataract extractions performed annually. Most cataract surgery patients are over age 65 and qualify for Medicare, the health insurance program for Americans receiving social security benefits. The guidelines were endorsed by the American Academy of Ophthalmology and the National Society to Prevent Blindness, but dissenting physicians suggested that the government was more concerned with reducing Medicare spending than with promoting proper cataract care.

☐ Julie Foreman

Reducing your risk of developing cataracts

There is no sure way to prevent cataracts, but recent studies suggest some steps people can take to reduce their risk:

- Don't smoke. People who smoke 20 or more cigarettes a day have about twice the risk for developing cataracts as nonsmokers, according to a 1992 study.

- Wear sunglasses that block 100 per cent of the sun's ultraviolet rays. Some studies have found higher rates of cataracts among people who work outdoors.

- Maintain a diet high in vitamins A, C, and E. A 1991 study found a lower rate of cataracts among people taking vitamin supplements.

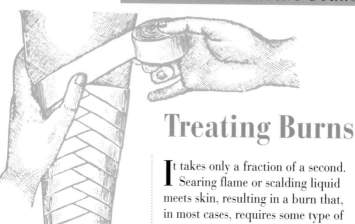

Treating Burns

It takes only a fraction of a second. Searing flame or scalding liquid meets skin, resulting in a burn that, in most cases, requires some type of treatment.

Each year in the United States, about 2 million people seek medical attention for burns, usually in a hospital emergency department or a physician's office. About 70,000 of these injuries are serious enough to require admission to a hospital, according to the American Medical Association. Fortunately, many burns, even though they are painful, can be treated at home with first-aid measures.

Hot liquids and steam cause scalds, which are some of the most common household burns. Bath water that is too hot can scald children. Or a parent may hold a child while drinking a steaming cup of coffee. The child squirms; the coffee spills. Or small hands may reach for the handle of a pot of soup, pulling down the simmering contents.

Flames also cause a large number of household burns, mostly in the kitchen, though summertime barbecues also pose a hazard. Not only are flames less contained in an outdoor grill than they are on a kitchen stove top, but overzealous chefs may be prone to using too much lighter fluid to ignite their charcoal. And people who smoke in bed risk an injury far more serious than a fingertip burn.

Flames and hot liquids are not the only culprits, however. Exposure to such chemicals as chlorine bleach or harsh cleaning products can burn the skin, as can gasoline. Contact with electric current—by touching a frayed electric cord, for example—can cause serious internal injuries while causing little visible damage to the skin. The treatment of burns caused by chemicals or by electricity is best left to medical professionals.

Burns affect the skin in much the same way that cooking affects an egg. Heat causes the protein in the egg white to thicken into an opaque mass. A similar process occurs when skin burns. Its protein thickens, increasing the skin's permeability. The injury also triggers the body's immune response, which releases chemicals such as histamine that are responsible for pain, redness,

Most common causes of household burns

- Hot water
- Irons
- Ranges or ovens
- Heaters or heating systems
- Cookware
- Chemical burns from bleach, batteries, and other sources
- Electric outlets or wiring

Source: U.S. Consumer Product Safety Commission.

and swelling. In extensive burns, damage to blood vessels can result in the loss of body fluid that, in turn, may damage internal organs.

Burns are classified as first, second, or third degree. These classifications describe the extent of damage to the three layers of the skin.

First-degree burns are the most common and the least serious. They can generally be treated without the aid of a medical professional, unless they cover a large area of the body or a particularly delicate area such as the face. Second-degree and third-degree burns are more serious and require medical attention.

Many people are familiar with first-degree burns in the form of sunburns. Like other first-degree burns, mild to moderate sunburns affect only the outer layer of skin. This tough layer, known as the epidermis, protects the body's internal organs from harmful elements in the environment, such as bacteria.

The common symptoms of a first-degree burn are pain, reddening of the skin, and skin that is warm to the touch. Slight swelling may also occur. The pain generally subsides in two or three days, and the damaged outer layer of skin may peel within a week.

Second-degree burns extend beyond the skin's outer layer, affecting the second layer, which is known as the dermis. This layer con-

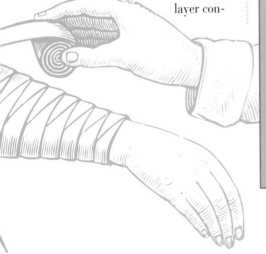

Treating minor burns

Minor burns affect a relatively small area and do no damage beyond the epidermis—the top layer of skin. They redden the skin but do not blister it or destroy tissue. Proper treatment can reduce pain and inflammation and help protect the burned area. More serious burns and burns from chemicals or electricity require medical attention.

Immediately run cold water over the burn to reduce pain and swelling.

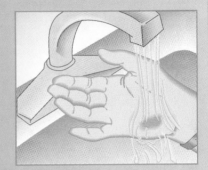

A towel or cloth wetted with cold water and pressed against the burn can also relieve pain and reduce inflammation.

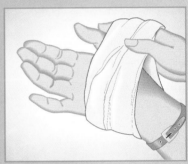

Jewelry and restrictive clothing should be removed from the burned area before swelling makes the removal impossible.

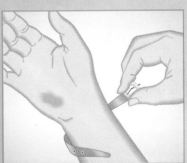

A clean dressing should be applied to the burn to protect the injured skin from infection.

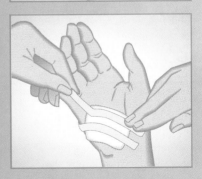

Source: The American Medical Association Encyclopedia of Medicine.

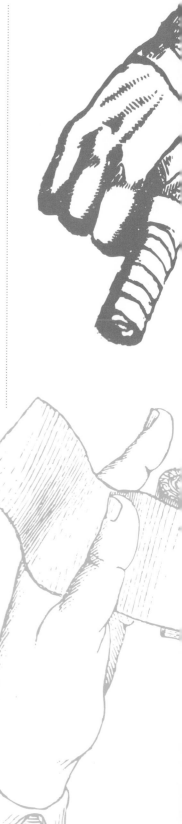

tains such vital structures as blood vessels, nerve endings, lymph vessels, sweat glands, and oil-secreting sebaceous glands. These structures are responsible for a number of the skin's crucial functions, including the regulation of body temperature and sensory responses to pressure, heat, and cold.

Common symptoms of second-degree burns are pain, redness, and blisters. Because second-degree burns damage the skin more deeply, it can no longer protect the body so well against infectious agents such as bacteria, and second-degree burns may be prone to infection as a result. But because the dermis isn't completely destroyed, it is able to regenerate new cells that grow vertically and horizontally to close the surface of the wound. Unless an infection develops, most second-degree burns heal in 10 to 14 days.

Third-degree burns are the most serious, destroying the entire thickness of the skin. Discoloration may range from chalky-white to brownish-gray. Muscle or bone also may be exposed. Such burns cause no pain because the nerve endings have been destroyed. Third-degree burns require immediate medical attention.

When treating minor burns at home, the first step is to place the burned area under cool, running water to help reduce swelling and relieve pain. Pressing a clean towel wetted with cold water against the burned area will also help relieve pain. Rinsing the injury with mild, nonirritating soap helps prevent infection. Remove any jewelry that may be retaining heat against the

skin or that may be difficult to take off should swelling set in. A clean, flat dressing, such as a washcloth, should be applied to the burned area. Elevating the injured area also helps reduce swelling.

Experts stress that any type of irritating substance applied to a burn can slow healing. Butter was once a popular choice in treating household burns. Although it may appear to act as a moisturizer, butter is animal fat containing salt and fatty acids that irritate burned skin. Similarly, antiseptic agents such as rubbing alcohol or iodine as well as topically applied steroid creams, such as hydrocortisone, can further irritate tender, burned skin.

Deciding whether to seek medical treatment for a burn is often a matter of common sense: If the burned area is extensive or deep, or the pain is intense, professional care should be sought. Burn-treatment experts also provide some decision-making pointers.

One rule of thumb concerns the area involved. If the burn covers an area of tissue larger than the backs of both hands, a medical professional should treat the burn. Another rule takes into account the part of the body that has been burned. Burns on the face, groin, and skin covering major joints, especially in the hands, should receive medical attention. With proper care, such complications as facial scarring, serious infection, and limited movement in the joints of the hands or other areas can be minimized or avoided.

Some burns may also be more serious than they first seem and require medical attention. Fluid-filled blisters may appear on a first de-

What NOT to do to a burn

- Never use adhesive dressings directly on a burn.
- Never apply butter, oil, or any greasy substance.
- Never apply lotions or creams.
- Never apply cotton or other fluffy material.
- Never break blisters.
- Never apply ice directly on a burn.

Source: The American Medical Association.

gree burn, or the skin in a more severe burn may become leathery and pale. A person should also seek medical evaluation if pain increases over several days or if the wound does not heal within 14 days. These symptoms may signal the presence of infection.

The circumstances surrounding the burn also play a role in determining whether medical attention is needed. For instance, a person who receives a minor, external burn in a house fire also may have breathed in carbon monoxide or other toxic products of combustion. Although the burn itself may not be serious, a medical evaluation is needed to determine if injury to the respiratory tract has occurred from inhaling toxins. The same rule applies if toxic chemical fumes have been inhaled. And anyone who loses consciousness after being burned should receive immediate medical care.

The age and health of the individual who has been burned are also important in determining whether to seek medical attention. Infants and young children, as well as older people, should receive medical attention, because their infection-fighting immune systems may not function fully. As a result, a burn can leave them especially vulnerable to infection.

Others who may also be susceptible to complications from burns include people in poor health, people who take drugs such as prednisone that suppress the body's immune system, or people who have an underlying condition such as diabetes that leaves them prone to infections. They, too, should see a medical professional.

The vast majority of burns are preventable. Again, common sense should prevail. People who smoke should never do so in bed. When cooking, turn pot handles away from curious children. Don't sleep with a heating pad at a high setting placed against your skin, and don't use lamps or electric appliances that have frayed cords.

Additional preventive measures include checking the hot water temperature in the home. Generally, the temperature of hot water should not exceed 120 °F (49 °C), to prevent scalds. The temperature should be lower for water used on infants. People who have diabetes, who are experiencing the aftereffects of a stroke, or who have other nerve damage that impairs skin sensation should check water temperature carefully. Because of their altered skin sensation, they may not recognize that water is too hot. Household plumbing should be checked so that cold water isn't diverted if a second faucet is turned on in another part of the home.

No burn is minor to the person who suffers it. Prevention is the best medicine, but in the absence of that, first aid is a simple and effective way to relieve the pain of a minor burn. ☐ Rebecca Voelker

Health Information by Phone

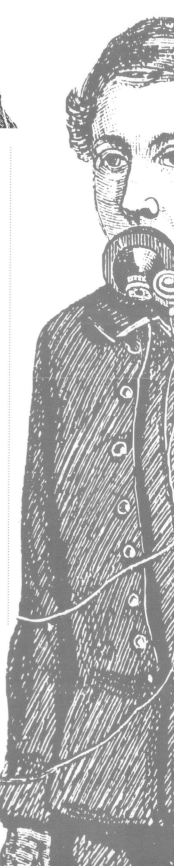

A wealth of health information is available by telephone. Listed below are some useful numbers.

AIDS

☎ **National AIDS Hot Line** (800-342-AIDS), operated by the Centers for Disease Control and Prevention, provides information and referrals 24 hours a day, 7 days a week. Spanish-language information is available at 800-344-7432. People who are hearing impaired can call 800-243-7889.

ALCOHOLISM AND DRUG ABUSE

☎ **National Council on Alcoholism** (800-NCA-CALL) provides written information and referrals 24 hours a day, 7 days a week.

☎ **Center for Substance Abuse Treatment** (800-662-HELP) refers callers to treatment centers and support groups weekdays from 9 a.m. to 3 a.m. and Saturdays and Sundays from noon to 3 a.m. Eastern time.

ALZHEIMER'S DISEASE

☎ **Alzheimer's Association** (800-272-3900) provides written information and referrals to local chapters weekdays from 8:30 a.m. to 5 p.m. Central time.

☎ **National Institute on Aging** (800-438-4380) provides information and referrals weekdays from 8:30 a.m. to 5 p.m. Eastern time. For information on other topics related to aging, call 800-222-2225.

ARTHRITIS

☎ **Arthritis Foundation** (800-283-7800) provides written information on treatment and refers callers to local chapters, which can recommend physicians and support groups, weekdays from 9 a.m. to 7 p.m. Eastern time.

ASTHMA AND LUNG DISORDERS

☎ **Lungline** (800-222-LUNG) provides written information and an opportunity to speak with registered nurses weekdays from 8 a.m. to 5 p.m. Mountain time.

CANCER

☎ **Cancer Information Service** (800-4-CANCER) of the National Cancer Institute answers questions and provides written information and referrals to treatment facilities and support groups weekdays during local business hours.

☎ **Cancer Response System** (800-ACS-2345) of the American Cancer Society (ACS) provides written information and referrals to local ACS programs and resources during local business hours.

CYSTIC FIBROSIS

☎ **Cystic Fibrosis Foundation** (800-824-5064) provides written information and referrals to local support groups weekdays from 8:30 a.m. to 5 p.m. Central time.

DIABETES

☎ **American Diabetes Association** (800-ADA-DISC) answers questions and provides written information weekdays from 8:30 a.m. to 5 p.m. Eastern time.

DOWN SYNDROME

☎ **National Down Syndrome Society** (800-221-4602) provides written information and referrals to local parent support groups weekdays from 9 a.m. to 5 p.m. Eastern time.

EPILEPSY

☎ **Epilepsy Foundation of America** (800-EFA-1000) provides written information and referrals weekdays from 9 a.m. to 5 p.m. Eastern time.

EYES AND VISION

☎ **Prevent Blindness America** (800-221-3004) provides information on eye health and safety weekdays from 8 a.m. to 5 p.m. Central time.

FOOD AND NUTRITION

☎ **Consumer Nutrition Hot Line** (800-366-1655) of the National Center for Nutrition and Dietetics answers questions and provides taped messages on nutrition topics. The line is staffed weekdays from 10 a.m. to 5 p.m. Eastern time.

☎ **Meat & Poultry Hot Line** (800-535-4555) of the U.S. Department of Agriculture answers questions on the proper handling, preparation, and storage of meat and poultry weekdays from 10 a.m. to 4 p.m. Eastern time. Taped messages are available 24 hours a day.

GENERAL HEALTH AND SAFETY

☎ **Auto Safety Hot Line** (800-424-9393) provides taped information on recalls, crash-test results, tire quality, and other automotive safety topics 24 hours a day, 7 days a week. Callers also can report auto safety problems.

☎ **Consumer Product Safety Commission Hot Line** (800-638-2772) provides taped information on product recalls, corrective actions, and other product safety questions 24 hours a day, 7 days a week. Callers also can file complaints about unsafe products.

☎ **National Health Information Center** (800-336-4797) maintains data on about 1,000 organizations that can provide current health in-

formation and refers callers to the appropriate agency weekdays from 9 a.m. to 5 p.m. Eastern time.

HEADACHE

☎ **National Headache Foundation** (800-843-2256) answers questions, provides written information, and makes referrals to doctors weekdays from 9 a.m. to 5 p.m. Central time.

HEARING

☎ **Hearing and Speech Help Line** (800-638-8255) provides information on speech, language, and hearing problems as well as referrals weekdays from 9:30 a.m. to 1 p.m. and 1:30 to 4:30 p.m. Eastern time.

HEART DISEASE

☎ **American Heart Association** (800-AHA-USA-1) provides written information on cholesterol and all aspects of heart disease as well as referrals to local chapters weekdays during local business hours.

MENTAL ILLNESS

☎ **National Alliance for the Mentally Ill** (800-950-6264) provides written information and refers callers to local chapters that in turn direct callers to local resources. The line is open weekdays from 10 a.m. to 5 p.m. Eastern time.

OSTEOPOROSIS

☎ **National Osteoporosis Foundation** (800-223-9994) provides written information 24 hours a day, 7 days a week.

PARKINSON DISEASE

☎ **National Parkinson Foundation** (800-327-4545) provides written information and referrals to neurologists weekdays from 8 a.m. to 5 p.m. Eastern time.

SEXUALLY TRANSMITTED DISEASES

☎ **National Sexually Transmitted Diseases Hot Line** (800-227-8922), operated by the Centers for Disease Control and Prevention, answers questions and provides information and referrals weekdays from 8 a.m. to 11 p.m. Eastern time.

Special Reports

Feature articles present in-depth information about
topics of current importance in health and medicine.

The Origin of New Diseases   44
by Robin Marantz Henig
Although many infectious diseases have been conquered, many
new ones are emerging—the result of crowding, the widespread
destruction of natural habitats, and other human activities.

Can Vitamins Help Prevent Cancer?   60
by John Grossmann
Researchers are looking at the disease-fighting powers of vitamins
and other nutrients in such everyday foods as broccoli and carrots.

Dr. Spock Talks About Raising Children Today   74
A conversation with the editors
America's foremost baby doctor talks about how problems parents face
have changed since the first edition of his best-selling *Baby and Child Care*.

Bagging the Ulcer Bug   88
by Robin Netherton
Medical researchers have found evidence that bacteria cause most
cases of ulcers and that antibiotics can cure these ulcers for good.

Exercise: The Gain Made Plain   102
by Richard Saltus
We've all heard that exercise is good for us, but just how does it
benefit the body—and how can you make the most of these benefits?

Getting a Good Night's Sleep   118
by Dianne Hales
Studies show that most Americans are not getting the sleep they need. Some
simple steps can improve both the quantity and the quality of your sleep.

See page 58.   See page 102.

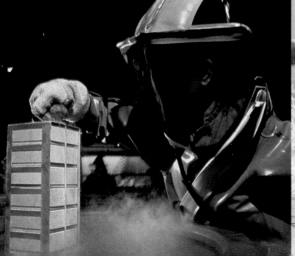

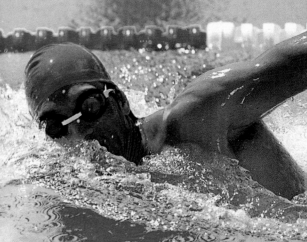

New Hope for Spinal Cord Injuries   132
by Richard Saltus

New drugs are helping many people overcome spinal cord injuries, and
researchers think that someday it may be possible to reverse paralysis.

Home, Safe Home   146
by Michael Woods

Each year, thousands of Americans die in home accidents. With planning
and vigilance, most home accidents and injuries can be prevented.

Understanding Type II Diabetes   160
by Mark Stolar

If not carefully treated, Type II diabetes can cause devastating complications.
The key to preventing them is the close control of blood sugar levels.

Medicines for the Mind   174
by Bernard Salzman

The widely prescribed antidepressant Prozac is only one of an
arsenal of drugs that can treat a range of psychiatric disorders—
disorders that affect millions of Americans each year.

When the World Turns: Dizziness and Its Causes   188
by Bruce H. Dobkin

Whether we feel just a little off-balance or as if we are spinning in space,
dizziness is an unsettling sensation with many different causes.

Coping with Alzheimer's Disease   202
by Donna Cohen

Alzheimer's disease robs a person of the very qualities that constitute
the self, and it can devastate families. But help is available.

See page 146.   See page 160.   See page 203.

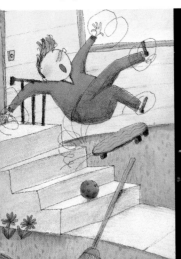
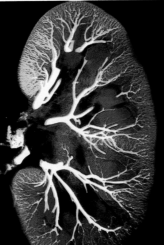
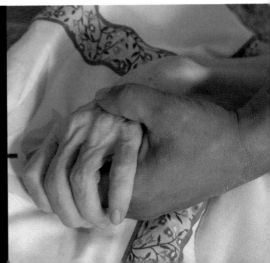

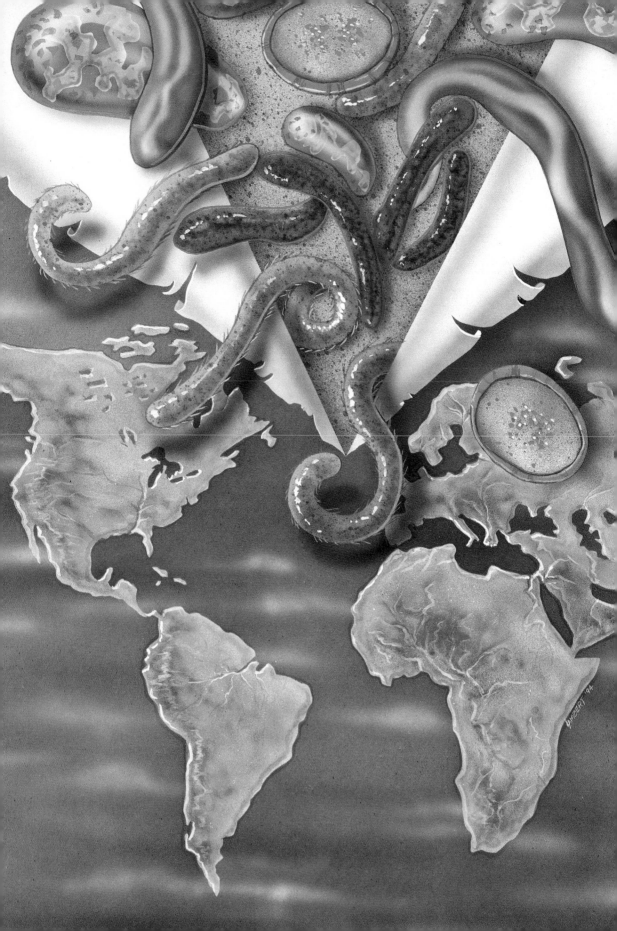

The Origin of New Diseases

By Robin Marantz Henig

Although many infectious diseases
have been conquered, many new ones
are emerging—the result of crowding,
the widespread destruction of natural
habitats, and other human activities.

In 1993, two frightening outbreaks of new infectious illnesses
occurred in the United States. Early in the year, more than 500
people in several Western states got sick, and 4 died, from eating fast-food hamburgers contaminated with a new strain of the
common bacterium *Escherichia coli*. And in the spring, a flulike
illness that progressed rapidly to respiratory failure erupted in
the Southwest. The disease was first noted among Navajo Indians in the Four Corners region—the juncture of Arizona, Colorado, New Mexico, and Utah. The malady, unofficially dubbed
Four Corners disease, was quickly traced to a microorganism
called a hantavirus.

The sudden appearance of those two illnesses was a reminder
that infectious disease is still a serious threat to human health
in the United States. Yet as recently as 1969, the U.S. surgeon
general had asserted that the war against infectious diseases had
been won, not only here but elsewhere in the world. And at the
time, it seemed to be true. Medical scientists had made dramatic
advances against infectious illnesses. Vaccines were on their way
to eliminating some killers, such as smallpox, and antibiotics
had defanged many others, including syphilis and tuberculosis.

But the surgeon general's victory speech was clearly premature. Since the late 1960's, we have witnessed the spread of a number of deadly infectious diseases, some of which have never been seen before. The emergence of new diseases has been due in large part to human activities, such as settlement in previously undisturbed natural habitats where unknown viruses and other microorganisms have been hidden for eons.

The most notorious new infection of recent years is AIDS. That disease, which destroys the body's immune system, seemingly materialized out of thin air in the United States in the early 1980's and was later traced to a virus, named HIV (human immunodeficiency virus). But before AIDS, there had been other surprises in the form of new bacterial illnesses. They included Lyme disease, a tick-borne infection that attacks the joints, named for the town in Connecticut where the first outbreak occurred in 1975; Legionnaire's disease, a form of pneumonia first noted in 1976 among American Legion members attending a convention in Philadelphia; and in the late 1970's, toxic shock syndrome, an illness caused by an infection that most often afflicts young women during their menstrual periods.

Although much of the media coverage of newly emerging diseases has focused on the United States, previously unknown diseases can crop up almost anywhere. The tropics are the greatest source of new infectious diseases because of their immense biological diversity.

One of the latest illnesses to emerge from a tropical region is a new strain of cholera, a disease contracted from a bacterium that is transmitted in human feces. The cholera outbreak began in 1992 in India and Bangladesh and soon spread to several other Asian countries. Perhaps the most deadly of the new tropical afflictions is Ebola hemorrhagic fever, a virus-caused disease that produces massive internal bleeding and is fatal in up to 90 percent of cases. The disease is named for the region around the Ebola River in Zaire, where the illness first broke out in 1976, sweeping through dozens of villages in a localized epidemic that left several hundred people dead.

Responding to the danger

With infectious diseases on the rise around the world, public health experts have become concerned about the possibility of a devastating plague that could kill millions of people. In 1992, the Institute of Medicine in Washington, D.C., an advisory body to the U.S. government, issued a report on emerging diseases. Warning that we can expect to see more new diseases in coming years, the institute recommended the development of a global surveillance system for spotting emerging infectious diseases anywhere in the world and preventing their spread.

In the meantime, scientists at many institutions have been

The author:

Robin Marantz Henig is a free-lance writer and the author of *A Dancing Matrix: How Science Confronts Emerging Viruses.*

New diseases in the United States

Several new illnesses have emerged in the United States since the early 1970's. The most deadly and widespread of those diseases is AIDS.

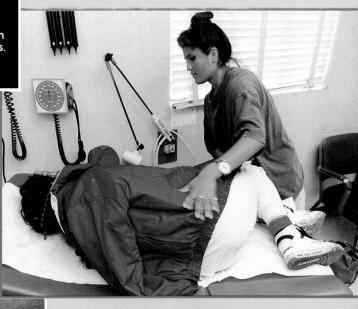

A victim of the so-called Four Corners disease, which first appeared in 1993 in the Southwest, is treated at an Arizona clinic, *right*. A skin rash is one sign of Lyme disease, *below*, named after the Connecticut town where a cluster of cases occurred in the early 1970's.

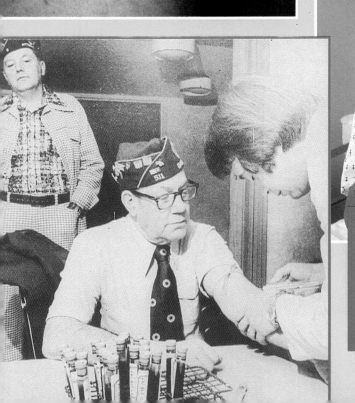

A patient with AIDS, a disease first identified in 1981, prepares a dose of a drug that suppresses symptoms, *above*. After the 1976 Legionnaires' disease outbreak in Philadelphia, a Legionnaire's blood is tested to see if he has been exposed to the bacterium that was found to cause the illness, *left*.

Disease	Time and place of emergence	Symptoms
AIDS	Early 1980's— United States	Severe infections, caused by normally harmless microorganisms, and the development of rare cancers— both resulting from a weakened immune system.
Cholera (new strain)	1992—India and Bangladesh	Diarrhea and vomiting, causing severe loss of body fluids; muscle cramps.
Ebola hemorrhagic fever	Mid-1970's— Africa	High fever, formation of clots in blood vessels, massive internal bleeding.
Four Corners disease	1993—Southwestern United States	Fever, abdominal pain, severe lung congestion.
Legionnaires' disease	1976—Philadelphia	A form of pneumonia, characterized by fever, headache, and diarrhea.
Lyme disease	1975—Lyme, Conn.	Skin rash, fatigue, chills, fever, muscle aches, pain in joints.
Toxic shock syndrome	Late 1970's— United States 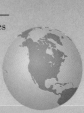	High fever, vomiting, diarrhea, skin rash. In severe cases, shock and kidney failure may develop.

A few modern plagues

New diseases that have emerged in recent years vary widely in their severity. Some can be treated successfully, while others resist treatment and are often fatal. AIDS and a devastating illness called Ebola hemorrhagic fever are among the most dreadful of the new crop of diseases.

	Cause, and mode of transmission	**Treatment and outcome**
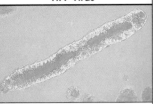 **HIV virus**	HIV virus. Transmitted through sexual contact with an infected person, through contact with infected blood, or from an infected pregnant woman to her unborn baby.	Other, resultant illnesses treated with drugs. The disease appears to be nearly 100 percent fatal.
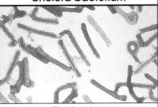 **Cholera bacterium**	*Vibrio cholerae* 0139 bacteria. Transmitted in food or water contaminated with the feces of an infected person.	Can be treated successfully with antibiotics and replacement of lost fluids. The disease can be fatal if left untreated.
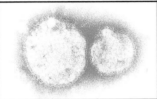 **Ebola virus**	Ebola virus. Transmitted through contact with the blood or body fluids of an infected person.	No effective treatment. The most virulent strain of the virus is fatal in up to 90 percent of cases.
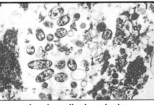 **Hantavirus**	Hantavirus. Transmitted in airborne particles of the dried urine and feces of infected deer mice; disease results from the inhalation of particles.	No effective treatment, though researchers are investigating several drugs. The disease is fatal in as many as 70 percent of cases.
Legionella bacteria	*Legionella pneumophilia* bacteria. Thought to be transmitted when a person inhales contaminated droplets from an air conditioning system or other source of stored water.	Can be treated successfully with antibiotics, though the disease can be fatal to older or unfit patients.
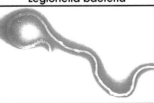 **Lyme disease bacterium**	*Borrelia burgdorferi* bacteria. Transmitted by the bite of an infected deer tick.	Can be treated successfully with antibiotics if diagnosed early. If untreated, can lead to inflamed joints, heart problems, and damage to the nervous system.
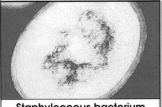 **Staphylcoccus bacterium**	*Staphylococcus aureus* bacteria, which are present in the environment. Prolonged use of highly absorbent tampons seems to promote the growth of the bacteria. Infection can also occur in older women, men, and children.	Treated with antibiotics and, if shock develops, intravenous fluids. Most patients recover fully if treated early, but the disease can be fatal.

learning as much as they can about new infectious illnesses as they are identified. They hope to develop vaccines that will protect people from deadly new microorganisms or at least to devise effective treatments for infections that do occur.

The nature of the adversary

Infectious diseases are caused by tiny microorganisms, often called microbes, that are invisible to the naked eye. Microbes that cause illness are also known as pathogens. The most common pathogens are various bacteria and viruses, though a number of other microorganisms, including some kinds of fungi and protozoa, also cause disease. An infectious disease is termed contagious if it is easily transmitted from one person to another.

An organism that a microbe infects is known as the host for that microbe. In many cases, a microorganism and its host live in perfect harmony. Such is the case for many tropical viruses and the insects, monkeys, or other animals in which they have lived and reproduced for thousands or millions of years. Because the microbes and their hosts have evolved together, the hosts have gradually become resistant to the microorganisms. But when a microbe jumps from a long-time animal host to a human being, it may cease being a harmless parasite and—simply because it is new to the human species—become a pathogen.

Eventually, a pathogen may adapt itself to its human hosts and cause a milder illness. It is in the microbe's best interest to do so, because if a disease is rapidly fatal, the host is likely to die before the microbe can get passed along to another host. But it takes time for a microbe and a new host species to get accustomed to each other, so an emerging pathogen may hit its earliest victims especially hard. It is usually in the first wave of a new disease that death rates are highest.

In the human host, the microorganism causes disease by either disrupting a vital body process or stimulating the immune system to mount a defensive reaction. An immune response against a pathogen, which can include a high fever, inflammation, and other damaging symptoms, can be more devastating than the direct damage caused by the microbe.

To survive and multiply, a pathogen needs not only a suitable host but also an exit route to infect a new host before the first one dies. Not every disease-causing microorganism is passed directly from one host to the next. Many pathogens are transmitted only with the aid of an intermediate organism, such as an insect. These intermediaries are known as vectors. A vector harbors a pathogen in its body with no ill effect and then passes it on to a human host through a scratch or bite. One of the most common vector-transmitted diseases is malaria, a tropical illness caused by one-celled parasites that are spread by mosquitoes.

In some cases, new diseases arise when *mutations* (genetic

changes) in microbes turn them into pathogens. For example, the new strain of the cholera bacterium that has been infecting people in much of Asia apparently resulted from a mutation. A reshuffling of genes known as genetic reassortment, which occurs when microorganisms acquire genetic material from other microbes, can also give rise to new pathogens. The creation of pathogens by these genetic processes are especially worrisome because the changes are random and unpredictable.

Four Corners disease

Occasionally, some natural phenomenon in the environment is responsible for a new disease. Such was the case with Four Corners disease.

The illness came to the attention of public health officials in May 1993 after a young Navajo man in New Mexico became deathly ill while traveling with his family in their car. He had come down with flulike symptoms a few days before, and in the car he started gasping for breath. The young man was rushed to a hospital, but he was already dead when he arrived. An X ray showed that his lungs were filled with fluid.

The circumstances surrounding this puzzling death set off alarm bells. At the time the young man was stricken, doctors learned, he had been on his way to the funeral of his fiancée. She had died the week before in just the same way. It appeared that an outbreak of some unfamiliar disease was brewing.

By early June, 18 people in the Four Corners area, most of them Navajos in their teens or 20's, had contracted the strange respiratory illness, and 11 of them had died. Tribal elders believed they had an explanation for the mysterious plague. They had noticed that, for the first time in memory, there had been sufficient rainfall to keep the piñon trees on the reservation in full flower for the entire year. Rodents that eat the sweet meat of the piñon nut had become fat and plentiful, their population boosted by the rich food supply as well as by ground that was moist and soft and good for burrowing.

The scientists who flocked to the area to investigate the outbreak soon supported the Navajos' theory. They concluded that the local rodents, especially one species known as the deer mouse, were harboring a previously unknown type of hantavirus. Anyone living in proximity to deer mice—which was more likely that year as the mice proliferated—was liable to become infected by inhaling dust particles that contained dried flecks of rodent urine or feces contaminated with the virus.

Scientists know of several varieties of han-

Spreaders of infection

A human being or other organism that a pathogen infects and within whose body it breeds is known as a host for that microbe. The deer mouse, *above*, is host to the Four Corners disease virus, though the mouse does not get sick. An organism that harbors a pathogen and transmits it from one host to another is a vector. The deer tick, *below*, is the Lyme disease vector.

tavirus, all of which are carried by rodents. The viruses have long been recognized as a source of disease in Asia and parts of Europe, but no disease-causing hantavirus had ever been found in North America. The Asian and European hantaviruses attack the kidneys, but those infections are usually not fatal. The Four Corners hantavirus, which was isolated in the laboratory in November, was far more lethal than its cousins and was the first hantavirus known to cause a respiratory illness.

Identification of the new hantavirus, combined with efforts to exterminate deer mice in the area and restrict contact between mice and humans, helped slow the spread of the Four Corners illness. Still, by November 1993, 45 hantavirus infections had been reported in 12 states, and by May 1994, the toll had risen to 72 in 17 states, including several on the East Coast. In more than half of those cases, the disease was fatal. A February 1994 report from the Centers for Disease Control and Prevention (CDC) in Atlanta, Ga., said that at least two of the hantavirus infections—one in Louisiana and the other in Florida—seem to have been caused by still other strains of the virus that biologists had been unaware of.

The human factor

The outbreak of the Four Corners disease was a freak of nature. With most new infectious diseases, however, some human action is involved, changing the environment so that an existing microbe can take up residence in a new ecological niche. Once that happens, a pathogen that had been confined to a remote habitat appears in a new or wider region, or a microbe that had infected only animals suddenly begins causing human disease.

Several human activities have led to the emergence and spread of new diseases:
- Encroachment on wildlife habitats. The construction of new villages and housing developments in rural areas brings people into contact with animals—and the microbes they harbor.
- Changes in agriculture. The introduction of new crops attracts new crop pests and the microbes they carry to farming communities, exposing people to unfamiliar diseases.
- Destroying rain forests. As tropical countries make use of their rain forests, building roads through forests and clearing areas for settlement or commercial ventures, people encounter insects and other animals harboring unknown microorganisms.
- Uncontrolled urbanization. The rapid growth of cities in many developing countries concentrates large numbers of people in crowded areas with poor sanitation, which foster the transmission of contagious diseases.
- Modern transport. Ships and other cargo carriers often harbor unintended "passengers," such as insects and rats, that can spread diseases to faraway destinations.

- High-speed globe-trotting. With international jet-airplane travel, people infected with a new disease can carry the disease to the far side of the world before their first symptoms appear.

The emergence and spread of AIDS

AIDS provides a textbook example of how a new infectious disease can appear and be spread far and wide. Although medical experts are still debating exactly when and how AIDS emerged, a widely accepted theory is that HIV—the AIDS-causing human immunodeficiency virus—came from a closely related virus that infects certain African monkeys. For some reason, that virus, known as SIV (simian immunodeficiency virus), made a cross-species jump and began infecting people in central Africa.

The transmission of SIV to a human being may have occurred when someone in an isolated rural village got a cut on the hand while butchering a monkey or was scratched or bitten by a pet monkey. In the human host, according to the theory, SIV mutated to become HIV. The newly lethal virus was then spread through sexual relations, and young people began dying of infections that their bodies could no longer fight off. But in the villages of Africa, dying of a mysterious illness is not uncommon, so the appearance of a new disease could have gone largely unnoticed.

Public health experts think that AIDS might have remained hidden in the rural areas of Africa had the continent not been transformed by social changes in the 1960's and 1970's. During that period, people began migrating to the cities in large numbers in search of work. As a result, the experts say, AIDS arrived in the cities and was soon poised to become a global menace.

AIDS seems to have spread beyond Africa in the late 1970's. Some researchers think it was brought to the Western Hemisphere by Haitians who had worked temporarily in Africa. The disease was first noted in the United States in the early 1980's among male homosexuals, who may have contracted the virus in Haiti. For several years, nearly all new cases of AIDS in the United States were seen in homosexual men and in abusers of intravenous drugs, who transmitted the virus with dirty needles. Increasingly, however, the virus is being contracted through heterosexual sex, which has long been the primary mode of transmission in Africa. Worldwide, about 75 percent of AIDS cases have been contracted through heterosexual relations.

Scientists now know of two AIDS viruses, designated HIV-1 and HIV-2. Furthermore, they have found that HIV-2, which causes most cases of AIDS in Africa, is more closely related to SIV than to HIV-1, the virus most common in the United States. That finding suggests that AIDS started from two separate SIV viruses. Researchers think HIV-2 got its start at least 100 years ago. HIV-1, they theorize, came along about 50 years later.

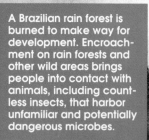
A Brazilian rain forest is burned to make way for development. Encroachment on rain forests and other wild areas brings people into contact with animals, including countless insects, that harbor unfamiliar and potentially dangerous microbes.

Human activity—the fount of most new diseases

Human activities are the primary cause of the emergence and spread of new diseases around the world.

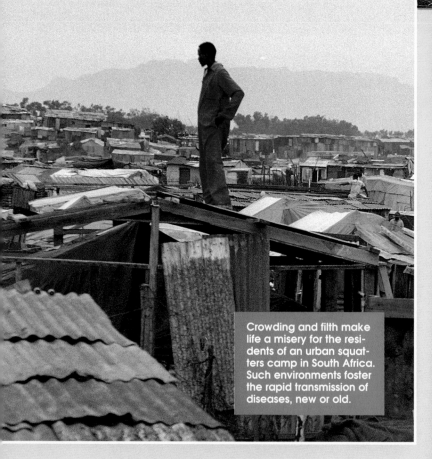
Crowding and filth make life a misery for the residents of an urban squatters camp in South Africa. Such environments foster the rapid transmission of diseases, new or old.

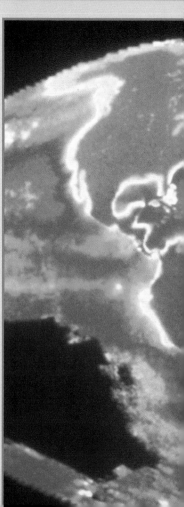

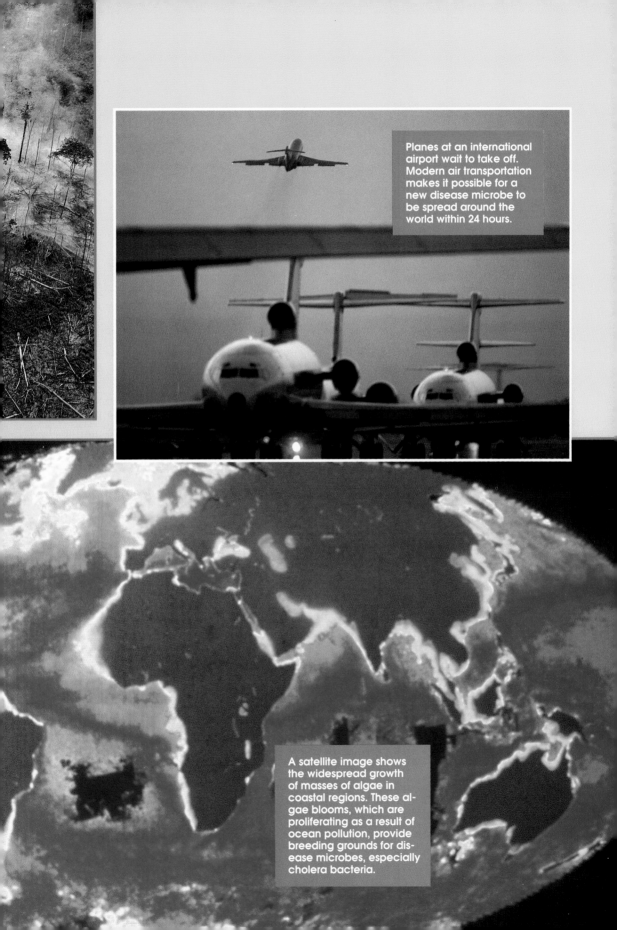

Planes at an international airport wait to take off. Modern air transportation makes it possible for a new disease microbe to be spread around the world within 24 hours.

A satellite image shows the widespread growth of masses of algae in coastal regions. These algae blooms, which are proliferating as a result of ocean pollution, provide breeding grounds for disease microbes, especially cholera bacteria.

Dengue—our next plague?

Although AIDS is the most infamous disease to reach the United States in this century, public health experts say that we can expect to see others in coming years. Many experts think that a tropical disease called dengue fever (pronounced *DEHNG gee* or *DEHNG gay*) and a related and much more serious illness called dengue hemorrhagic fever are the most likely candidates for the next American plague. The latter is an often-fatal sickness that mainly strikes children. There are four distinct viruses that cause dengue.

The stage was set for a U.S. dengue outbreak in 1975, when the so-called Asian tiger mosquito, a vector for the disease, was introduced into Texas in a shipment of tires from Japan. Since arriving in Texas, the mosquito has spread to 18 states, mostly in the South and Southwest. In many areas, it has replaced the *Aëdes aegypti* mosquito. That insect is also a dengue vector, but the tiger mosquito is a much more aggressive insect and would probably be a very efficient transmitter of the disease.

A handful of dengue cases are reported each year in the United States among travelers returning from the tropics, but no cases are known to have arisen here. Public health officials caution, however, that with tiger mosquitoes increasing in number across the southern half of the nation, it may be just a matter of time. The arrival in the United States of a sufficient number of people carrying the infection could ignite a dengue epidemic, with tiger mosquitoes spreading the infection to other people. No vaccine for the disease is yet available.

Lyme disease

For now, the most prevalent vector-transmitted illness in the United States is Lyme disease. As with most new maladies, Lyme disease took doctors completely by surprise.

In the summer of 1975, at least five young children in the town of Lyme, Conn., were diagnosed with juvenile rheumatoid arthritis (JRA), a progressive and debilitating disease of the joints. The children suffered from swollen knees, aching joints, and difficulty walking. The children's mothers, though, were skeptical of the diagnosis. It made no sense to them that so many youngsters from the same community would be suffering from an illness that is quite rare. Two of the women took their concerns to the state health department, and through persistence they convinced the professionals that something strange was happening in the town of Lyme.

Scientists began to investigate the supposed outbreak of JRA in Lyme, looking into every possible explanation for the clustering of cases: a pollutant in the air, radiation from a nearby nuclear power plant, contaminants in the water supply. But the most relevant clues, they concluded, were that most of the vic-

Antibiotics—losing the battle against infection?

Beginning in the early 1940's, when penicillin, the first antibiotic, became widely available, many bacterial infections were transformed from potential killers to mere inconveniences. But now some infections are again presenting potentially life-threatening hazards. That turnaround is occurring because the bacteria causing those infections are becoming resistant to the antibiotics that once vanquished them.

Drug resistance occurs because in any crop of bacteria, a few bacteria out of millions will acquire *mutations* (genetic changes) that, by chance, give those microbes resistance to one or more antibiotics. When a particular antibiotic is used against a bacterial infection, the few bacteria resistant to that drug will survive.

In most cases, the body's immune system will destroy those remaining bacteria. But if a person's immune system is weak, the leftover bacteria may remain and may even transfer their drug resistance to other bacteria already in the body. The next time the individual is infected by one of those microorganisms, the antibiotic that halted the previous bacterial onslaught may no longer be effective. Unless the new infection can be stopped with a different antibiotic, the patient's life may be in danger.

The more that antibiotics are used, the more prevalent drug-resistant strains of bacteria become. Doctors have tended to overprescribe antibiotics, often at their patients' insistence.

Farming practices may also be contributing to the problem. Antibiotics are widely used to treat infections in farm animals and are routinely added to animal feed as a preventive measure. The antibiotics encourage the growth of resistant strains of bacteria, which often lodge in the animals' flesh and are still there when the animals are slaughtered and sent to market. People can pick up the resistant microbes by eating undercooked meat and poultry.

The ability of bacteria to transfer antibiotic resistance to other bacteria is an especially worrisome phenomenon. A mutation conferring drug resistance is passed to other microbes in bits of genetic material called plasmids. Because it is common for several kinds of bacteria to mingle on the skin, on soiled bandages, and elsewhere, opportunities abound for a mutation to spread.

Already a number of serious infections are becoming increasingly difficult to treat with existing antibiotics. Drug-resistant illnesses include some *salmonella* (food poisoning) infections and typhoid fever.

Antibiotic resistance also underlies the resur-

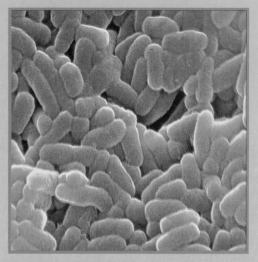

Tuberculosis (TB) bacteria, *above*, are becoming a major health threat because some strains have developed a resistance to antibiotics. TB, which has been on the rise since the mid-1980's, now kills more people around the world than any other infectious illness.

gence of tuberculosis (TB), which is becoming a major public health threat some 40 years after it seemed to have been conquered. TB now kills more people throughout the world than any other infectious disease. Drug-resistant strains of TB, with death rates as high as 75 percent, have been reported in at least 17 states.

Altogether, drug-resistant infections cause nearly 15,000 deaths each year in U.S. hospitals. Some health experts believe, in fact, that an antibiotics crisis is developing. Already, about 10 percent of infections from *Streptococcus pneumoniae*, the most common cause of bacterial pneumonia, and an even higher percentage of infections from *Staphylococcus aureus*, the bacterium that causes toxic shock syndrome and a number of other conditions, are resistant to every known antibiotic except one, vancomycin. If those strains were to become resistant to vancomycin as well, deaths from infections would undoubtedly soar.

Researchers are working to develop new drugs against infections, possibly including vaccines, to prevent such a nightmare. In the meantime, health officials say, doctors need to be more judicious in their use of antibiotics, and patients should temper their demands for the drugs. In addition, hospitals should be on the lookout for new strains of antibiotic-resistant bacteria and take quick action to contain them.   [R. M. H.]

tims lived near heavily wooded areas, had been stricken during the summer months, and had developed a round skin rash resembling an insect bite before their other symptoms began. To the researchers, the evidence indicated that the outbreak was an infectious disease spread by an insect, spider, or tick.

They were right, though the puzzle wasn't completely solved for another seven years. In 1977, scientists identified the vector as the deer tick, a tiny parasite whose favorite host is the white-tailed deer. And in 1982, as the disease spread throughout the Northeastern United States, investigators finally identified the microbe that the deer tick carries. It was a tiny spirochete, a corkscrew-shaped bacterium. And luckily, it could be killed with antibiotics. Treated early, Lyme disease is usually completely curable. But if left untreated for too long, the illness can cause not only joint inflammation but also damage to the heart and nervous system.

Lyme disease had been an affliction just waiting to happen. During the first half of the 1900's, the dense forested regions of the Northeastern United States were cleared to make room for farms and later for suburbs. This profound change in the region's ecology cleared the area of white-tailed deer, which had been plentiful. It also eliminated the wolves and other animals that were the deer's predators. Eventually, some of the forest

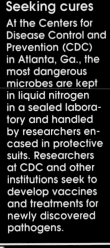

Seeking cures
At the Centers for Disease Control and Prevention (CDC) in Atlanta, Ga., the most dangerous microbes are kept in liquid nitrogen in a sealed laboratory and handled by researchers encased in protective suits. Researchers at CDC and other institutions seek to develop vaccines and treatments for newly discovered pathogens.

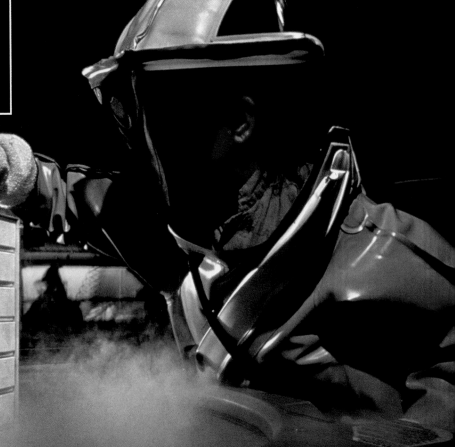

grew back, and the deer returned. But their predators did not. As a result, the deer population grew, and with it the population of deer ticks. And as the ticks proliferated, the more likely it became that a person would get bitten by an infected tick.

Preparing for future outbreaks

As human activities continue to impinge upon the natural world in the United States and other countries, the introduction of other new diseases into the human race is all but inevitable. Scientists worry that when the next strange outbreak occurs, we won't be any more ready for it than we were for AIDS.

But awareness of the danger is spurring action. In 1993, the global surveillance system urged by the National Academy of Sciences moved closer to reality with plans to establish an international effort named ProMED (Program for Monitoring Emerging Diseases). ProMED, which is expected to be up and running by 1997, is being coordinated by the World Health Organization, an arm of the United Nations, with the CDC also playing a central role. The program will establish a global network of "sentinel outposts" to alert scientists to environmental changes that could be setting the stage for an emerging disease.

Meanwhile, at the CDC and elsewhere, researchers are seeking vaccines and cures for diseases that have already burst upon the scene. Some of the pathogens they are studying, such as the Ebola virus, are so dangerous that they must be confined in ultrahigh-security laboratories, where they are kept frozen most of the time. Investigators working with these lethal microorganisms are not allowed into the laboratory until they have donned protective garments resembling space suits, and they must go through a special cleanup procedure before they leave.

As we step up the battle against emerging infectious illnesses, the biggest danger, scientists say, is a return to complacency. Just as we already learned that the fight against infectious disease had not been won, we must now understand that it is probably not even winnable. We may find vaccines or treatments for many new diseases, but we will never completely tame nature.

But in this battle, we have one weapon that has always served humanity well: our intelligence. As scientists learn more about how new diseases emerge and spread, we should—with proper diligence—be able to keep one step ahead of the microbes that threaten humanity's precarious perch in the natural world.

For further reading:

Henig, Robin Marantz. *A Dancing Matrix: How Science Confronts Emerging Viruses*. Vintage Books, 1994.

Levins, Richard, and others. "The Emergence of New Diseases." *American Scientist*, January/February 1994.

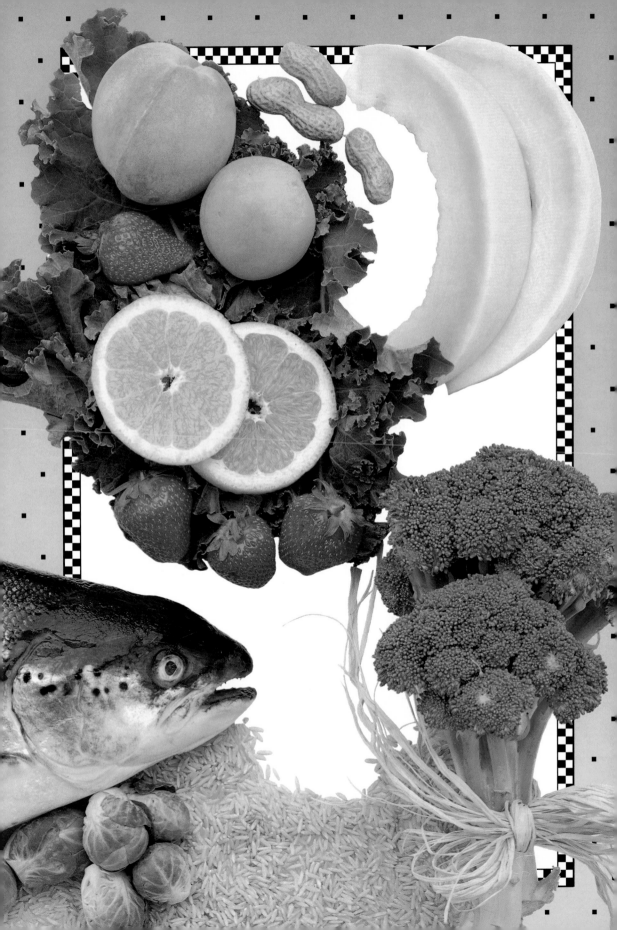

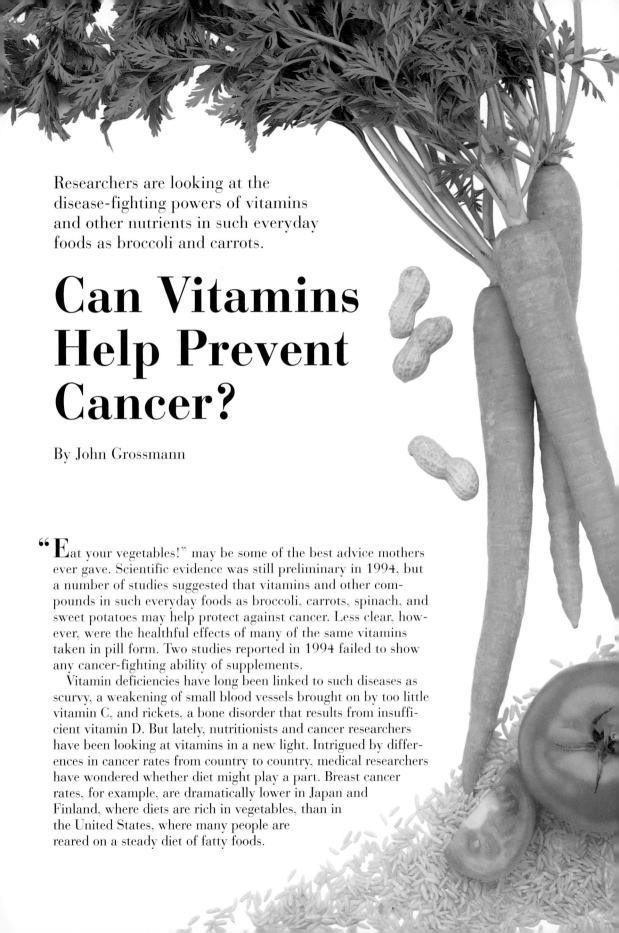

Researchers are looking at the disease-fighting powers of vitamins and other nutrients in such everyday foods as broccoli and carrots.

Can Vitamins Help Prevent Cancer?

By John Grossmann

"Eat your vegetables!" may be some of the best advice mothers ever gave. Scientific evidence was still preliminary in 1994, but a number of studies suggested that vitamins and other compounds in such everyday foods as broccoli, carrots, spinach, and sweet potatoes may help protect against cancer. Less clear, however, were the healthful effects of many of the same vitamins taken in pill form. Two studies reported in 1994 failed to show any cancer-fighting ability of supplements.

Vitamin deficiencies have long been linked to such diseases as scurvy, a weakening of small blood vessels brought on by too little vitamin C, and rickets, a bone disorder that results from insufficient vitamin D. But lately, nutritionists and cancer researchers have been looking at vitamins in a new light. Intrigued by differences in cancer rates from country to country, medical researchers have wondered whether diet might play a part. Breast cancer rates, for example, are dramatically lower in Japan and Finland, where diets are rich in vegetables, than in the United States, where many people are reared on a steady diet of fatty foods.

Many studies are still needed to better understand which components of foods may fight which cancers and how they might do so. But some researchers are optimistic that they have established a beachhead. "We know that if you eat plenty of fruits and vegetables you get less cancer—30 to 50 percent less, a significant difference," says Peter Greenwald, director of cancer prevention and control at the National Cancer Institute (NCI) in Bethesda, Md.

To be sure, if your diet leans toward fruits and vegetables, you will have less room on your plate and in your stomach for such high-fat foods as cheeseburgers and French fries. But many researchers also see a more direct effect. They believe that vitamin-bearing produce provides the body with powerful compounds that suppress cancer growth by taming molecules called free radicals. Dubbed molecular Jack the Rippers, free radicals rank high on medicine's most wanted list. Current theories put them at the scene of a number of serious diseases, though their link with disease has yet to be proved.

The free radical theory

Just what is this marauding molecule? A free radical is an unstable molecule that reacts readily with another molecule or compound nearby. Free radicals form in the body as a result of chemical reactions involving oxygen. The chemical reaction that creates oxygen free radicals is called oxidation, and it occurs during *metabolism*—the process in cells that turns nutrients into energy. When the oxygen free radicals react with other compounds in the cell, they can cause serious damage.

Herbert Pierson, a specialist in pharmaceutical sciences and founder of a National Cancer Institute (NCI) project that is investigating cancer-preventing chemicals in foods, offers an explanation. "Imagine you're driving down a highway in your car doing 55 miles per hour, behind other cars also doing 55. Suddenly, a fancy sports car passes you doing 125 miles per hour, weaving in and out of traffic. The sports car nudges a car that hits another car, which bumps another, and so on, setting off a chain reaction of multicar collisions. The sports car represents a free radical."

The damaging chain reactions set off by free radicals occur because the oxygen atom in the free radical is "hungry" for electrons. Oxygen atoms, like all atoms, consist of a nucleus surrounded by orbiting electrons. The oxygen atom "wants" eight electrons in its outer orbital shell. To stabilize itself, an oxygen free radical with fewer than eight electrons in its outer shell borrows an electron from a nearby molecule. If the free radical reacts with DNA (deoxyribonucleic acid), the molecule of which genes are made, the reaction can cause *mutations* (changes in DNA) that may lead to cancer.

The author:

John Grossmann is a freelance writer based in Pennsylvania.

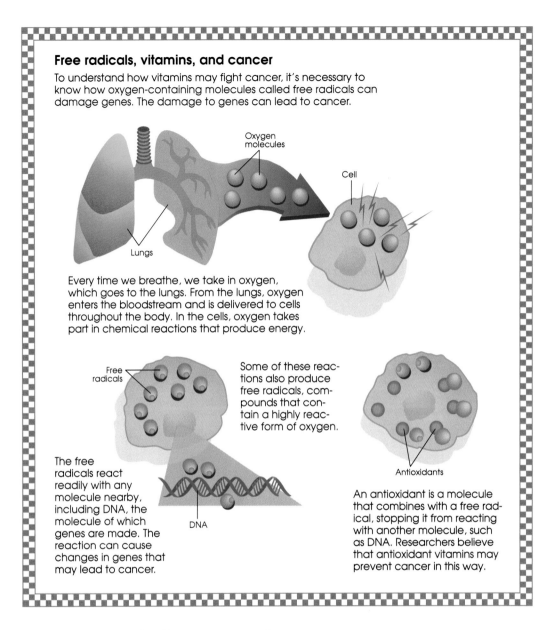

Free radicals, vitamins, and cancer

To understand how vitamins may fight cancer, it's necessary to know how oxygen-containing molecules called free radicals can damage genes. The damage to genes can lead to cancer.

Oxygen
molecules

Cell

Lungs

Every time we breathe, we take in oxygen, which goes to the lungs. From the lungs, oxygen enters the bloodstream and is delivered to cells throughout the body. In the cells, oxygen takes part in chemical reactions that produce energy.

Free radicals

Some of these reactions also produce free radicals, compounds that contain a highly reactive form of oxygen.

The free radicals react readily with any molecule nearby, including DNA, the molecule of which genes are made. The reaction can cause changes in genes that may lead to cancer.

DNA

Antioxidants

An antioxidant is a molecule that combines with a free radical, stopping it from reacting with another molecule, such as DNA. Researchers believe that antioxidant vitamins may prevent cancer in this way.

Potential cancer-fighting compounds

Compounds called antioxidants, researchers theorize, come to the rescue. Using Pierson's example, antioxidants cause reactions that resemble the effect of police cars arriving and making the sports car slow down and stay in its own lane. Vitamins C and E and beta carotene, which the body converts to vitamin A, are antioxidants. They donate extra electrons to free radicals, restabilizing them and ending the reaction.

It's also possible that vitamins form cancer-fighting teams. Studies conducted at the Research Center for Advanced Technology at the University of Tokyo in Japan suggest there is a co-operative effect of vitamins C and E. Vitamin C, which dissolves

Some foods that may fight cancer

Certain foods are especially good sources of the antioxidant vitamins C and E and of beta carotene, which the body turns into vitamin A. Studies suggest that diets rich in these foods may help prevent cancer. Vitamin D and folate, though not antioxidants, have also been linked to a reduced risk of certain cancers.

Compound	Fruits	Vegetables	Other sources
Beta carotene	Apricots Cantaloupe Mangoes Nectarines Papaya Peaches	Asparagus Broccoli Brussels sprouts Carrots Kale Pumpkin Spinach Sweet potatoes Winter squash	
Folate	Oranges Pineapple	Asparagus Black-eyed peas Lentils Lima beans Spinach	Liver Oatmeal Peanuts Sunflower seeds Wheat germ
Vitamin C	Blackberries Cantaloupe Grapefruit Honeydew melon Kiwi Oranges Pineapple Raspberries Strawberries Tomatoes	Asparagus Broccoli Brussels sprouts Cabbage Cauliflower Kale Peppers	
Vitamin D			Egg yolks Fortified milk Liver Salmon Sardines, fatty fish Tuna
Vitamin E	Olives Peaches Prunes	Asparagus	Brown rice Margarine Mayonnaise Nuts Oatmeal Peanut butter Safflower oil Wheat germ

Source: National Institutes of Health.

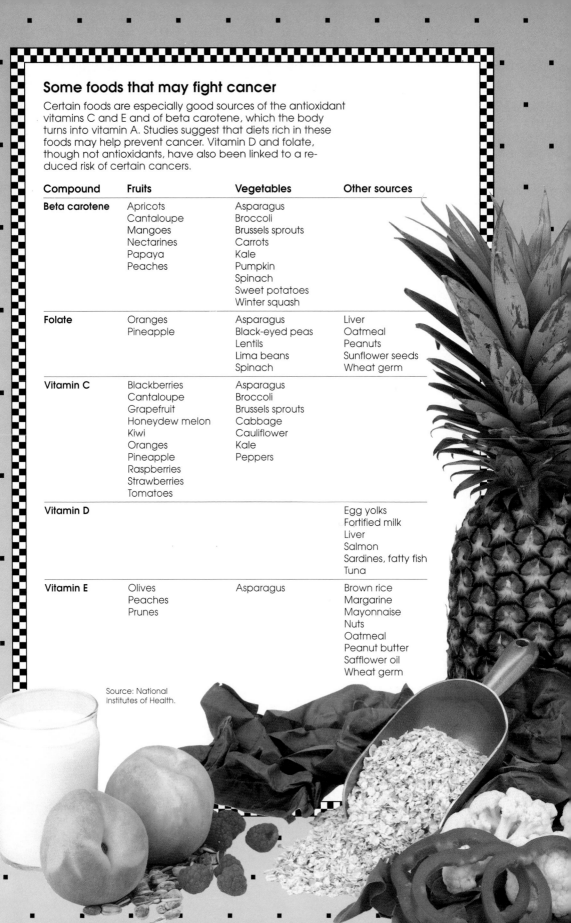

in water, reacts with free radicals in body fluids. Vitamin E, on the other hand, dissolves in fat and reacts with free radicals in fatty tissue, such as cell membranes. Findings reported by the Japanese researchers in December 1991 indicate that the addition of vitamin C to test samples of blood prolongs the free radical scavenging ability of vitamin E molecules at the surface of the cell membrane, where fatty tissue and fluid meet.

Scientists from Children's University Hospital in Heidelberg, Germany, reported in April 1993 that a compound called genistein, though not a vitamin, may have anticancer properties. In laboratory experiments, it appears to halt the growth of beginning tumors by blocking the development of small blood vessels needed to nourish a growing tumor. The scientists identified significant levels of genistein in the urine of people who eat a Japanese-style diet rich in soybeans and vegetables. Their genistein levels were at least 30 times higher than average genistein levels in Europe and North America. Might this be the reason, scientists speculate, why breast cancer and prostate cancer are much more prevalent in Europe and the United States than in Japan? Might it also explain why prostate cancer rates rise among Japanese men who have worked in Europe or the United States for many years?

Another possible cancer-fighting substance making headlines in 1994 was sulforaphane, a compound in broccoli, Brussels sprouts, and kale. A researcher at Johns Hopkins School of Medicine in Baltimore, who identified the substance, found in laboratory studies that sulforaphane triggers the formation of an enzyme that disarms free radicals before they can damage DNA. Tests on human subjects are needed to determine whether sulforaphane can block tumor formation.

Chances are, most researchers say, there is no single vitamin or compound, no magic bullet, that would prevent cancer. Instead, studies point to an array of beneficial substances in food, some of which are better suited than others to fighting specific kinds of cancers.

Evidence from China

One of the most widely reported studies of 1993 found that adding beta carotene, vitamin E, and the mineral selenium to the diet of people in rural China helped lower the death rate from cancers of the stomach and esophagus. The study involved nearly 30,000 men and women in Liaoning Province, a region in northern China with an especially high rate for those two cancers—as much as 100 times higher than that of the United States. The researchers theorized that the high rates for cancers of the stomach and esophagus might be related to the region's low consumption of foods rich in antioxidant compounds.

The study participants who took daily supplements of beta

carotene, vitamin E, and selenium (which also acts as an antioxidant) from 1986 to 1991 reduced their risk of dying of cancer of the stomach or esophagus by 13 percent. Deaths as a result of cancer of the esophagus fell by about 4 percent; stomach cancer deaths dropped by 21 percent.

Thinking yellow, orange, and leafy green

Closer to home, researchers studying the eating habits of nearly 90,000 women nurses in the United States announced that eating foods rich in vitamin A, such as carrots, cantaloupe, spinach, and sweet potatoes, could help some women reduce their chances of developing breast cancer. The eight-year study divided the women into four levels of vitamin A consumption, ranging from a low of less than 6,630 international units (IU) per day to a high of more than 17,640 IU per day.

Over the study period, 1,439 women developed breast cancer. There was no difference in breast cancer rates among the three groups with the highest levels of vitamin A consumption. But women in the group that averaged less than a serving a day of foods rich in vitamin A had about a 20 percent greater risk of developing breast cancer than the women in the other groups. Thus, if vitamin A has a protective effect against breast cancer, it might well kick in at a fairly low level of intake.

Deficiency of another nutrient, the B vitamin folate, appears to predispose women to cervical cancer, according to nutrition researchers at the University of Alabama at Birmingham. "We found a fivefold increase in risk of developing cervical dysplasia, a precancerous stage of cervical cancer [among women with low blood levels of folate]," says Douglas C. Heimburger, director of the university's division of clinical nutrition.

He and his colleagues do not know precisely how folate might help protect against this particular form of cancer, but they speculate that antioxidant protection of the cell's genetic material may be involved. The dietary message is clearer: Folate is abundant in leafy green vegetables such as spinach, broccoli, and Brussels sprouts. Think leafy green, nutritionists suggest.

Vegetables may also play a role in reducing the risk of the leading cancer killer of all: lung cancer. Although smoking has been implicated in the majority of lung cancer deaths, some 15 percent of lung cancer fatalities—about 22,350 each year—occur among people who never smoked. This number might be cut by some simple dietary changes, researchers at the Yale Cancer Center of the Yale School of Medicine in New Haven, Conn., reported in January 1993. "According to our findings, if people were to add 1½ servings of raw fruits and vegetables to their normal daily diet, then they would reduce their risk of lung cancer by 40 percent," says Susan T. Mayne, program director for prevention at the Yale Cancer Center.

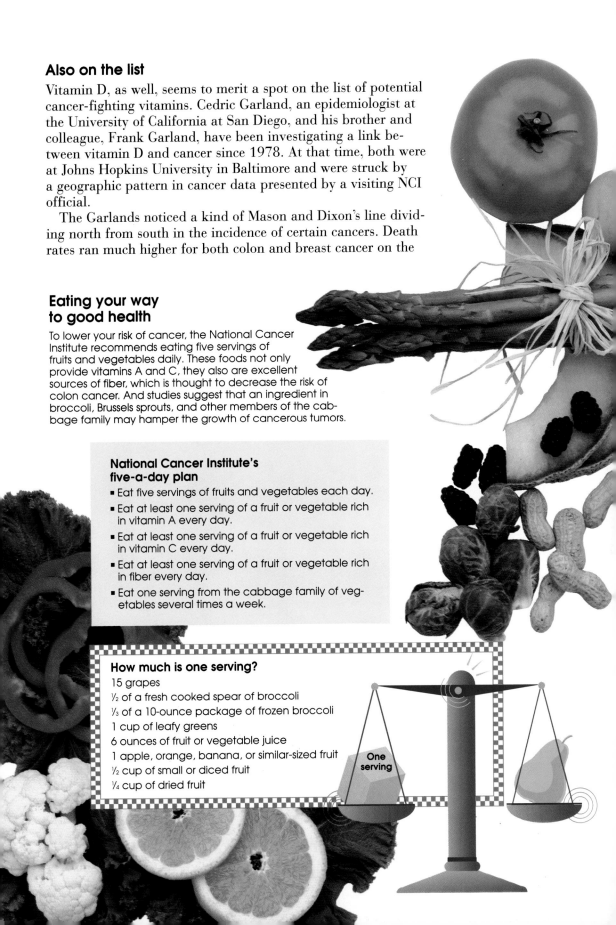

Also on the list

Vitamin D, as well, seems to merit a spot on the list of potential cancer-fighting vitamins. Cedric Garland, an epidemiologist at the University of California at San Diego, and his brother and colleague, Frank Garland, have been investigating a link between vitamin D and cancer since 1978. At that time, both were at Johns Hopkins University in Baltimore and were struck by a geographic pattern in cancer data presented by a visiting NCI official.

The Garlands noticed a kind of Mason and Dixon's line dividing north from south in the incidence of certain cancers. Death rates ran much higher for both colon and breast cancer on the

Eating your way to good health

To lower your risk of cancer, the National Cancer Institute recommends eating five servings of fruits and vegetables daily. These foods not only provide vitamins A and C, they also are excellent sources of fiber, which is thought to decrease the risk of colon cancer. And studies suggest that an ingredient in broccoli, Brussels sprouts, and other members of the cabbage family may hamper the growth of cancerous tumors.

National Cancer Institute's five-a-day plan
- Eat five servings of fruits and vegetables each day.
- Eat at least one serving of a fruit or vegetable rich in vitamin A every day.
- Eat at least one serving of a fruit or vegetable rich in vitamin C every day.
- Eat at least one serving of a fruit or vegetable rich in fiber every day.
- Eat one serving from the cabbage family of vegetables several times a week.

How much is one serving?
15 grapes
½ of a fresh cooked spear of broccoli
⅓ of a 10-ounce package of frozen broccoli
1 cup of leafy greens
6 ounces of fruit or vegetable juice
1 apple, orange, banana, or similar-sized fruit
½ cup of small or diced fruit
¼ cup of dried fruit

One serving

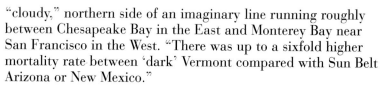

Vitamin E and heart disease

Cancer isn't the only chronic disease that might be thwarted by antioxidant vitamins. Recent studies suggest that vitamin E may play a role in preventing heart attacks.

In two large studies reported in May 1993, researchers at the Harvard School of Public Health and Brigham and Women's Hospital, both in Boston, found a lower risk of coronary artery disease in middle-aged men and women who took at least 100 international units (IU) of vitamin E in daily supplements for at least two years. The men's risk fell by 37 percent and the women's by 46 percent, compared with people who obtained vitamin E through diet alone.

The studies, which included almost 40,000 men and more than 80,000 women, supported a theory that vitamin E blocks the damaging effects that oxygen-containing molecules called free radicals have on low-density lipoprotein (LDL), the so-called bad cholesterol. Researchers suspect that the effect—the oxidation of LDL cholesterol—is an early step in *atherosclerosis*, a condition in which fatty deposits build up on artery walls. This artery-clogging build-up hampers blood flow, forces the heart to work harder, and can eventually lead to a heart attack.

In December 1993, researchers at the University of Texas Southwestern Medical Center at Dallas reported on the effectiveness of larger doses of vitamin E, alone and in combination with other vitamins, in preventing the oxidation of LDL cholesterol. "We've found that 800 IU of vitamin E was just as safe and effective in limiting the susceptibility of LDL cholesterol to being oxidized as was a vitamin 'cocktail' containing 800 IU of vitamin E, 1 gram of vitamin C, and 30 milligrams of beta carotene," said Ishwarlal Jialal, the study's principal investigator.

The 36 men in the study were divided into three groups. One group took the vitamin E supplement only; the second took the vitamin cocktail; and the third, a *placebo* (pill with no active ingredients). After three months, the investigators found that LDL oxidation in the first two groups was cut by about 50 percent. The findings prompted Jialal to recommend vitamin E supplements for a narrowly defined group: people under age 50 with heart disease but with no other risk factors for heart disease, such as high blood pressure. "They may have more to gain than to lose by taking antioxidants while we await more clinical trials," he said.   [J. G.]

"cloudy," northern side of an imaginary line running roughly between Chesapeake Bay in the East and Monterey Bay near San Francisco in the West. "There was up to a sixfold higher mortality rate between 'dark' Vermont compared with Sun Belt Arizona or New Mexico."

The Garlands theorized that vitamin D, which the body manufactures in response to sunlight, somehow offered protection against these two common cancers. Subsequent studies have borne out the link between vitamin D and cancer. Added support for the role of vitamin D in preventing colon cancer came most recently from an analysis of frozen blood samples drawn as far back as 1974 from 25,000 residents of Washington County in Maryland. Garland notes, "The higher the level of vitamin D in the blood, the lower the incidence of cancer." Those who ranked in the upper half in terms of vitamin D levels had about half the risk of developing colon cancer.

Vitamin D may work its anticancer magic by enhancing the body's absorption of calcium, a substance that helps prevent uncontrolled cell growth. That theory would make milk fortified with vitamin D an excellent line of defense against colon and breast cancers—especially since exposure to the sun carries its own cancer risk: an increased incidence of skin cancer. Vitamin D is one nutrient plants cannot provide us. Other sources besides sunlight include salmon, tuna, liver, and eggs.

Some studies suggest vitamin C may have value in a supporting role, if not as a primary cancer fighter. Oxidative heart damage is a common side effect of the cancer-fighting drug adriamycin. Some research has shown that vitamin C helps prevent damage to the heart from oxidation. Still, many scientists remain skeptical about claims made for vitamin C.

The need for more information

The possibility of preventing some cancers with everyday foods excites many scientists. Nonetheless, their optimism remains guarded. Not only is the study of antioxidants still young, but scientists are just beginning to understand the complex ways in which the hundreds of different nutrients in food interact within the body. And many questions remain unanswered. For example, does the same carrot plant grown in two different soils have the same cancer-preventing compounds? Is a boiled or microwaved carrot less beneficial than a raw carrot?

Moreover, the nature of most of the research to date necessarily casts most findings in a preliminary rather than a conclusive light. The bulk of the studies have looked at interactions of

Vitamins and cancer research

A growing number of studies suggest that vitamins and other compounds found in food may fight cancer. But scientists are only beginning to understand the connection between diet and disease.

Compound	Cancer
Beta carotene	May lower the risk of cancers of the breast, cervix, lung, stomach, and mouth.
Folate	May lower the risk of cancer of the cervix.
Vitamin C	May lower the risk of cancers of the mouth, larynx, esophagus, pancreas, stomach, rectum, breast, cervix, and lung.
Vitamin D	May lower the risk of cancers of the colon and breast.
Vitamin E	May lower the risk of cancers of the breast, cervix, lung, mouth, pancreas, stomach, colon, rectum, and urinary tract.

Source: National Cancer Institute.

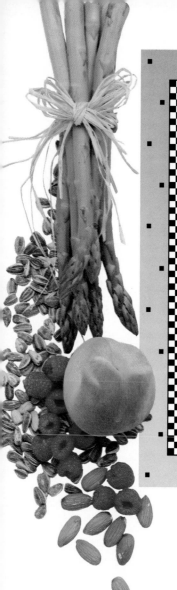

Recommended daily dietary allowances

Compound	Recommended dietary allowance	Dangers of high intake
Beta carotene	No official recommendation apart from vitamin A. For vitamin A, the recommen–dation is 800 to 1,000 micrograms.	High doses may turn skin yellow.
Folate	180 to 200 micrograms	High doses may cause digestive problems, sleep problems, and nervousness.
Vitamin C	50 to 60 milligrams	Huge doses—10,000 milligrams a day—may cause diarrhea and nausea.
Vitamin D	5 to 10 micrograms	High doses may deplete bones of calcium and phosphorus.
Vitamin E	8 to 10 milligrams	None known up to 80 times recommended daily allowance.

Source: U.S. Food and Drug Administration;
Food and Nutrition Board of the National Academy of Sciences.

molecules in test tubes or at effects on laboratory animals, both less-than-perfect stand-ins for the human body. And those studies that have focused on human beings have generally relied upon statistical correlations—comparisons of cancer rates in different population groups—rather than on controlled studies that attempt to demonstrate a cause-and-effect relationship.

Even the much-publicized Liaoning study in China came with a disclaimer about the relevance of the results to populations outside the region. William J. Blot of the NCI said that because the Liaoning population has chronic dietary deficiencies and because not many types of cancer are prevalent in the region, the applicability of the findings to well-nourished populations and to all types of cancer may be limited.

What is needed is information from clinical trials in Europe and North America. In these trials, researchers zero in on an antioxidant by giving specific amounts to volunteers in certain groups and then comparing disease rates in those groups to disease rates in so-called control groups who receive a *placebo* (a pill with no active ingredients). Such trials are now underway.

An investigation of the cancer-preventing potential of beta carotene has been made part of the Physician's Health Study of

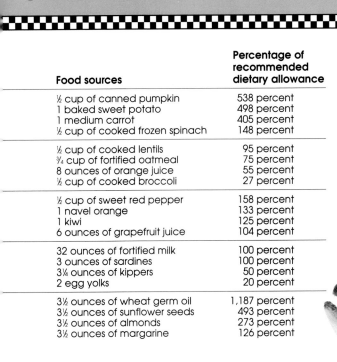

Food sources	Percentage of recommended dietary allowance
½ cup of canned pumpkin	538 percent
1 baked sweet potato	498 percent
1 medium carrot	405 percent
½ cup of cooked frozen spinach	148 percent
½ cup of cooked lentils	95 percent
¾ cup of fortified oatmeal	75 percent
8 ounces of orange juice	55 percent
½ cup of cooked broccoli	27 percent
½ cup of sweet red pepper	158 percent
1 navel orange	133 percent
1 kiwi	125 percent
6 ounces of grapefruit juice	104 percent
32 ounces of fortified milk	100 percent
3 ounces of sardines	100 percent
3¼ ounces of kippers	50 percent
2 egg yolks	20 percent
3½ ounces of wheat germ oil	1,187 percent
3½ ounces of sunflower seeds	493 percent
3½ ounces of almonds	273 percent
3½ ounces of margarine	126 percent

male doctors begun in 1980 by the Harvard Medical School in Boston. Some of the 22,000 doctors in the study are now taking beta carotene, while others receive a placebo. Cancer rates in the two groups will be compared after the study ends in 1995.

Women are receiving attention in the Women's Health Study, an even larger, five-year study begun in 1992 by the Harvard Medical School and Brigham and Women's Hospital, also in Boston. The preventive effects of beta carotene and vitamin E on cancer and heart disease will be monitored among some 40,000 study participants aged 45 and older.

The long-awaited results of a study in Finland on antioxidant benefits for smokers took many people in the cancer-prevention field by surprise. The Finnish study, reported in April 1994, found no reduction of lung cancer among some 29,000 male smokers aged 50 to 69 who were given beta carotene, vitamin E, or both antioxidants over a period of five to eight years. The men in the study who took beta carotene alone, in fact, had an 18 percent higher incidence of lung cancer and a somewhat higher risk for prostate cancer than did the other groups. On the other hand, the men who took vitamin E had a somewhat lower risk for prostate cancer than those who did not take it.

Several aspects of the Finnish study have come under scrutiny. Some researchers have pointed out that the doses of vitamin E were low—50 milligrams a day. Other studies that have shown a benefit from vitamin E have involved daily doses of 100 milligrams or more. Other critics have said that the study period was too short. Considering that cancer of the lung takes years to develop, they felt it was unrealistic to expect a few years of taking vitamins to counteract the damage from years of smoking. The men in the study continued to smoke every day.

Researchers were also caught off guard by a second study on vitamins and cancer in 1994. The four-year study reported in July that the antioxidant vitamins C and E and beta carotene, taken as supplements, failed to reduce the chances of developing precancerous growths in the colon. Cancer researcher E. Robert Greenberg of the Dartmouth-Hitchcock Medical Center in Hanover, N.H., the director of the study, said the negative results could mean that fruits and vegetables may contain other substances that help reduce the risk of cancer. It could also be that the antioxidant supplements were not taken long enough or at high enough levels to have an effect. More studies will be needed to resolve these questions.

What about vitamin supplements?

Meanwhile, Americans are still reaching for vitamin supplements. Seven in 10 Americans were taking vitamin supplements in 1993, according to a poll taken by *Newsweek* magazine, and 15 percent of daily users reported they had begun taking supplements within the last year. Some physicians are recommending vitamin E supplements, especially to older patients, because of findings that vitamin E may help ward off heart disease. Vitamin E is not as readily available in food as are other antioxidants. See VITAMIN E AND HEART DISEASE on page 68.

Even before the results of the Finnish and Dartmouth studies were reported, most nutritionists and cancer experts were recommending a whole-foods approach to vitamins, for several reasons. For one thing, it is not yet clear whether vitamins and nutrients supplied in pills perform the same antioxidant feats as those provided in food. Moreover, researchers are still a long way from pinpointing how much of a specific vitamin works best against a particular cancer. Finally, there are hundreds of different nutrients in fruits and vegetables, many of which researchers are just beginning to study.

The federal government has taken a cautious approach in its consumer information policy regarding vitamins. The 1990 Nutrition Labeling and Education Act allows for foods and supplements to carry health claims regarding vitamin content and the possibility that certain vitamins may reduce the risk of some cancers. In mid-1994, the U.S. Food and Drug Administration

(FDA) was beginning to approve sample labeling for foods that claimed anticancer benefits thanks to vitamins A or C. But the FDA had not yet allowed any such claims on vitamin supplement pills. In fact, recommended dietary allowances (RDA's) for various vitamins had become somewhat contentious.

Since 1941, RDA's for vitamins and minerals have been set by the Food and Nutrition Board of the National Academy of Sciences, an advisory group to the federal government. Some medical researchers feel that many of the values may be outdated.

When addressing such fundamental health matters, officials move very cautiously. The chief concern is that larger doses of antioxidant vitamins may have harmful side effects, especially in the megadoses (doses 5 to 10 times the RDA) that some individuals take in the belief that more of a good thing can only be better. On the contrary, excess vitamin A can cause headaches, liver damage, bone damage, diarrhea, and, in pregnant women, birth defects. High doses of vitamin C have been linked to kidney damage and bladder problems.

More fruits and vegetables

Most doctors recommend the plate ahead of the pill as the preferred way of supplying the body with antioxidant vitamins. In addition to recommending regular exercise and reiterating that smokers quit their deadly habit, the NCI strongly advises consumers to adopt its Five-a-Day for Better Health Program. This program promotes eating five or more servings of fruits and vegetables each day to reduce the risk of cancer. Most Americans eat only three servings a day.

A 6-ounce glass of fruit or vegetable juice with breakfast provides one serving. A half cup of cut-up fruit also equals one serving, as does an apple. The Five-a-Day plan carries with it the added health benefits of increasing dietary fiber. And by curbing the appetite with healthy offerings, the plan cuts down the intake of foods high in artery-clogging fat and cholesterol.

In short, a promising way of fighting cancer is easily doable. What is more, the "medicine" actually tastes good, too.

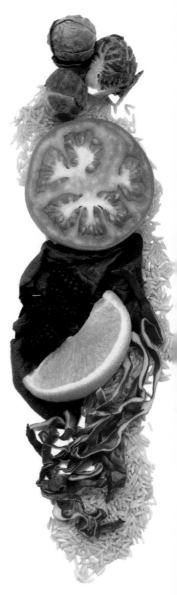

For additional information:

For information and publications on diet and cancer, call the Cancer Information Service of the National Cancer Institute, 1-800-422-6237.

Diet, Nutrition, & Cancer Prevention: A Guide to Food Choices. National Institutes of Health Publication No. 87-2878.

Eat More Fruits & Vegetables. National Institutes of Health Publication No. 92-3248.

Eat More Salads for Better Health. National Institutes of Health Publication No. 92-3250.

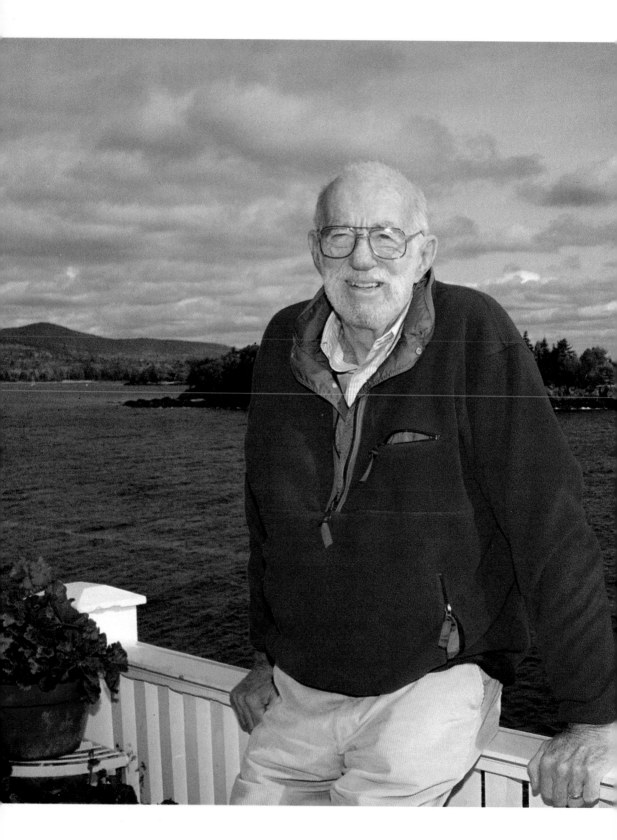

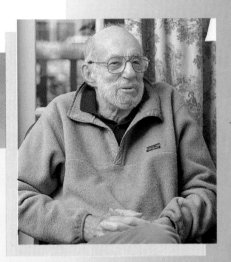

America's foremost baby doctor talks about how the problems that parents face have changed since the first edition of his best-selling *Baby and Child Care* appeared in 1946.

Dr. Spock Talks About Raising Children Today

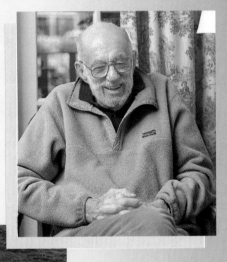

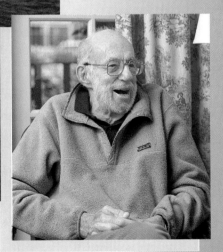

Health & Medical Annual: Your book *Baby and Child Care*, which first appeared in 1946, and the books, magazine articles, and newspaper columns that followed, have had a profound influence on the way parents raise their children. In nearly 50 years of giving advice to parents, you've obviously seen a number of changes in child-rearing problems and practices. Is raising a child harder today than it used to be?

Dr. Spock: I think so, because what parents worry about has changed. When I started pediatrics practice in 1933, parents worried about diseases: Is the ear infection going to spread to the mastoid? Is the cold going to turn into pneumonia? Will the polio epidemic on the West Coast spread to the East Coast, and so should we keep children out of the swimming pool now? Antibiotic drugs now cope efficiently with pneumonia, ear infections, and many other common infections. And more and more vaccines are available.

Parents now have to worry about the so-called drug scene, teen-age pregnancy, and how to make a child behave. I think that it's harder to worry about these than to worry about disease. But what parents worry about the most depends on the individual family. There's plenty to worry about.

H&MA: How can parents make their job easier?

Spock: I think the biggest problem the average parent faces on a daily basis is getting a child to behave cooperatively, and that's often because parents are afraid to provide firm, clear leadership. They're always wondering whether they should or shouldn't interfere.

I think of the example of 8-year-old Charlotte, who has been watching television in the living room, while her mother reads. When the mother suddenly says, "Charlotte, dear, it's half an hour after your bedtime," Charlotte, instead of being apologetic, says, "None of my friends have to go to bed at this hour. Besides, last week you let me stay up till an hour after my bedtime."

Instead of insisting, "Charlotte, it's time for bed," the mother acts perplexed, goes back to her book, and Charlotte goes on watching television for another half-hour. When the mother then says, "Charlotte, it's now *an hour* after your bedtime," Charlotte again objects strenuously.

H&MA: I don't imagine this would have happened when you were a child or when you started pediatrics practice.

Spock: No, it didn't. Parents knew what they expected of a

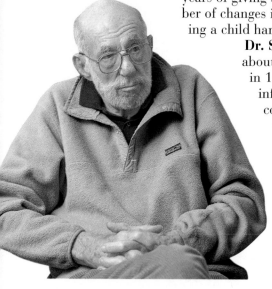

❝ I think the biggest problem the average parent faces on a daily basis is getting a child to behave cooperatively, and that's often because parents are afraid to provide firm, clear leadership. **❞**

child and asked for it without hesitation. Today, a lot of parents go wrong in thinking they've either got to be disagreeable or let the child do what the child wants to do. But this isn't so. Requiring cooperation and politeness from a child doesn't mean being disagreeable. Parents need to know what they expect of a child and to ask for it in a very friendly way. The friendlier their tone, the more likely it is that the child will do what they ask. Children like to have parents who are clear about what they expect and have no qualms about saying so.

H&MA: It's clear that not exercising authority can make life difficult for the parents. What effect is this having on children?

Spock: I think it makes children pesky. They become used to arguing every point, and they expect to intimidate the parents at least two-thirds of the time. When they succeed, of course, it encourages them to keep on objecting to what the parent asks.

H&MA: What's led to this erosion of parental authority in your opinion?

Spock: I think part of the explanation lies with all the "experts" like myself who have muscled into child-rearing and have written books on the subject. Parents get used to thinking, "Let's see what Spock says, or [Arnold L.] Gesell, or [T. Berry] Brazelton, or Penny Leach." If you go into a bookstore nowadays and ask for the books on raising children, you find a 25-foot shelf. When my book came out [in 1946], there were only about three books.

We disconcert parents, even parents who have a lot of self-assurance, so that they no longer trust their own instincts. And there are also a lot of parents who grew up without much self-assurance because their parents were overly bossy, and this can make parents hesitate to exercise authority.

I think mobility is another factor. Parents today rarely bring up their children in the same household or on the same block as the grandparents. But in simpler societies, beginning parents normally take their cues from the grandparents.

H&MA: There are some who have claimed that you contributed to this erosion of parental authority by encouraging permissiveness in child-rearing. How do you respond to that charge?

Spock: That accusation was first made in 1968—22 years after my book first came out—when supporters of then-President

> 66 Parents need to know what they expect of a child and to ask for it in a very friendly way. The friendlier their tone, the more likely it is that the child will do what they ask. 99

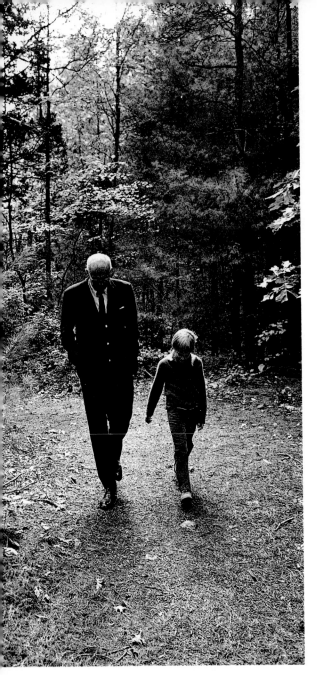

> **❝** [As a parent], it never occurred to me that I had to instill values. I thought all you had to be was a decent person and an educated person, and a child would fall into line. I still think that that's the most important thing. But I think that parents need to reinforce their values by discussing them. **❞**

Richard M. Nixon were upset by the fact that so many young people had decided that the war in Vietnam was abominable and that they were not going to be coerced into fighting in it. Conservatives saw this as lack of patriotism, and lack of self-discipline, and lack of courage, and lack of principles.

About a week or two after I had been indicted by the federal government along with four other people for my vigorous, outspoken opposition to the war, Norman Vincent Peale, a conservative clergyman and friend of Nixon, got the idea there was a connection between the student protests and the way the protesters had been reared. Peale said in a sermon that the trouble was that my book had persuaded parents to give these youths instant gratification as babies. I don't think I was ever permissive. I have always said parents should give firm, clear leadership and ask for cooperation and politeness.

H&MA: In fact, your books discuss the responsibilities of parents to instill values in children. What values do you think are the most important to communicate?

Spock: I'm putting more and more about values into each revision, and I'm also writing a book about values and spirituality. Many people think that by spiritual values you mean religion, and although religion is one of the greatest sources of spiritual values, I talk primarily about values that are not connected with religion. I think of such simple, everyday things as respect for your parents and respect for your children. I think of kindliness and of encouraging your children to be helpful, kind, and loving. These values could all come under the heading of love.

H&MA: And parents are failing on this score?

Spock: I think so. When I was raising my sons during the 1930's and 1940's, it never occurred to me that I had to instill values. I thought all you had to be was a decent person and an educated person, and a child would fall into line. I still think that that's the most important thing. But I think that parents need to reinforce their values by discussing them. I don't mean stern lectures all the time. There's nothing worse than that.

H&MA: What effect do you think television is having on children's values?

Spock: With many parents having so little time to spend with their children, children are learning their ideals from television. That means they're basically learning brutality, greediness, and the power of wealth. Television is potentially one of the greatest educational tools that's ever been invented and is recognized as such in many countries. Television could be teaching children and adults about the rest of the world and about scientific developments. But instead, it's mostly violence and silly stuff.

H&MA: Do you think that violence on television is having a disruptive effect on children?

Spock: I think it's having a horrible effect. It's clear that we're one of the most violent nations in the world, and we're becoming more violent. And yet we're teaching children violence by letting them watch it on television. It's been calculated that the average American child has watched 18,000 murders on television by the time they reach adulthood.

It's not that we're training well-brought-up children to be thugs. It doesn't go that far. But anytime that a child or an adult watches brutality, it brutalizes them to a slight degree. It desensitizes them. They start out with horror at the idea of brutality, but they get used to it just the way soldiers get used to the brutality of the war. And kids who are brought up without any particular ideals or who have been abused are being trained to use brutality to solve problems.

H&MA: You have spoken out against war toys. Does refusing to give little boys guns really work? Won't they just pick up a stick and use it for a gun?

Spock: You have to know that a boy will pick up sticks if he lives in an average community where other kids have guns and holsters. If someone gives your son a toy gun, I don't advocate that you snatch the gun away from him, and I don't advocate that you grab the stick away from a child when he's using it in gun play with other children. But I do think that parents can say, "I don't want to buy you a gun because there's too much killing in the world. We have got to love other people." In that way, parents can counteract to a degree the joy and the brutality of gun play.

I say the same thing to parents who say, "But if I don't let him watch television programs, he sneaks over to his friend's house." Again, the attitude of the parents will be highly influential, even though it's not enough to keep the child from these things.

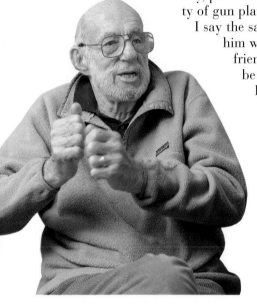

66 I believe very strongly that during the first three years of life, a child's view of the world is being solidified. It's not that this outlook can't be changed later, but it's a job to change it later. . . . the influence of the person who is taking care of the child is very great. **99**

H&MA: Families have undergone a number of changes since your book first came out. Many more children are now raised in single-parent households. How do you expect them to fare?

Spock: I think the first thing that should be said is that children can be raised very successfully by single parents. But it also should be said that it's much more difficult to raise a child as a single parent. It's good to be able to consult with a spouse and to have someone who says, "Dear, don't you think you're overdoing vitamins?" or politeness or whatever. Two people can strike a balance. And it's good for children to have both a male and a female parent because men and women tend to look at things somewhat differently.

H&MA: You offered advice to working mothers in the very first edition of *Baby and Child Care.* Has that advice changed?

Spock: I said in the first edition that if mothers knew how important the child's earliest years were, they might be willing to put off going to work for a year or so, until the child's outlook on the world and the family had a chance to crystallize. I believe very strongly that during the first three years of life, a child's view of the world is being solidified. It's not that this outlook can't be changed later, but it's a job to change it later.

H&MA: Some mothers have to work, whether they want to or not. Wouldn't that advice make them feel guilty?

Spock: Several mothers told me that my advice had made them feel very guilty. I don't think you should make parents feel guilty, and so in subsequent editions I pulled my neck in. I said that the influence of the person who is taking care of the child is very great. That's where children get their character and their outlook on life.

If a parent has to work—and I dropped the issue of whether

the parent should or shouldn't work—the important thing is to put the child in the care of somebody who has the same point of view as the parents. Parents ought not to hire anybody on short notice. They should have several long talks with the person and be present at least part of the time for the first week or two so they can see what the approach of the sitter is.

H&MA: Enrollments in day-care centers have been on the rise. What do we know about the benefits and the drawbacks of day care?

Spock: There have been conflicting reports on day care. You obviously get the best results when day care is run by a university department of child development and all the teachers are well-trained and dedicated to developing the best in children. I think we know now that such care is almost as beneficial as good parental care. On the other hand, day care can be no good if it is run by people who don't understand children or think that discipline is their most important job, or if there are too many children per teacher or day-care worker.

In recent editions of *Baby and Child Care*, I conclude that parents should look very carefully for high-quality day care. And I encourage them to work to elect Presidents, members of Congress, governors, and mayors who believe in the importance of good day care. I feel strongly that the government ought to subsidize high-quality day care.

H&MA: Do you see fathers taking a greater role in raising children?

Spock: Yes, and I think it's wonderful that fathers are finding child-rearing an inspiring thing to do. But it's still a minority of fathers. Our society doesn't think of child-rearing as the proper work for a father. Only in the evening or on weekends is he expected to participate. I think that fathers can be just as good nurturers, aside from breast-feeding, as mothers can be. We should get over this prejudice that only mothers really know how to care for children and that fathers can only be helpers to mothers.

For the father to do a good job, both parents must think of him as an equal partner in the care of the children, not as a helper. His wife has got to recognize him as having as much authority and as much good judgment as she has. Many times, when the husband tries to participate or help, the wife says, "No, no. You shouldn't do it that way." That response discourages the father and also sends the child the wrong message.

H&MA: Women also are having children later and later. What effect do you think this has on children and on parents?

Spock: It used to be said, have your children when you're young and resilient and you understand children better because you're closer to them in age. Then a study by a well-known psychologist showed that older parents are generally more understanding, more patient, and more tolerant. That's not to say

Baby doctor to the millions

The name Dr. Spock came to be synonymous with child-rearing in America after World War II. The first edition of Benjamin Spock's *The Common Sense Guide to Baby and Child Care* appeared in 1946, and its calm, friendly, reassuring tone made the book an immediate favorite with parents. Rather than telling parents what to do, Spock explained to them in a friendly, readable manner what children were like at different stages and what parents could expect. Each edition began with the words, "Trust yourself. You know more than you think you do." That advice was a far cry from the prevailing child-care wisdom, which prescribed strict adherence to rigid schedules and training.

The sixth edition of Spock's best-selling *Baby and Child Care* appeared in 1992. And at age 91, he was at work on a new book exploring how we can make the world a better place for our children.

Benjamin McLane Spock was born in New Haven, Conn., in 1903. He was the oldest of six children born to Benjamin Ives Spock, a lawyer, and Mildred Stoughton Spock. Spock credits his mother and her love of babies and small children with inspiring his own love of children. His mother was a stern disciplinarian, however, and Spock felt that there had to be more agreeable ways of bringing up children.

Spock graduated from Yale University in 1925. The year before, as an oarsman on the Yale eight-oared rowing team, he won a gold medal in the Olympic Games in Paris. Spock received his M.D. in 1929 from Columbia University's College of Physicians and Surgeons.

Before entering practice, Spock completed residencies in medicine, pediatrics, and psychiatry. As a resident, he noted that the advice many pediatricians gave had no sound psychological basis and was sometimes cruel. Thumb-sucking, for example, was considered a bad habit, and the sooner you interfered with a child's bad habit, the better your chances of squelching it.

Spock was horrified to see that babies in hospitals were routinely spread-eagled, their wrists tied to crib slats to prevent them from sucking their thumbs. The children, Spock realized, were miserable because they were sick, miserable because they were separated from their parents, and the most natural thing was to suck their thumbs. He felt that physicians ought to have a sound basis for encouraging or discouraging thumb-sucking and that there must be better ways of doing so.

The residency in psychiatry gave Spock the idea that training in the theories of Sigmund Freud, the founder of psychoanalysis, might provide some answers about thumb-sucking, feeding problems, and other issues that troubled mothers. And so, at the same time that he set up a pediatrics practice in 1933, he began psychoanalytic training. Out of this combined training in pediatrics and psychoanalysis came the book that made Spock famous.

The publisher, in Spock's telling, was looking for a physician who had studied the emotional side of child-rearing. He overcame Spock's initial hesitation with the assurance that the book

that they're all that way. Some are very cranky. Of course, the job can be well done by young parents and by older parents, just as it can be done not so well by young parents or old parents. There's nothing that tells you now is the right time to have a child.

H&MA: Have ideas about the ideal spacing between children changed?

Spock: I have often been asked what's the ideal spacing. I know that any spacing can be successful or unsuccessful. Many people seem to think about two years between the first child and the second is about right. But there's plenty of ferocious jealousy that comes out at two years of age. And if parents

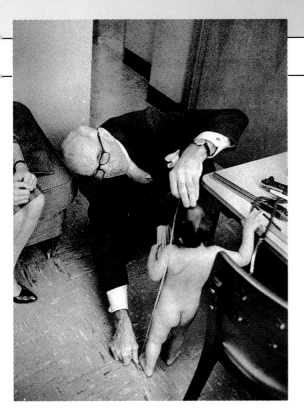

1951, when he became a professor of child development at the University of Pittsburgh. In 1955, Spock moved to Cleveland, where he was professor of child development at Western Reserve University (now Case Western Reserve University) and supervising pediatrician at the university's family clinic. He retired from Western Reserve in 1967.

Spock notes that as a pediatrician, he had a tendency to "whoop it up" with children. His concern for his young patients was reflected in a contraption he rigged up in his office: To reach the examining table, a child had to climb a short enclosed staircase and crawl through a trapdoor.

Spock's concern for children—and the world we were creating for them—led to his involvement in the peace movement during the 1960's. He served as co-chairman of the National Committee for a Sane Nuclear Policy, a group that advocated bans on nuclear testing. Later, he joined protests against the war in Vietnam. Spock was indicted in 1968, along with four others (including William Sloane Coffin, the chaplain of Yale University), for conspiracy to promote resistance to the military draft. His conviction was later overturned. In 1972, Spock ran for President as the candidate of the People's Party, receiving 79,000 votes in 10 states.

Spock has two sons from his first marriage to Jane Cheney and four grandchildren. In 1976, he married political activist Mary Morgan. The two collaborated on *Spock on Spock*, published in 1989, in which the world's most famous baby doctor relates episodes from his life story.

didn't have to be very good: At 25 cents a copy, they could sell 10,000 copies a year. By 1994, 40 million copies were in print. *Baby and Child Care* had outsold every book but the Bible.

Spock practiced pediatrics in New York City from 1933 to 1947, with a two-year interruption for service in the U.S. Navy during World War II. He taught child psychiatry at the Mayo Clinic and the University of Minnesota from 1947 to

space their children very far apart, then teen-age children may be quite miffed by the idea that their mother is involved in such a thing.

H&MA: You became a stepfather to an 11-year-old girl in 1976, when you married your second wife, Mary Morgan.

Spock: Right. Being a stepfather was one of the most unsuccessful things I ever did, at least for a number of years. In the first place, I hadn't had any experience with daughters. I had helped to raise two sons, and I discovered that girls can be quite different from boys.

Mary's daughter, Ginger, could hardly stand the looks of me. When she'd come back from school, she wouldn't acknowledge

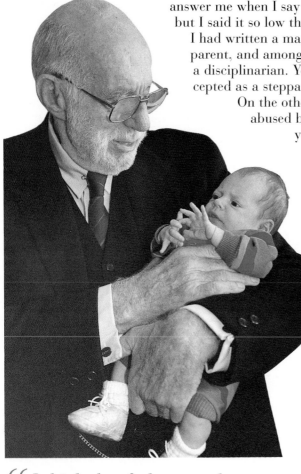

my presence. I would say, "Hi, Ginger," and she would never reply. I asked her once in exasperation, "Why is it you never answer me when I say 'hello'?" And she replied, "I said it, but I said it so low that you didn't hear it."

I had written a magazine article on how to be a stepparent, and among other things, I said, "Don't try to be a disciplinarian. You'll have enough difficulty being accepted as a stepparent without being a disciplinarian. On the other hand, you shouldn't let yourself be abused by the child. You should stand up for yourself and insist on reasonable politeness. But don't go out of your own corner to try to correct the child."

H&MA: But that advice didn't work?

Spock: I found that it might have been good advice for somebody, but it didn't do me any good at all. I was so angry that I couldn't follow my advice to not become a disciplinarian. Ginger was having her teeth straightened at considerable expense, and she refused to put her braces on or wear her retainer. It bothered me so to see Ginger not being considerate of her father, who was paying the bills, that I couldn't help saying, "Aren't you going to put on your braces?" And my interfering made her furious. It gives the child the chance to say, "You're not my parent, and so I don't have to do what you say." And it buttresses their defiance.

H&MA: What should the parent do? Did Mary intervene?

Spock: Mary said she felt she was being pulled apart by Ginger tugging her one way and me tugging her the other. The parent's position is a very awkward one. I used to say, "Mary, can't you make her be civil to me?" But Mary didn't want to be in the position of scolding Ginger into being nominally polite to me. It's a tough job to be the biological parent, and you owe loyalty to both your new spouse and your children.

H&MA: What finally changed things?

> 66 I think that fathers can be just as good nurturers, aside from breast-feeding, as mothers can be. We should get over this prejudice that only mothers really know how to care for children and that fathers can only be helpers to mothers. 99

Spock: Very, very gradually our relationship improved. When Ginger was graduating from high school, she arranged for me to give the commencement address, which I felt was a triumph.

We were on a television show together once. And the interviewer happened to ask, "What made you feel better about your stepfather?" And Ginger without hesitation replied, "I was having an angry argument with my mother, and my stepfather took my side." And I thought, now this is a practical piece of advice. This isn't just theory. We're very good friends now.

H&MA: How did your experience change the advice you gave?

Spock: I tell stepparents to take it easy. Keep out of the discipline situation, but don't let yourself be abused. Don't expect too much, and don't condemn yourself as a stepparent because you're not succeeding right away. In some cases, it seems hardly to take any time at all. But in other cases, it seems to take forever.

H&MA: The first generation of "Spock babies" are about to become grandparents. Does Dr. Spock have any advice for grandparents?

Spock: I have always told grandparents, from my own experience, don't interfere. I have explained that it will annoy them at times to see things being done that they don't approve of: for example, so-called feeding on demand. The switch from extremely rigid feeding schedules to self-demand horrified some grandparents. It can be agony for grandparents, especially if child-rearing customs have changed, and these customs always are changing in America. But I tell grandmothers that it's really none of their business unless the mother asks. The wise grandmother is one who can listen, and having the grandmother listen can be a great comfort to a young mother.

A grandmother once wrote to me and said, "Will you write to my daughter and tell her to put more clothes on the child when the weather is cold." I've wondered what a young mother would think if she got a letter from me saying, "You aren't putting enough clothes on your child. Your mother told me so."

H&MA: From the other side, what should parents do when grandparents have different ideas about child-rearing?

Spock: I think it's good for young parents to recognize that the grandparents have a natural and wholesome interest in how their grandchildren are brought up. Even when the advice is unwanted, the mother can at least listen to the grandmother. She doesn't have to do what the grandmother recommends, and

> **❝** I tell stepparents to take it easy. Keep out of the discipline situation . . . . and don't condemn yourself as a stepparent because you're not succeeding right away. **❞**

she can respond in a matter-of-fact, cheerful way, "I was discussing that with the pediatrician, and he said he believes such and such."

H&MA: How do you feel we are doing by our children as a society?

Spock: Let's sum it up by saying that Americans are child-centered when it comes to their own children. They'll give them orthodontia and piano or ballet lessons. But the majority of Americans are relatively insensitive to the needs of other children. This is why we have such poor schools in many deprived neighborhoods. And that's why we have such cruel facilities for handling so-called delinquent children.

H&MA: You participated in the 1924 Olympics and won a medal for rowing. In this year's games, the attack on ice-skater Nancy Kerrigan gave us a sense of how far competitiveness can go. What's happened to sportsmanship?

Spock: Participation in sports tends to be evaluated in terms of the money to be earned or the fame that opens the doors to earning money. I think that's a great mistake. Sports should be one, for fun; two, for learning skills; and three, for learning team play. And winning, especially winning money, should be played down.

H&MA: How do you feel about the desire of some parents to raise "superkids"?

Spock: I don't think that's the fault of parents. I think it's the fault of our society, which is excessively competitive. And new parents feel it's their duty to keep their children from falling behind: If other children are learning to read at the age of three in a day-care center, then why isn't our day-care center teaching reading and writing?

H&MA: There's also a push to teach children how to use computers. Is a child who learns to play computer games at age 3 going to want to read?

Spock: It may be that the computer helps children learn to read and in the long run is a boon. But I can't help worrying that it will get people off the track. Anything that artificializes or depersonalizes education I think is potentially dangerous. The fundamental motivation behind learning seems to be a good relationship between student and teacher. You want to learn because you like the person doing the teaching.

There is an intense drive in all children, especially at the ages of 3, 4, and 5, to be like the parent, and this is what makes children want to learn. I think you can judge educational pro-

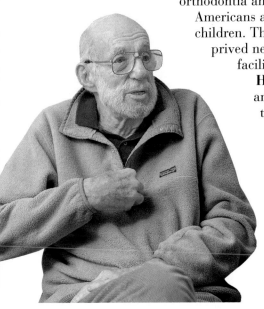

❝ There is an intense drive in all children, especially at the ages of 3, 4, and 5, to be like the parent, and this is what makes children want to learn. **❞**

grams by asking: Does it retain the importance of the good relationship? I don't think you get that out of a machine.

H&MA: Which areas of child rearing are now undergoing scrutiny? What might be new topics in your next edition?

Spock: Well, I'm writing a book called *A Better World for Our Children*. It's primarily an inquiry into whatever happened to our idealism and our spiritual values. Why is America more and more violent? Why is America more and more materialistic? What's happened to the spiritual values that we used to have, the emphasis on lovingness, kindliness, helpfulness?

I'd like to use Christmas as an example. I certainly did the wrong thing as a parent. And I have seen people ever since doing what I think is wrong: giving children everything that they ever thought of for Christmas. Children go to see Santa Claus to enlist his help in getting what they want, and on Christmas Day, they indulge in an orgy of greed. And if a present isn't something that they wanted very much, they just put it aside. There is no obligation to thank anybody.

At Christmastime, children should be making presents, even of a very simple kind, for their grandparents, aunts and uncles, and cousins. Or at least they should be making Christmas cards and paper chains for Christmas tree decorations, instead of assuming that the mother will buy the tinsel and the ornaments.

The emphasis on spiritual growth should extend beyond Christmas. Children love to be given responsibility and jobs. I think two-year-olds should be helping to set the table and to carry the flatware out to the kitchen afterward. And children through later stages of childhood should have appropriate duties imposed not by disagreeable, scolding parents but by parents who recognize that the most valuable thing they can do for a child is to encourage the child's natural helpfulness.

For further reading:

Spock, Benjamin, and Rothenberg, Michael. *Dr. Spock's Baby & Child Care*, 6th edition, NAL Dutton, 1992.

Spock on Spock: A Memoir of Growing Up with the Century. Pantheon, 1989.

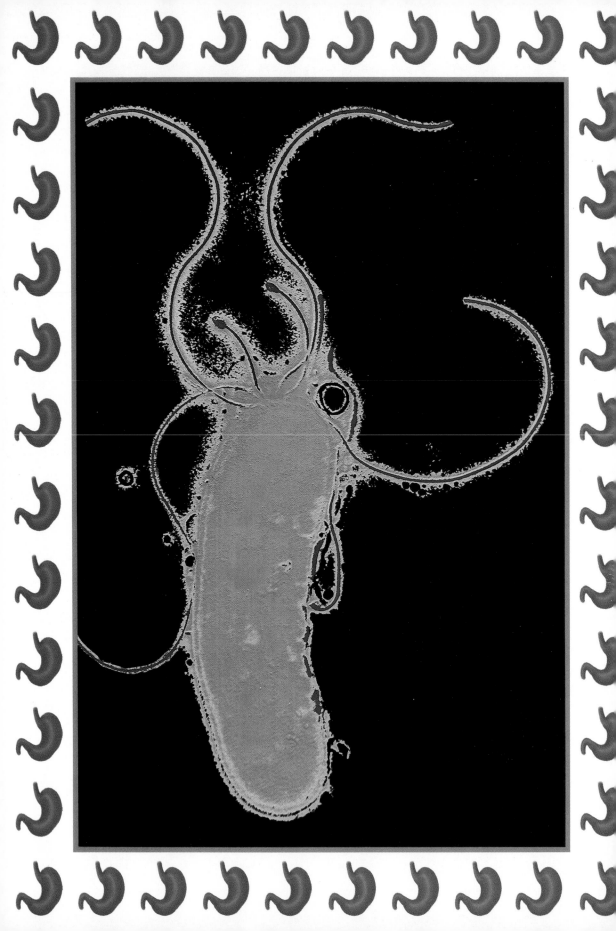

Bagging the Ulcer Bug

By Robin Netherton

Medical researchers have found
evidence that bacteria cause most
ulcers and that antibiotics can
cure these ulcers for good.

For decades, ulcers have been an unpleasant fact of American
life. After all, *peptic ulcers*—painful irritations of the stomach
or small intestine—strike as many as 1 in 10 Americans.

And no wonder. The habits long blamed for ulcers—eating
spicy foods, drinking coffee and alcohol, and smoking—were
those Americans too often indulged in, as doctors reminded
their patients. And didn't the prime suspect in triggering ulcers—stress—go hand in hand with the American way of life?

Whatever the cause, most ulcer sufferers learned that they
would probably have to live with the condition. Expensive drugs
might curtail an attack, but the problem frequently recurred.

So went the conventional wisdom. Over the past decade, however, medical researchers have overturned these long-established
beliefs about ulcer disease. In many cases, the real culprit appears to be a bacterium, *Helicobacter pylori* (*H. pylori* for
short). Moreover, by treating *H. pylori* infection, physicians can
usually banish a patient's ulcers for good.

In February 1994, an independent advisory panel of 14 medical experts, meeting at the National Institutes of Health (NIH)

Medical researchers be-
lieve that infection with
the bacterium *Helico-
bacter pylori, opposite
page,* causes most di-
gestive tract ulcers.

in Bethesda, Md., recommended treating ulcers with a two-week course of common antibiotics meant to cure *H. pylori* infection. This approach raises the prospect that many ulcers may someday be no more than an occasional, curable nuisance.

The new consensus represents a revolution in ulcer treatment—and a hard-won revolution at that. In the early 1980's, when two Australian physicians identified *H. pylori* and suggested that it caused ulcers, most *gastroenterologists* (doctors who specialize in diseases of the stomach and intestines) understandably had their doubts. The link between ulcers and various other conditions, particularly psychological stress, had been medical common sense for years. In fact, the ulcer had become an example of the harmful physical effects of tension-filled modern life—even though researchers did not know the precise mechanism by which stress caused ulcers.

Scientists have long understood how an ulcer grows. The stomach is a hostile place, home to hydrochloric acid, which helps dissolve the food we eat. Not surprisingly, an acid that can break down a sirloin steak is also strong enough to damage human tissue—including the lining of the stomach itself. What keeps this acid from digesting its surroundings is a protective layer of mucus that coats the inside of the stomach and the nearby *duodenum* (the upper part of the small intestine).

When something creates an opening in the mucous layer, the digestive acid can attack the exposed tissues. Extensive exposure to hydrochloric acid can form the wound known as an ulcer. About 80 percent of peptic ulcers are located in the duodenum and thus are called duodenal ulcers. These ulcers are most common in people aged 30 to 50. About 20 percent of peptic ulcers are gastric ulcers, located in the stomach. They are most likely to appear in people over age 60.

Symptoms of an ulcer

The first sign of an ulcer is commonly stomach pain, usually a dull aching or burning in the upper abdomen. Additional symptoms can include bloating, nausea, vomiting, lack of appetite, or weight loss, though these symptoms can also accompany various other digestive tract ailments. The pain may come and go daily, occur between meals or with them, or wake a person in the middle of the night.

In serious cases, an ulcer may bleed, leading to a loss of blood either in vomit—which may be bright red, or brown like coffee grounds—or in the stool, which may look red, or tarry and black. An ulcer may also create an obstruction in the digestive tract, blocking the movement of food out of the stomach and causing profuse vomiting. In a very few instances, the ulcer may *perforate* (eat through) the wall of the stomach or intestine, causing severe pain and requiring emergency surgery. Any of

The author:

Robin Netherton is a freelance writer and editor.

Peptic ulcer: An open sore

An ulcer is an open sore on the skin or on a mucous membrane. Ulcers on mucous membranes most commonly form in the digestive tract. A gastric ulcer develops in the lining of the stomach; a duodenal ulcer, in the *duodenum* (upper part of the small intestine). Digestive tract ulcers are also called peptic ulcers.

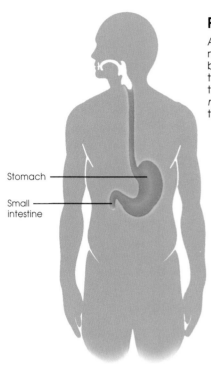

Stomach

Small intestine

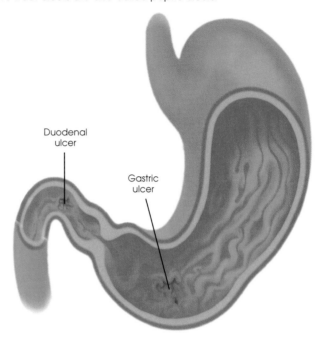

Duodenal ulcer

Gastric ulcer

these complications can be life threatening. Each year about 6,000 Americans die from ulcer complications, according to the National Center for Health Statistics (NCHS), a branch of NIH.

Far many more live with their ulcers. Perhaps as many as 10 percent of Americans alive today—25 million people—will develop ulcers at some point in their lives. About 4.4 million people in the United States suffered from ulcers in 1992 alone, the latest year for which statistics are available from NCHS.

Known and suspected culprits

Although scientists worked out the process of an ulcer's development long ago, they have been less successful at pinpointing the reasons most ulcers occur in the first place. Some cases pose no mystery. Extended use of aspirin or related painkillers called *non*steroidal *anti-in*flammatory *d*rugs (NSAID's) has been implicated in at least 10 percent of duodenal ulcers and 20 percent of gastric ulcers in the United States. For more information about NSAID's and ulcers, see ULCERS THAT WON'T RESPOND TO ANTIBIOTICS on page 100.

In addition, certain rare conditions—such as Zollinger-Ellison syndrome, which involves excess secretion of stomach acid—make a person prone to ulcers. Tumors of certain glands near the thyroid may also be associated with ulcers. Conditions such as these account for about 3 percent of duodenal ulcers and 10 to 15 percent of gastric ulcers, according to the NIH.

But for most ulcers, the cause has been less straightforward. Over the years, doctors have suggested many different irritants as possible culprits, including certain foods, alcohol, cigarettes, and coffee. Still, studies never produced conclusive evidence that these substances had more than a contributing effect—if that—on ulcer development.

Even as experts debated the importance of such factors, few disputed one seemingly obvious cause of most ulcers: psychological stress. The theory has been that people under stress may produce more stomach acid and thereby dispose themselves to ulcers. The stress hypothesis gradually became widely accepted.

Another reason experts at first doubted the theory that bacteria could cause ulcers was the fact that very few bacteria can live in the stomach. Although other parts of the human digestive tract normally harbor various microorganisms, both helpful and harmful, the stomach's high acid content creates an environment extremely hostile to microbes.

So at a 1983 meeting, when gastroenterologist Barry J. Marshall of Royal Perth Hospital in Australia described a new bacterium that his colleague J. Robin Warren had isolated from patients' stomach tissues and suggested that the organism caused ulcers, an international audience of scientists thought he was mistaken. Perhaps, said skeptics, the microbe was a contaminant that had tainted the laboratory specimens. And even if it were possible that the bacterium lived in people's stomachs, that didn't mean it caused ulcers. Maybe it was a harmless colonizer normally found in the digestive tract, or simply a visitor that moved in only after an ulcer formed.

A dangerous experiment and a new theory

But Marshall was certain that his new bacterium was a stomach dweller, and a nasty one at that. Desperate for proof, he conducted a daring, and dangerous, experiment. In June 1984, Marshall brewed a broth of *H. pylori* and drank it. It tasted, he said afterward, like "swamp water."

A few days later, Marshall woke up vomiting. He hadn't developed an ulcer, but he did have a bad case of *gastritis* (stomach inflammation). Laboratory tests showed that his stomach was teeming with *H. pylori*. By comparison, tests he had taken before drinking his microbial cocktail had shown him free of infection. His experiment demonstrated that *H. pylori* could live in the stomach, and that it did cause illness. Because *chronic*

How an ulcer forms

Medical researchers believe that most peptic ulcers form as a result of infection with the bacterium *Helicobacter pylori*. *H. pylori* acts in combination with gastric acid, a powerful digestive juice secreted by glands in the stomach.

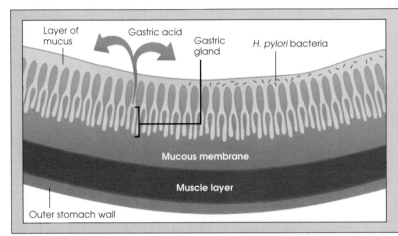

Layer of mucus

Gastric acid

Gastric gland

H. pylori bacteria

Mucous membrane

Muscle layer

Outer stomach wall

H. pylori can live in the digestive tract for years without causing serious problems.

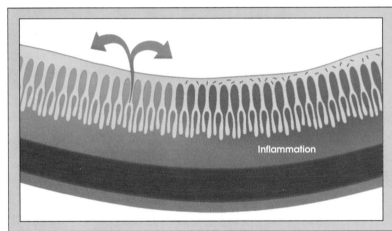

Inflammation

Infection with *H. pylori* can lead to *gastritis*—inflammation of the stomach lining. The inflammation reduces the ability of the stomach's coating of mucus to protect against the corrosive action of gastric acid.

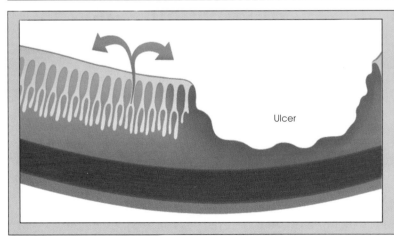

Ulcer

Over time, the wounded area may develop into an ulcer.

(long-term) gastritis is often a precursor to more serious stomach disorders—including ulcers—the stunt lent some credence to his theory.

Marshall named the new bacterium *Campylobacter pyloridis*, thinking it was a relative of the *Campylobacter* bacteria responsible for some kinds of food poisoning. (The word *pyloridis* refers to the pylorus, the entrance to the duodenum, where Marshall and his colleague Warren had found the bug.) In 1989, scientists renamed the bacterium *Helicobacter*, after realizing that it differed sufficiently from *Campylobacter* to constitute a separate group. The new name refers to the bacterium's *helical* (corkscrew) shape—a shape that may enable *H. pylori* to spiral rapidly through stomach acid and burrow into the mucous layer.

In the mucous layer, scientists now believe, *H. pylori* latches onto cells of the stomach lining by binding to chemicals on the surfaces of these cells. As *H. pylori* multiplies, it releases substances that damage the surrounding tissue. Scientists are still piecing together what happens next, but it seems that as the body attempts to fight off the infection, the stomach lining becomes inflamed, causing gastritis. Over time, if the infection remains unchecked, the damaged area may develop into an ulcer.

During the 1980's, other researchers conducted their own experiments. As research progressed, the evidence of *H. pylori*'s role in the formation of ulcers mounted. The most convincing data came from studies of ulcer treatments. Researchers found that their ulcer patients were infected with *H. pylori*—and that if treatment could eliminate the infection, it almost always rid patients of their ulcers as well.

The standard ulcer treatment

Traditional treatment of ulcers typically consists of a four-week to eight-week regimen of a drug that helps heal ulcers by reducing the body's production of stomach acid. Such drugs—called histamine H_2-receptor antagonists, or H_2-blockers—include cimetidine (sold under the trade name Tagamet), ranitidine (Zantac), famotidine (Pepcid), and nizatidine (Axid). Another group of drugs that work to cut acid production are known as proton-pump inhibitors. The most commonly prescribed of these drugs is omeprazole (Prilosec).

Such treatment rarely constitutes a lasting cure, however. The great majority of patients develop new ulcers within two years after they stop the standard drug treatment. Long-term use of H_2-blockers can keep ulcers from recurring. But these drugs cause side effects, the most common of which are headaches, diarrhea, and nausea. And the drugs are expensive. A year's supply of Tagamet or Zantac can cost as much as $800 to $1,000. These drugs have, however, reduced the need for surgery to re-

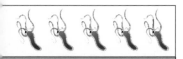

Symptoms of an ulcer

Some ulcers may persist for years with few symptoms. But when symptoms do appear, they can include:

- Dull aching or burning between the abdomen and the lower chest, often occurring between meals or in the middle of the night.
- Nausea and vomiting.
- Abdominal bloating.
- Red or black stool.
- Loss of appetite or weight loss.

pair ulcers that fail to heal. Although surgery was quite common for ulcer patients 20 years ago, before the drugs became widely available, fewer than 2 percent require it today.

Other recommendations under the standard procedure might include taking an over-the-counter antacid, such as Maalox or Mylanta, to neutralize acid in the stomach. Ulcer patients were also advised to eat frequent small meals, because food in the stomach can lessen the effects of stomach acid. And, of course, they were told to avoid the standard suspects: stress, smoking, alcohol, and coffee, and any foods that supposedly brought on ulcer symptoms. Although doctors once told patients to drink milk to soothe ulcers, they know now that milk actually increases acid production in the stomach.

The new ulcer treatment

The NIH consensus statement outlines different treatments for ulcers, based on findings from studies of *H. pylori*. While doctors are still experimenting with various treatments, experts generally recommend a two-week course of two antibiotics—for example, metronidazole and tetracycline—to wipe out the *H. pylori* infection. The use of two antibiotics simultaneously is designed to prevent *H. pylori* from developing a resistance to the drugs. A few of the bacteria in a person's stomach might survive treatment with any single antibiotic, but it is far less likely that they could resist two different drugs at once.

The new treatment may also include two medications that were frequently used for ulcers in the past: omeprazole to cut acid production and bismuth. Bismuth, best known as an ingredient in the over-the-counter medicine Pepto-Bismol, has antimicrobial properties. Finally, along with the antibiotics, the patient may be instructed to take a traditional ulcer drug such as ranitidine to help the existing ulcer heal.

Eradicating *H. pylori* is not easy. The antibiotics cause such side effects as nausea, vomiting, and diarrhea in perhaps 15 percent of patients, and the standard ulcer drugs may prompt their usual side effects as well. Also, taking so many pills—often more than a dozen each day—may be difficult or inconvenient for many patients. But the treatment only lasts two weeks, and the entire course of pills typically costs less than $100. This is less than treatment with traditional ulcer medications and far less than long-term maintenance with those drugs.

The strongest case for the new treatment, however, is its effectiveness, as demonstrated by recent research. For example, in May 1992, gastroenterologist David Y. Graham at Veterans Affairs Medical Center in Houston reported the results of a study involving 83 duodenal ulcer patients and 26 gastric ulcer patients, all infected with *H. pylori*. He found that 95 percent of duodenal ulcer patients treated with a traditional ulcer drug

Diagnosing an ulcer

To diagnose an ulcer, physicians may use an *endoscope*—a narrow, flexible tube that has a tiny video camera at one end. After threading the endoscope down the patient's esophagus, the physician can view the inside of the stomach or duodenum. An ulcer (inset) appears as a raw, wounded area.

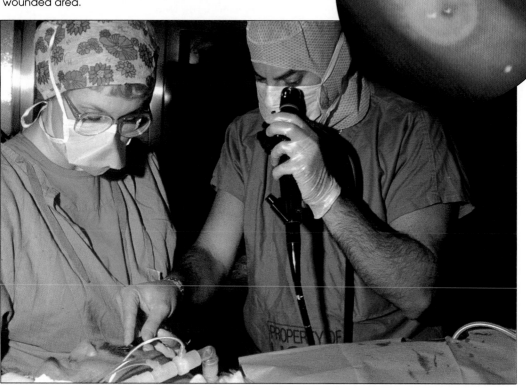

suffered a recurrence within a year. By contrast, ulcers recurred in only 12 percent of the duodenal ulcer patients who received the traditional drug plus antibiotics to fight *H. pylori*. Among gastric ulcer patients in the study, ulcers returned in 74 percent of those who took only the traditional drug, compared with 13 percent of those who followed the experimental regimen.

A team of scientists in Vienna, Austria, reported similar results in February 1993. Standard treatment with a common ulcer drug healed 75 percent of 52 patients with *H. pylori* infection and duodenal ulcers, but 86 percent of these patients suffered recurrences within a year. In 52 other patients, however, the same ulcer drug combined with antibiotics healed 92 percent, and only 8 percent experienced recurrences.

Tidy as the theory is, *H. pylori* infection cannot account for all ulcers, because not all ulcer patients are infected with the bacteria. Even so, among those patients whose ulcers cannot be attributed to NSAID use or other diseases, more than 90 percent of those with duodenal ulcers and 80 percent of those with stomach ulcers are infected, according to the NIH panel. That leaves a small number of ulcers that are not associated with *H. pylori* infection.

By the same token, although *H. pylori* infection often causes stomach inflammation, it does not guarantee that a person will develop an ulcer. *H. pylori* infection, it turns out, is far more common than are ulcers. About 20 percent of Americans have *H. pylori* living in their stomachs by age 20, and some 60 percent of 60-year-olds are infected. The fact that most people who are infected never develop an ulcer suggests that other factors must be involved in ulcer development.

The NIH panel concluded that unknown conditions—such as other characteristics of the patient or the particular *strain* (subtype) of *H. pylori*—may figure into ulcer development. It is also possible that stress and other factors once blamed for ulcers do indeed play a contributing role, even if they are not the primary cause. In any case, it is fairly evident that smoking and drinking alcohol or coffee can aggravate ulcers once they have formed. Smoking, in particular, seems to interfere with ulcer healing.

Now that researchers know to look for *H. pylori*, they are

Treating an ulcer

The traditional ulcer treatment relieves symptoms with drugs that minimize the ulcer's exposure to gastric acid. In February 1994, an expert panel recommended treating ulcers caused by *H. pylori* infection primarily with antibiotics that destroy the bacteria.

Traditional treatment

Type of drug	Effect
▪ H$_2$-blocker, such as Tagamet or Zantac	▪ Promotes healing by reducing the production of gastric acid.
▪ Proton-pump inhibitor, such as Prilosec	▪ Same as H$_2$-blocker.
▪ Antacid	▪ Helps neutralize gastric acid.
▪ Sucralfate	▪ Coats the ulcer to shield it from irritation by gastric acid.

Newly recommended treatment

Type of drug	Effect
▪ Antibiotics	▪ Kill *H. pylori* bacteria in the stomach and duodenum.
▪ H$_2$-blocker	▪ Promotes healing by reducing the production of gastric acid.
▪ Antacid	▪ Helps neutralize gastric acid.

The *H. pylori*-stomach cancer connection

Recent research suggests that the *H. pylori* bacterium that contributes to the development of ulcers may be linked with a far more serious condition: stomach cancer. Each year, stomach cancer kills about 14,000 Americans and strikes 24,000 more, according to the National Institutes of Health. Of all cancers worldwide, only lung cancer is more common and more deadly.

Researchers have built an increasingly strong case linking *H. pylori* with stomach cancer. Several studies have found that stomach cancer patients are more likely than people without the disease to be infected with *H. pylori*. For example, researcher Julie Parsonnet at Stanford University in Palo Alto, Calif., examined blood samples taken as part of a medical study in the 1960's from 186 people who later developed stomach cancer. In October 1991, she reported that 84 percent showed signs of *H. pylori* infection, compared with 61 percent of an equivalent cancer-free group.

Other scientists have found that high rates of *H. pylori* infection correspond to high rates of stomach cancer around the world. In May 1993, a team of researchers representing 14 countries reported the results of a study in which they compared the prevalence of stomach cancer in 17 groups of volunteers from Europe, Japan, and the United States. The researchers found high rates of stomach cancer in countries where infection with *H. pylori* was high and lower rates of the cancer in countries where infection was low.

Medical researchers have yet to prove, however, whether—or how—*H. pylori* causes can-cer. Some researchers theorize that long-term inflammation from *H. pylori* infection may damage *genes* (blueprints for cell function) in stomach cells, leading over many years of infection to cancer.

Bolstering this argument is the fact that stomach cancer rates are highest in developing countries, whose residents tend to be infected with *H. pylori* as children. This suggests that the longer people carry the infection, the more likely they will develop cancer. By comparison, in the United States, where *H. pylori* infection seems to occur increasingly later in life, stomach cancer is declining.

Still, no one can explain why some *H. pylori*-infected patients get gastritis or ulcers, while others develop stomach cancer. At the same time, some uninfected people get stomach cancer. Obviously, other factors must play a part.

For now, the *H. pylori* link points to new and promising treatments for stomach cancer. For instance, in September 1993, doctors in London reported that very early stomach tumors became smaller in five of six patients treated with antibiotics to eliminate *H. pylori*. This treatment was only experimental. Much work remains to be done before scientists can claim they have a cure, or even a treatment, for stomach cancer.

But if researchers find that eradicating *H. pylori* greatly reduces a person's risk of developing stomach cancer later in life, it is possible that doctors might work more aggressively to diagnose and treat the infection in people who have not developed this disease. [R. N.]

finding it nearly everywhere. In fact, experts have called it the most common chronic human bacterial infection. Infection is as common in other developed countries as it is in the United States, with people living in poorer households showing a higher rate of infection than people of higher socioeconomic status. Infection is even more prevalent in developing countries, where as many as 90 percent or more of residents are infected, often in childhood.

That pattern offers clues to another question scientists have yet to answer: How is *H. pylori* transmitted? The evidence seems to point to person-to-person contact—perhaps by means of an infected person's feces or saliva. Infections transmitted in this way are more likely to occur in developing countries or poor communities, where sanitation may be inadequate and living conditions may be overcrowded. Indeed, a 1992 study in London showed that people were more likely to carry *H. pylori* as adults if their childhood homes were crowded and lacked a hot-water supply, which influences the level of household hygiene.

The identification of an infectious "ulcer bug" may also help explain why ulcers sometimes run in families. Genetic traits may explain some of the familial connection. But if *H. pylori* can be transmitted easily among people who live together—as is likely—then perhaps people, in a sense, really do get ulcers from their spouses, parents, and children.

Not everyone who is exposed to *H. pylori* is destined to remain infected. When Barry Marshall infected himself deliberately, his body's defenses conquered the gastritis, and the infection, within a few weeks. But many people do develop long-lasting infections. If chronic stomach problems result, it takes medical treatment to find the bacteria and wipe them out.

Diagnosing *H. pylori* infection and ulcers

A blood test almost always reveals the presence of an *H. pylori* infection by detecting *antibodies* (disease-fighting molecules of the body's immune system) against *H. pylori*. Because such antibodies remain in the blood for years, a blood test can be positive even if someone who was infected is now free of the bacteria. Some researchers use a breath test in which the patient drinks a special liquid that promotes a response by the bacteria in the stomach. This response, in turn, produces chemicals that can be measured in the breath. However, breath tests are not yet widely available in the United States.

The most definitive test is a *biopsy* (tissue sampling), but it is also the most complicated and expensive. In a procedure called

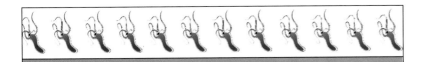

What to avoid when you have an ulcer

- **Smoking.** Smoking irritates the lining of the stomach. It may also lower the level of certain digestive juices that neutralize acid.

- **Aspirin, ibuprofen, and other nonsteroidal anti-inflammatory drugs taken on an empty stomach.** These drugs can aggravate an ulcer by irritating the lining of the stomach. They can also cause an ulcer to form.

- **Excess alcohol, coffee, and tea.** These beverages may aggravate an ulcer by stimulating the production of digestive acids.

Ulcers that won't respond to antibiotics

Scientists believe that infection with the bacterium *H. pylori* causes most cases of *peptic ulcers* (ulcers of the stomach or small intestine), but not quite all. Of the remainder, most result from long-term or frequent use of painkillers called *nonsteroidal anti-inflammatory drugs*, or NSAID's. Among these is aspirin, which can penetrate the acid-resistant layer of mucus that protects the stomach lining. Other common NSAID's include ibuprofen (sold as Motrin, Advil, and Nuprin) and naproxen (sold as the prescription drugs Anaprox and Naprosyn and approved for nonprescription sale as Aleve).

Most people who use these drugs realize that the pills can irritate the stomach lining, causing stomach pain, heartburn, nausea, or even bleeding. But once NSAID's reach the bloodstream, they deliver a second punch to the gut. The same chemical mechanism that enables the drugs to fight headaches and body pain can also diminish the stomach lining's ability to resist damage by stomach acid. In some cases, repeated use of the drugs can lead to *gastric* (stomach) ulcers.

While most people need not worry about getting ulcers from occasional doses of aspirin or related drugs, ulcers pose a serious threat to people who must take NSAID's daily over long periods of time. According to the U.S. Food and Drug Administration, 1 in 100 people taking NSAID's regularly for 3 to 6 months develops ulcers, gastrointestinal bleeding, or *perforations* (holes in the stomach wall). As many as 4 in 100 people develop such problems during the course of a year's treatment.

Regular NSAID users may gain some protection from the drug misoprostol (sold as Cytotec), which suppresses gastric acid, restores a body chemical depleted by NSAID use, and protects the stomach lining from damage. As a rule, anyone who takes aspirin or other NSAID's should eat food or drink water along with the pills, to buffer the drug's impact on the stomach.

Of course, someone using NSAID's can still develop an ulcer caused by *H. pylori* infection. For that reason, physicians recommend that ulcer patients who use NSAID's be tested for *H. pylori* and treated with antibiotics if an infection is found. [R. N.]

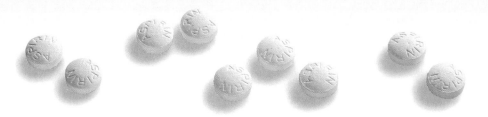

endoscopy, a doctor views the lining of the stomach or duodenum by passing an *endoscope* (a thin, flexible tube with a miniature video camera at one end) down the patient's throat to the stomach. The doctor can then thread a cutting tool through the tube to snip out a small bit of tissue for laboratory analysis.

Even if there were a test that was accurate, cheap, and easy, doctors would probably not routinely screen patients for *H. pylori* infection, simply because so many people carry the bacterium without developing problems that require treatment. Therefore, doctors are unlikely to call for any of these tests until they suspect the presence of an ulcer or related problem.

In diagnosing an ulcer, doctors may use endoscopy, which enables them to see the ulcer itself. Or they may use a series of X rays called an upper gastrointestinal (GI) series. For this, the patient drinks a chalky liquid containing barium, a substance that shows up in X rays. The liquid coats the lining of the stomach and duodenum, and any abnormality in the lining, such as an ulcer, appears highlighted in the X rays.

While the discovery of *H. pylori* only adds a step to diagnosis, it calls for a major change in ulcer treatment. The NIH panel found the evidence convincing enough to endorse antibiotic treatment for all *H. pylori*-infected patients with gastric or duodenal ulcers, whether they have a new ulcer, are suffering from a recurrence, or are taking ulcer drugs for long-term maintenance. The panel also recommended that patients who suffered from bleeding ulcers, which are potentially life threatening, continue on standard maintenance therapy for added protection against recurrence, until studies confirm that it is not necessary. Of course, not every ulcer should be treated with antibiotics. Patients who do not test positively for *H. pylori*, or whose ulcers are due solely to NSAID use or other disorders, are unlikely to benefit from antibiotics.

Still, not all doctors agree with the consensus panel's recommendation, and none are required to follow it. Some view the antibiotic regimen as experimental or difficult, prescribing it only for patients who pose complications or don't respond to standard ulcer drugs. After all, most ulcers do heal with traditional treatment, and some even resolve without treatment—though there is no guarantee that the problem will not recur.

Finally, because the findings on *H. pylori* are so new, some doctors may simply be unfamiliar with the new approach. As with any condition, patients should not hesitate to discuss treatment options with their doctor. They may also wish to seek a second opinion.

But for now, medicine has accomplished a great deal just by holding out the promise of curing a condition that brings misery to millions of people. For ulcer sufferers—not to mention people who once lived in fear that their stressful lives would bring on the malady—a simple treatment can now spell relief for good.

For further reading:

Chazin, Suzanne. "The Doctor Who Wouldn't Accept No." *Reader's Digest*, October 1993, pp. 113-124.

Monmaney, Terence. "Marshall's Hunch." *The New Yorker*, Sept. 20, 1993, pp. 64-72.

The report *Helicobacter Pylori in Peptic Ulcer Disease* can be obtained free from the National Institutes of Health by calling (800) 644-6627 or faxing a request to (301) 816-2494.

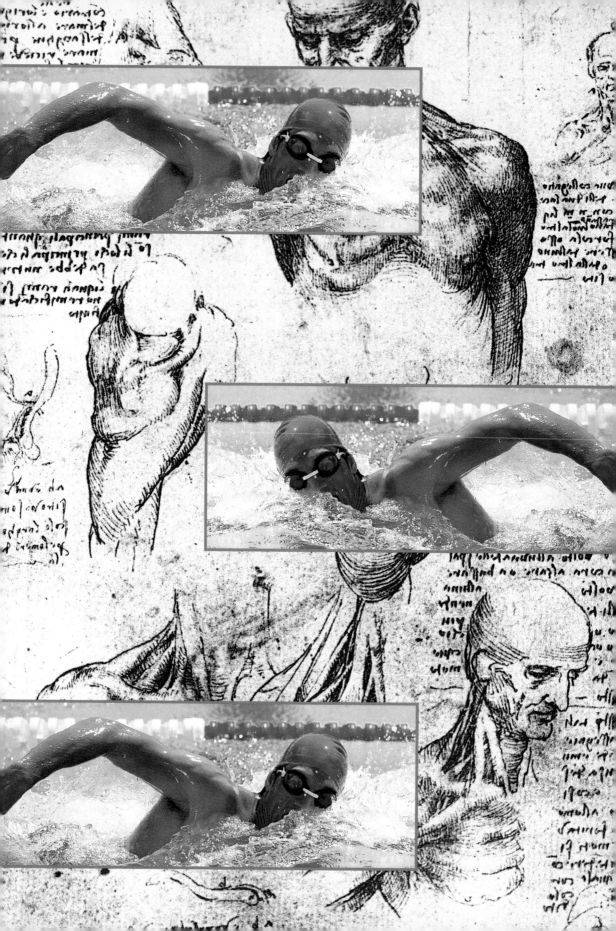

We've all heard that exercise is good for us, but just how does it benefit the body—and how can you make the most of these benefits?

Exercise: The Gain Made Plain

By Richard Saltus

"**W**henever I feel like exercise," quipped Robert Maynard Hutchins, an American educator, "I lie down until the feeling passes." Today, most Americans would probably agree in principle that exercise is good for them, but their actions suggest that they share the sentiments of Hutchins.

Although surveys found some upswing in leisure-time fitness activities from the 1960's to the 1980's, that trend has since leveled off. The proportion of people saying they had a mainly *sedentary* (inactive) life style stayed at about 60 percent from 1986 to 1990, according to a health-risk survey carried out by the Centers for Disease Control and Prevention (CDC) in Atlanta, Ga. And only about 10 percent of the respondents engaged in what is considered a minimum amount of exercise to keep the heart fit—20 minutes of pulse-raising activity at least three times a week.

Concerned about this trend, the American Heart Association in 1992 began listing a lack of physical exercise as one of the risk factors for heart disease. And the CDC in 1993, recognizing that many people will not maintain a rigorous exercise routine, made an effort to at least get Americans up off the couch. The CDC suggested that people try to fit in 30 minutes of physical

The skeletal muscles

The muscles that attach to bones and enable us to move are known as skeletal muscles. Even when we are standing still, the skeletal muscles are at work holding our body upright. Because these muscles are under our conscious control, they are sometimes called voluntary muscles. The muscles of the heart and internal organs such as the intestines are involuntary.

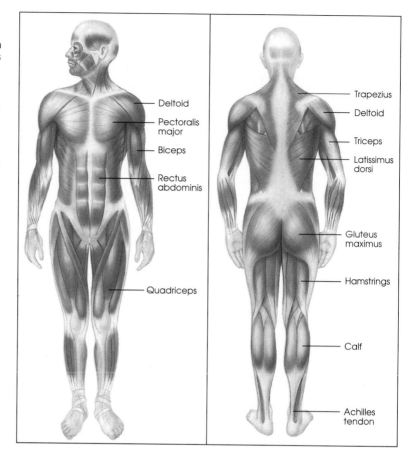

Deltoid
Pectoralis major
Biceps
Rectus abdominis
Quadriceps

Trapezius
Deltoid
Triceps
Latissimus dorsi
Gluteus maximus
Hamstrings
Calf
Achilles tendon

The author:

Richard Saltus is a science writer for the *Boston Globe.*

activity every day. This activity could include climbing stairs, gardening, pushing a stroller, dancing, or any other form of exertion.

The three kinds of muscle and the work they do

To understand the benefits of exercise—and why physicians recommend exercise—it's necessary to know something about how muscles work and what effect exercise has on them. We're all aware of using our muscles to dash up the stairs or run for the bus. But lots of activities we take for granted also depend upon muscles: the beating of the heart, the digestion of food, the intake of air. Exercise helps maintain these muscles.

The more than 600 muscles in the human body are grouped into three categories—skeletal, smooth, and cardiac. Skeletal muscles support the bones and, by pulling them, enable us to move. These muscles are attached to bones by tough, flexible tissues called tendons. Skeletal muscles are sometimes called voluntary muscles because we can control their movement.

Smooth muscle makes up the walls of such organs as the

stomach, intestines, and uterus as well as the walls of veins and arteries. Smooth muscle contracts slowly and rhythmically—though not under our conscious control, which is why these muscles are also called involuntary.

Cardiac muscle, found only in the heart, forms that organ's pumping chambers. Steady contractions of this involuntary muscle create the heartbeat and push blood through the bloodstream.

Exercise has noticeable effects on skeletal and cardiac muscle. Physiologists suspect it may help maintain smooth muscle as well. These benefits arise from the nature of muscle tissue itself.

How muscles do the work they do

All muscles consist of fibers that are held together by connective tissue. Blood vessels embedded in that tissue supply muscle fibers with the oxygen and nutrients they need for energy. Nerves also run through the connective tissue, carrying signals from the brain that tell the muscles to contract and relax.

Contractions of the skeletal muscles produce the many actions that the human body performs, from the blink of an eye to the leap of a pole vaulter. Even when we are sitting or standing still, some of our muscles remain in a state of semicontraction to support the body and maintain its upright posture.

Like any power generator, muscles require fuel that they can convert into energy. Much of this fuel is stored in the muscles in the form of a starchlike substance called glycogen. The body produces glycogen from the food we eat, especially *carbohydrates* (starches and sugars). Because carbohydrates are such a good source of glycogen, athletes often eat large quantities of them before an athletic event.

Within the muscle fibers, glycogen is broken down to help make a compound called adenosine triphosphate (ATP), which supplies the energy for the muscle contraction. Most contractions of skeletal muscles occur when the thin strands called filaments that make up each muscle fiber slide past one another and shorten the muscle.

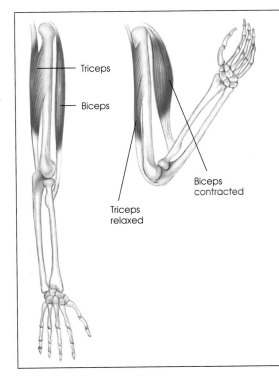

Triceps

Biceps

Biceps contracted

Triceps relaxed

How muscles move a limb

Skeletal muscles are capable of two actions—contraction, which shortens them, and relaxation, which restores their original length. These muscles work in opposing pairs to move limbs. For example, the arm bends when the biceps muscle in the upper arm contracts. To straighten the arm again, the opposing muscle—the triceps—contracts, and the biceps muscle relaxes.

A warm-up is important before undertaking more strenuous exercise. Warm muscles are more elastic and less likely to become injured. The same exercises can be used to cool down, easing the body to a lower level of activity after a workout.

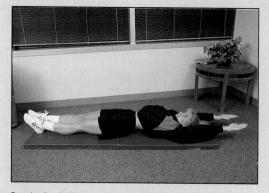

Begin flexibility exercises with the elongation stretch. Extend hands and legs as far as possible. Hold for 10 seconds. Repeat three times.

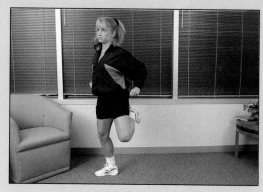

In the step leg curl, shift your body weight from side to side to as you lift one leg and then the other. Extend arms out and back in.

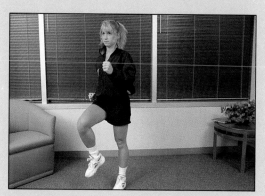

Marching in place helps increase blood flow to the muscles. You may raise your legs and arms higher or lower, as you feel comfortable.

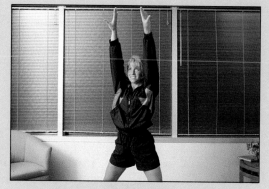

Deep breathing brings oxygen to the muscles. Breathe in as you reach upward, breathe out while bringing arms down in front.

The simplest muscle contractions are called twitches. Each skeletal muscle is made up of a mixture of fast-twitch and slow-twitch fibers, which differ in the way they produce ATP. Fast-twitch fibers contract quickly, creating the explosive power used for jumping, sprinting, weightlifting, and other exercises done at high intensity for a short time. The chemical reactions that power fast-twitch fibers are called *anaerobic* (not oxygen-dependent), because they do not use oxygen in producing ATP molecules. Muscles using anaerobic power tire quickly.

Slow-twitch fibers contract less quickly. Their power relies upon the release of energy from ATP in *aerobic* (oxygen-dependent) chemical reactions. Slow-twitch fibers use glycogen

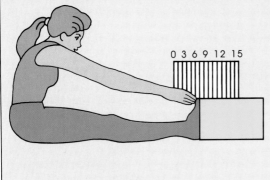

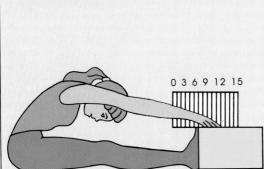

	Men (inches*)	Women
High	14+	15+
Above average	11-13	12-14
Average	7-10	7-11
Below average	4-6	4-6
Low	3 or less	3 or less

*These figures are for people in their 20's. Subtract 1 inch for each decade after that. For example, a 40-year-old woman would score high if she could reach 13 inches or more.

and oxygen steadily and continuously, providing muscles with the stamina needed in long-distance running, bicycling, cross-country skiing, and other endurance events.

What is fitness?

Most people have some sense of whether they are fit or not. If they feel sluggish, weak, or lacking in endurance they may say, "I'm really out of shape." Physiologists, who study how the body works, have a more comprehensive definition of fitness, however. They define fitness as the ability to perform moderate to vigorous levels of physical activity without undue fatigue and the capacity to maintain that ability through life. More simply, fitness is the ability to perform work with a minimum of effort.

Exercise specialists agree on four basic measures of physical fitness: flexibility, strength, muscular endurance, and cardiorespiratory endurance. Some physiologists consider the proportion of fat and muscle in the body, which is known as body composition, to be a fifth measure of fitness.

Improving flexibility

Flexibility is the ability to move easily at the joints and to use muscles through their full range of motion. Muscles that are not exercised become tight and lose their elasticity. As a result, they are more prone to pulls and tears. Exercises that stretch the muscles and rotate bones at the joints improve flexibility.

Exercises that improve flexibility

Flexible muscles move easily and are less vulnerable to pulls and tears. To increase flexibility, hold the stretches shown for 10 to 30 seconds; then relax and repeat three to five times.

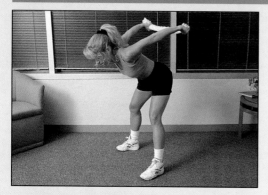

With legs apart, holding a towel behind your back, bend forward to stretch the upper arms and shoulders. Stand straight and repeat.

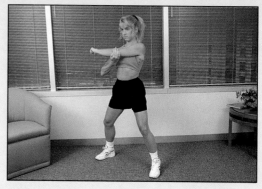

With back straight, pull your elbow across the chest toward the opposite arm to stretch upper arms and back. Reverse and repeat.

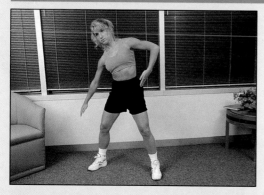

With back straight and legs apart, extend one hand toward your knee to stretch the side muscles. Repeat on other side.

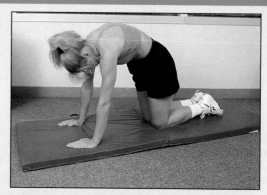

To stretch back muscles, kneel on a mat with palms down and arch your back like a cat. Return back to flat position and repeat.

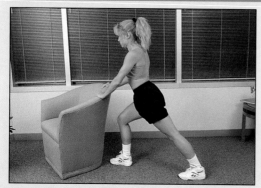

To stretch the calf, place rear foot flat with toes straight, and lean forward, holding onto a chair and bending the front leg. Reverse legs.

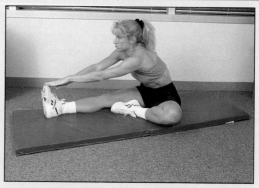

To stretch the hamstrings, bend one leg in and straighten the other. Reach both hands as far as you can toward the toes. Reverse legs.

Many health experts suggest that people over age 35 who have been inactive, or people suspecting a medical problem, obtain their doctor's approval before beginning a vigorous exercise program.

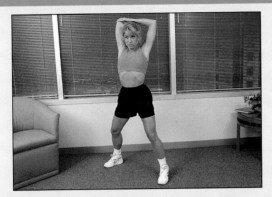

Lift your arm and bend; pull elbow toward the opposite arm to stretch your arms and sides. Reverse arms and repeat.

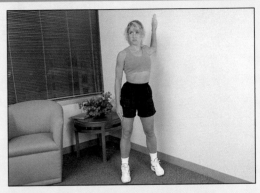

With one palm and lower arm against the wall, keep feet still and turn the upper body away from the wall. Reverse sides.

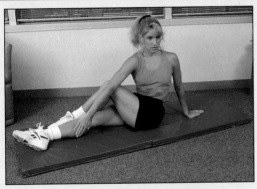

Seated on a mat, cross one leg over the other and turn your torso. Support yourself on one hand and reach other hand to knee. Reverse.

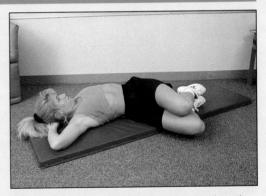

Lie on your back. With hands under your head, pull your knees together and bend. Drop the knees to one side and then the other.

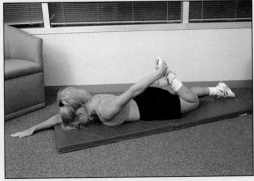

To stretch the quadriceps, lie face down on a mat with one arm out straight. Pull one foot as far as possible toward the hips. Reverse legs.

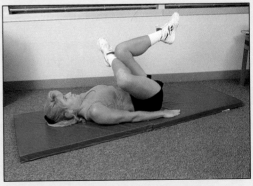

Lying on a mat with arms at sides, cross one leg over the other. Lift bottom leg, pulling against top leg for gluteal stretch. Reverse.

Stretching exercises also increase blood flow to the muscles and help prevent injury during heavier exertion.

Muscles whose flexibility is important to bodily motion include the calves, hamstrings, and quadriceps. The calf muscles, on the back of the lower leg, are essential for walking, running, and jumping. The hamstrings, a group of three muscles on the back of the upper leg, are used in nearly every sport and physical activity. The quadriceps, four thigh muscles, supply power for forward movement such as jumping, running, skipping, or kicking. The flexibility of muscles in the lower back, which enable us to bend and lift, is also crucial to physical fitness.

Building strength

Strength is a muscle's ability to exert force for a short time. Muscles gain strength by adding bulk, which occurs through enlarging individual muscle fibers. In response to such exercises as weightlifting, fast-twitch fibers add new filaments. The extra filaments give muscles their increased bulk and strength.

Muscles increase in size and strength after contracting while they overcome resistance. This happens when a person lifts weights or pushes and pulls against the resistance created by an exercise machine. According to exercise physiologists, muscles gain strength fastest if exercised according to the overload principle—that is, when they contract repeatedly against increasingly greater resistance.

The most direct way to build strength and increase muscle bulk is through weightlifting, according to exercise experts. In describing strength-building exercises, trainers refer to one completed movement, such as lifting and lowering a weight, as a repetition. A group of repetitions, with pauses for rest between them, is a set.

At the beginning, trainers advise people to choose a weight that they can move through four to eight repetitions for three sets. The person should work at this level until able to complete 10 to 12 repetitions per set. As the muscles become stronger, the 10 to 12 repetitions become easier—a signal that it's time to shift to the next heavier weight. After gradually working up to 10 or 12 repetitions with that weight, the person again moves up to a heavier weight. Physiologists recommend that people work muscles in this way three or four times a week if they want to build their strength.

For people who are not concerned with achieving maximum muscle bulk but rather with attaining a level of strength to keep themselves fit, the principles used in weightlifting still apply. Many household tasks and recreational activities—toting a child or working in a garden, for example—involve carrying, lifting, and moving objects. Many such activities also involve pushing and pulling against resistance.

You can test your stength with these three simple exercises. The ratings apply to men in their 20's. To determine your own rating, subtract 15 percent for each decade of age after that. Women, who have less muscle mass, generally perform at a rate 20 to 25 percent below men.

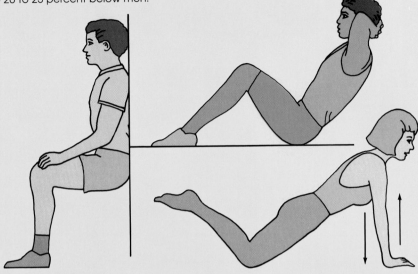

Wall sit
Lean against a wall with your knees bent. How long you can maintain this position provides a measure of your lower body strength.

90 seconds ....High
60 seconds ....Average
30 seconds .....Below average
Less than 30 seconds ....Low

Source: Excerpted from *The Wellness Guide to Lifelong Fitness*, © Health Letter Associates, 1993.

Abdominal hold
With your knees bent and your hands behind your head, sit up at a 45-degree angle. How long you can hold this position provides a measure of your middle body strength.

25 seconds ....High
15 seconds ....Average
5 seconds ....Below average
Less than 5 seconds ....Low

Pushup
The number of pushups you can complete provides a measure of your upper body strength. Women, who have less upper body muscle than men, can do a modified, bent-leg version of the standard pushup.

25 ....High
15 ....Average
5 ....Below average
Fewer than 5 ....Low

Developing endurance

Muscular endurance is the ability of muscles to contract repeatedly or to apply force continuously. Endurance depends on the amount of glycogen stored in the muscles and the efficiency with which the muscles convert this fuel to energy. Aerobic exercise—exercise that uses oxygen to produce ATP—improves endurance by altering the chemistry of slow-twitch fibers. As a result of aerobic exercise, the muscle fibers are able to store more glycogen and produce more ATP. These changes enable athletes engaged in intense, continuing motion to keep going longer.

Cardiorespiratory endurance is a measure of how well the heart and lungs deliver oxygen to the muscles. The more fit a person is, the more oxygen the lungs can take in and the more oxygen-rich blood the heart can deliver to the muscles. The aerobic exercises that promote muscular endurance promote

Exercises that build strength

Muscles develop strength by having increasingly greater demands placed on them. Start slowly with a few repetitions of each exercise. Gradually work up to 3 sets of 10 repetitions.

Upper body

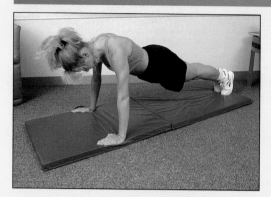

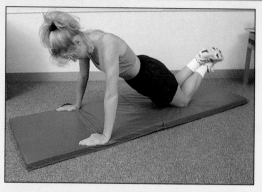

The traditional pushup builds strength in the chest and upper arms. Bend the arms to lower the body close to, but not touching, the floor.

A modified pushup with legs bent is less strenuous but also builds strength. Lower face close to, but not touching, the floor.

Middle body

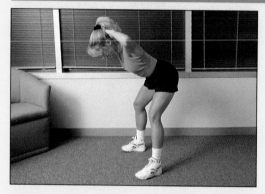

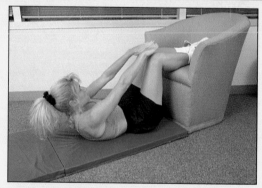

With hands placed on back of head and legs apart, bend knees, keep back straight, and lean forward. Stand straight and repeat.

The crunch firms stomach muscles. With back on mat and feet on chair, reach hands as far as possible toward feet. Relax and repeat.

Lower body

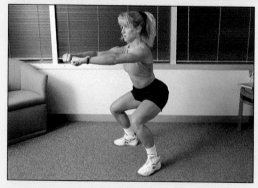

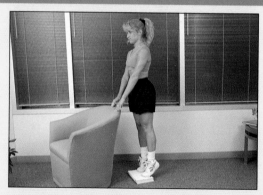

With back erect and knees positioned over the toes, extend arms, bend knees, and squat. Straighten and repeat.

Calves can be strengthened by tiptoeing close to the edge of a book placed on the floor. Bring heels to the floor and repeat.

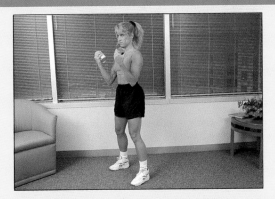

To strengthen biceps, hold soup cans tightly and curl arms up toward shoulders. Lower your arms gently to your sides and repeat.

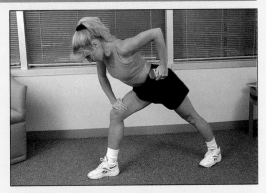

Lean forward with one arm on bent front leg. Clutch a soup can in the other hand and move arm in a rowing motion. Reverse sides.

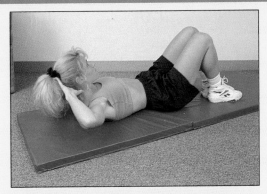

In this stomach crunch, the feet stay on the floor and the hands under the head. Lift the torso up as far as you can. Relax and repeat.

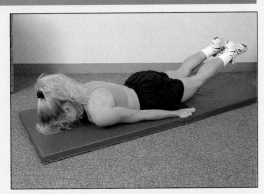

The rear leg lift helps lower-back muscles. Lie face down on the mat, arms at your sides, and lift your feet off the floor as far as possible.

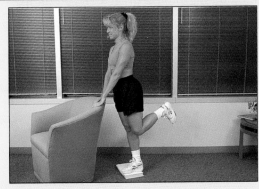

Standing on book, keeping knees together, lift one lower leg back. Straighten leg, allowing foot to return to side of book but not to floor.

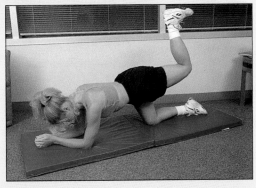

To strengthen gluteal muscles, support yourself on your elbows, face to the mat, bend one leg, and lift it high. Repeat on the other side.

Building muscular endurance

Muscular endurance is the ability of skeletal muscles to contract repeatedly. Activities that build muscular endurance include

- Basketball
- Bicycling
- Football
- Gymnastics
- Hiking
- Ice skating
- Jogging
- Roller skating
- Running
- Skiing
- Swimming
- Wrestling

Building cardiorespiratory endurance

Cardiorespiratory endurance is the ability of the heart and lungs to take in oxygen and deliver it to the muscles. Activities that build cardiorespiratory endurance include

- Aerobic dancing
- Bicycling
- Cross-country skiing
- Jogging
- Rowing
- Running
- Skating
- Skipping rope
- Swimming
- Walking briskly

cardiorespiratory endurance as well, by improving the heart's pumping ability.

With thicker and stronger chambers, the heart can pump more blood with each beat and therefore handle a normal blood flow with fewer beats. As a result, the cardiorespiratory system of an aerobically fit person does not have to work as hard during everyday activities or during exercise. In addition, aerobic exercise promotes the formation of new capillaries—the body's smallest blood vessels, which deliver oxygen to the muscles. The extra capillaries boost the amount of oxygen that reaches the muscles.

When the cardiorespiratory system cannot supply sufficient oxygen during exercise, the muscles are forced to produce ATP through anaerobic processes. This can create a sensation of burning and fatigue in the muscles.

Personal fitness: Less pain, more gain

All benefits of exercise and all forms of physical fitness depend on regular, sustained exercise. If exercise becomes less regular or less intense, the gains are gradually lost. The changes within the muscle fibers that promote endurance return to pretraining levels. Extra capillaries that built up during exercise shut down, and the muscle filaments added during strength training deteriorate from disuse.

On the positive side, according to the American College of Sports Medicine (ACSM), a fit person can skip an occasional aerobic or strength-training session, or even cut back on the number of sessions per week, for as many as 15 weeks without slipping backward on the fitness ladder. Although a person loses aerobic capacity when not exercising, muscles seem to "remember" the training they once had. For reasons not clear to physiologists, when a person starts training after a lapse, it is easier than it was when the person first began.

Exercise carries risks as well as benefits. Experts say that many of the people who recognize the benefits of exercise are less aware of the potential for injury. High-impact exercises that involve running and jumping carry a greater risk of injury than do low-impact activities, such as walking or jogging. Even walking and jogging, however, put repeated stress on feet, legs, and knees and can lead to injuries. Beginners are advised not to jog more than three days a week and not longer than 30 minutes at a time.

A key to avoiding injury to muscles and joints is to warm up for 5 to 10 minutes at the start of a workout. Good warm-up exercises include jumping jacks, jogging in place, or skipping rope. These exercises raise the heart rate, thereby increasing blood flow to the tissues and raising the temperature of the muscles. Warm muscles and tendons have more flexibility than

Raising the heart rate strengthens the heart muscle and helps maintain cardiovascular fitness. The American College of Sports Medicine recommends training at an intensity that reaches at least 50 percent and not more than 85 percent of your maximum heart rate, a range called the target heart rate. If you exceed the highest target rate, you are working too hard and should slow down. If you fall below the lowest target rate, you should work harder. To calculate your target heart rate:

1. Subtract your age from 220 to determine your maximum heart rate in heartbeats per minute.

2. To find your maximum target rate, calculate 85 percent of your maximum heart rate.

3. To find your minimum target rate, calculate 50 percent of your maximum heart rate.

4. These two numbers provide highest and lowest heart rates you should strive for during a cardiovascular workout.

5. To determine your heart rate as you exercise, locate your pulse at your neck or wrist and count the beats for 10 seconds. If you multiply that number by six, you will know how many times your heart is beating in one minute.

To determine the target heart rate for a 42-year-old person, for example:

1. 220 - 42 = 178 (maximum heart rate for age 42)

2. 178 x 0.85 = 151 (maximum target rate)

3. 178 x 0.5 = 89 (minimum target rate)

If your age is:	Your range is:
25	166—98
30	162—95
35	157—93
40	153—90
45	149—88
50	145—85
55	140—83
60	136—80
65	132—78
70	128—75
75	123—73

cold ones and are therefore less likely to sustain injury. Stretches that loosen up the neck, shoulders, lower back, thighs, and calves also help protect against injuries.

Cool-down exercises are as valuable as warm-ups. Cool-down activity eases the body's return to a lower level of activity at the end of a workout. During a workout, blood rushes into the arms and legs where it is needed, and breathing becomes rapid to increase the body's supply of oxygen. Cool-down exercises help restore normal breathing and allow blood to return to the heart.

During exercise, the muscles produce lactic acid as a waste product of turning glycogen into energy. When a person suddenly stops strenuous exercise, lactic acid can build up in the muscles and cause pain. A gradual slowdown allows the muscles to convert lactic acid back to glycogen. Rubbing muscles brings in blood to carry off excess lactic acid and relieve the pain.

Walking is a good cool-down activity. Stretching exercises similar to warm-up exercises are also good for cooling down. Moreover, muscles are at their most elastic when warm from heavy exercise. Further stretching at this point can help increase muscle flexibility.

Athletes generally incur injuries from the intensity of their activity, whereas lack of fitness renders beginners susceptible to injuries. Both athletes and beginners suffer similar kinds of injuries: sprains, strains, cramps, and tendinitis.

A sprain is a tearing or twisting of ligaments, tissues that hold bones in position at the joints. Sprains most often occur at the wrist and the ankle, and they can be extremely painful. A strain, often called a pull, is an overstretching of the fibers within a muscle, causing tenderness and pain. Tendons also can become strained or torn.

Minor sprains and strains can be treated using a four-part guideline abbreviated as RICE. *R*est is important to prevent further injury. *I*ce contracts blood vessels, limiting bleeding from injured capillaries. *C*ompression, by wrapping the injured area firmly but not too tightly with an elastic bandage, helps decrease swelling, which occurs from fluid leakage in damaged tissue. *E*levation of the injured part uses the force of gravity to drain excess fluid from the area and limit swelling. It's important to seek medical help if the RICE program fails to relieve pain and swelling.

Tendinitis, an inflammation of a tendon, most frequently occurs in the knees, shins, forearms, and the Achilles' tendon above the heel. Tendinitis is often recognizable by pain upon awakening that lets up during the day. It is treated with rest and mild stretching exercises to relieve tight muscles.

A cramp is a prolonged contraction of a muscle that fails to relax. Muscle cramps have a number of causes, and massaging or stretching the muscle can help relieve the cramp. A stitch in the side is another common annoyance during exercise. Doctors do not know for certain what causes side stitches, though some physiologists believe they result when blood rushes from the internal organs to the skeletal muscles. Deep breathing can sometimes relieve stitches.

A reasonable level of fitness

To minimize risk and sustain benefit, a proper schedule of exercise is crucial. Sports physiologists are seeking to design simple, efficient training programs that meet the minimum requirement needed to maintain fitness. After reviewing many studies on health and fitness, the American College of Sports Medicine in 1990 issued a statement on the type and amount of exercise an average adult needs to do to maintain fitness. The group recommended that:

- A healthy adult should exercise three to five times a week for 20 to 60 minutes each time.
- The exercise should be sufficiently intense to make the heart beat at 60 percent to 90 percent of its maximum rate. For information on this rate, see DETERMINING YOUR TARGET HEART RATE on page 115.
- The length of a workout should depend on its intensity. An activity of lower intensity should be performed longer than one of high intensity. For nonathletic adults, activities of low

to moderate intensity are recommended, to avoid injury and discouragement.

- Exercise should involve large muscle groups working in a continuous, rhythmic, and aerobic manner. Examples include cycling, cross-country skiing, dancing, jogging, running, rowing, skating, skipping rope, stair climbing, swimming, and brisk walking.

- A fitness program should include strength training of moderate intensity that works the major muscle groups at least two days a week. The recommended minimum is a routine of 8 to 10 different exercises, with each exercise repeated 8 to 12 times.

How much gain a person can expect from exercise depends in part on age, but recent studies show that people can receive some benefit at any age. A 1990 study by researchers at the Harvard Medical School in Boston found that nursing-home residents over age 90 who worked out for just eight weeks showed a significant increase in muscle mass, muscle strength, and walking speed.

Exercise physiologists say that the people who can benefit most from becoming more active are those who are least fit. These are also the people who have the hardest time overcoming their inertia. With this in mind, the ACSM made a distinction in a 1993 report between physical activity to achieve fitness and physical activity to improve health. The group said that exercise below the level recommended to achieve fitness has been shown to provide health benefits.

A brisk walk, a bicycle ride or a swim, a waltz around the room, taking the stairs rather than the elevator, working in the garden—all these activities provide health benefits. Not only can such exertion make you feel more relaxed and energetic, when done on a regular basis, it can help lower blood pressure and improve cholesterol levels. Recent studies have found that even a minimum of exercise can help stave off heart disease. So find an activity you enjoy and think about the benefits you'll reap.

For further reading:

American College of Sports Medicine. *ACSM Fitness Book*. Human Kinetics Publishers, 1992.

University of California at Berkeley Wellness Letter Editors. *The Wellness Guide to Lifelong Fitness*. Rebus Incorporated, 1993.

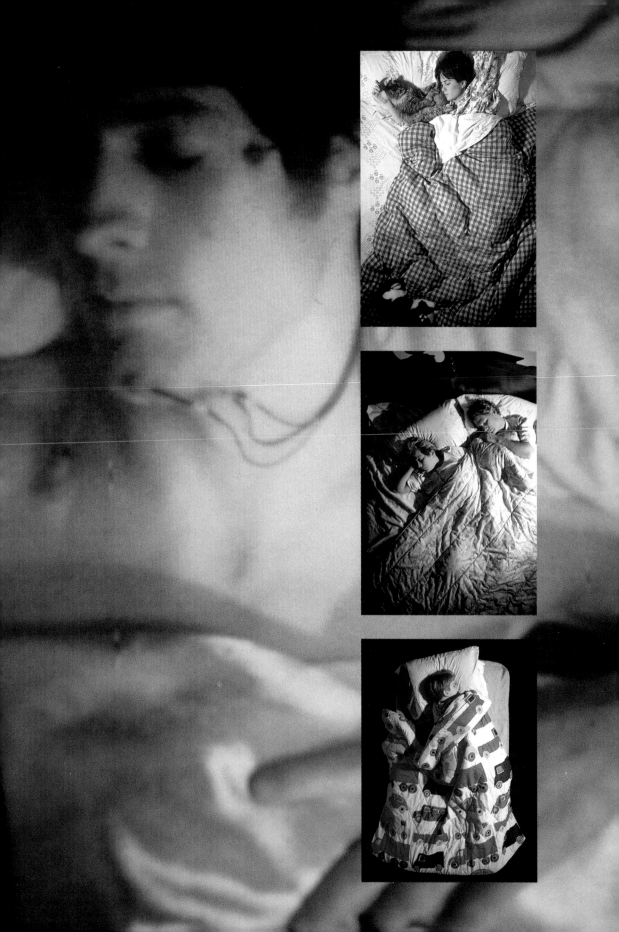

Studies indicate that most Americans
are not getting the sleep they need.
Some simple steps can help improve
both the quantity and the quality of
your sleep.

Getting a Good Night's Sleep

By Dianne Hales

We spend one-third of our lives sleeping—more time than we devote to any other pursuit or pleasure. From birth to death, sleep is so essential that we can go without food or water more easily than without rest.

Despite the importance of sleep, it appears that Americans are not getting enough of it. Within the last 100 years, Americans have cut their average nightly sleep time by more than 20 percent, from about 9½ hours to 7½ hours, according to sleep researchers. The result, say the researchers, is a silent epidemic of daytime drowsiness. "Most Americans no longer know what it feels like to be fully alert," says the father of modern sleep research, psychiatrist William Dement of Stanford University in California. "A substantial number, perhaps the majority, are functionally handicapped by sleep deprivation on any given day."

Recognizing that sleep-related problems had long been ignored, the United States Congress in 1993 established a National Center for Sleep Disorders Research as part of the National Institutes of Health in Bethesda, Md. And since 1980, the number of centers for the study of sleep and the treatment of sleep disorders in the United States has risen from about 25 to more than 220.

Although philosophers and poets for centuries have mused about what happens in this silent state, sleep has emerged as a scientific topic only since the 1950's. The development of machines to monitor brain waves, eye movement, and muscle activity enabled researchers for the first time to peer into the sleeping body, chart the stages of sleep, and distinguish between normal and abnormal sleep. Sleep has now become a medical subspecialty. Doctors who study sleep usually have psychiatry, neurology, or internal medicine as their primary specialty.

Despite the progress they have made, sleep specialists have not found an answer to one of biology's most tantalizing riddles: Why do we sleep? Does sleep allow our bodies to repair the wear and tear of daytime activity? Is it a means of conserving energy or a time for processing the mental activity of our waking moments? No one can say for sure, and it may well be that sleep serves many varied purposes.

The sleeping body

Many of us think that the body and brain shut down during sleep, like a car parked for the night. But as we sleep, muscles tense and relax. The body's pulse, temperature, and blood pressure rise and fall. The flow of digestive juices varies. Key hormones ebb and flow. The brain, like a motion-picture director, conjures up the fantastic stories—complete with plot, characters, and action—that we call dreams.

A normal night of sleep consists of several distinct stages, which scientists have identified with the help of an *electroencephalograph (EEG)*, an instrument that measures and records electrical waves given off by the brain. We move in and out of these stages of sleep, which are divided into two major types. An active state when we dream is called REM sleep after the *rapid eye movements* that occur during it. A quiet state is called non-REM or NREM sleep. There are four stages of non-REM sleep.

- Stage 1 is a twilight zone between full wakefulness and sleep. EEG's show that the brain produces small, rapid, irregular waves during this stage. The muscles of the body relax, and breathing is smooth and even.
- Stage 2 is characterized by larger brain waves punctuated by occasional sudden bursts of electrical activity that can occur spontaneously or in response to a stimulus, such as a sound. The eyes no longer respond to light, and bodily functions continue to slow.
- Stages 3 and 4 constitute our deepest states of slumber, during which the brain produces slower, larger waves. This stage is sometimes called *delta* or *slow-wave* sleep.

Sleepers enter REM sleep after spending about an hour in the

The author:

Dianne Hales is the author of *The Complete Book of Sleep* and *How to Sleep Like a Baby*.

four stages of non-REM sleep. During the REM stage, brain waves are small and fast, resembling those of wakefulness more than those of quiet sleep. The large muscles of the torso, arms, and legs become paralyzed and cannot move—possibly to prevent sleepers from acting out their dreams. The fingers and toes may twitch, breathing is quick and shallow, blood flow through the brain speeds up, and men may have erections.

Early in the night, the deep stages of non-REM sleep dominate, with REM periods gradually lengthening from less than 10 minutes to 30 minutes by morning. During a typical eight-hour night, most adults spend a total of about two hours in REM and about six hours in non-REM sleep. Sleep researchers have also observed that an individual deprived of REM sleep one night spends much more time than usual in REM sleep the next night. No matter how much REM sleep we get, we tend to recall only what was happening in our dreams in the minutes before waking up.

How much sleep we need

Over the course of a lifetime, sleep needs and patterns change dramatically—in both quantity and quality. Infants sleep more than twice as much as adults. Children spend much more time in REM and the deepest stages of non-REM sleep than grown-ups do. By their 30's, men spend less time in stages 3 and 4 of non-REM sleep. Women begin to sleep less deeply in their 50's. By age 65, people of both sexes spend half as much time in deep sleep as they did when they were 20. They may waken, if only for a few seconds, more than 100 times a night. Many older people make up for sleeping less at night by napping during the day.

Every individual seems to have an inborn sleep "appetite" that is as much a part of the person's makeup as are hair color, height, and skin tone. Average sleep time is 7½ hours a night, but anywhere from 5 to 10 hours can be considered normal. Some people—perhaps 1 or 2 in 100—are natural "short sleepers" who require less than 6 hours of rest a night.

Facts about sleep

- One of three Americans has problems sleeping.
- According to the National Commission on Sleep Disorders Research, 40 million adults suffer from a specific sleep disorder, such as chronic insomnia or obstructive sleep apnea. An additional 20 million to 30 million people have occasional sleep difficulties.
- Over the last century, Americans have cut their average nightly sleep time by more than 20 percent, from about 9½ hours to 7½ hours a night.
- In a poll sponsored by the National Sleep Foundation, only 5 percent of the people who complained of sleep difficulties had ever sought their doctor's advice.
- Effective treatments for sleep problems could help 3 out of 4 poor sleepers.
- By age 65, people typically spend only half as much time in deep sleep as they did at age 20.
- A healthy man of age 75 averages 153 wakenings during a seven-hour sleep period, while a 25-year-old will waken only 10 times.
- As many as 40 percent of women over age 40 may suffer from insomnia.
- Drowsiness is second only to alcohol as a factor in motor vehicle accidents. It plays a role in 200,000 to 400,000 collisions each year that claim as many as 6,500 lives.

Sources: National Commission on Sleep Disorders Research; National Sleep Foundation.

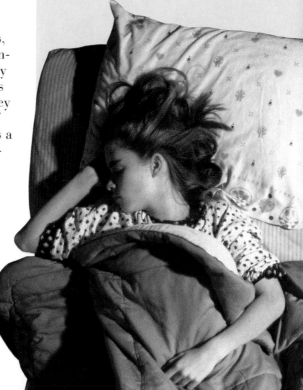

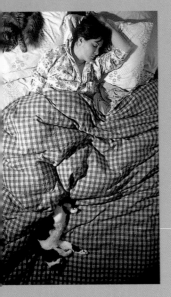

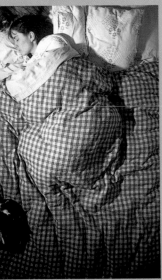

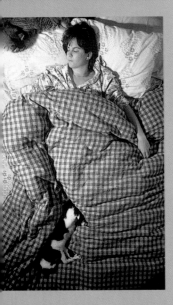

The stages of sleep

The billions of nerve cells in the brain communicate through electrical impulses. Scientists can measure and record this activity with an instrument called an electroencephalograph. Short, frequent waves represent increased brain activity, and long, slower waves appear when the brain is less active. On the basis of the waves produced, researchers have classified sleep into two types: REM (rapid eye movement) and non-REM, which consists of four stages.

Brain waves	Stage	The body
	Awake	The person is alert.
	Stage 1	This is the onset of sleep and lasts about five minutes. The heart and breathing rates begin to drop, and the eyes roll slowly from side to side.
	Stage 2	The eyes are generally still, and the heart and breathing rates drop further.
	Stage 3	Heartbeat and respiration continue to drop. Blood pressure and body temperature drop.
	Stage 4	This is the deepest stage of sleep. Heart and breathing rates drop 20 to 30 percent below those in the waking state. Muscles are completely relaxed. The sleeper does not move and is difficult to awaken.
	REM	REM is the time for dreaming. The heart and breathing rates pick up and become irregular. The eyes move rapidly back and forth under the eyelids. The body is still except for some face, leg, and finger twitches.

Source: Sleep-Wake Disorders Center, Montefiore Medical Center, New York City.

An equal number of "long sleepers" regularly sleep 10 hours or more each night.

Most people feel and function best when they're satisfying their natural sleep appetite, whether it's for 6 or 10 hours a night. One simple method of determining whether you are getting enough sleep is to keep your wake-up time the same every morning but vary your bedtimes. Are you groggy after six hours of shut-eye? Does an extra hour or two give you more stamina? Since too much time in bed can make you sluggish, don't assume that more is always better. Listen to your body's signals and adjust your sleep schedule to suit them.

You also might try keeping a simple sleep log for a week or two. Every night, before going to bed, jot down the time and how sleepy you feel. Use a 10-point scale, with 1 signifying that you're wide awake and 10 that you're dead on your feet. In the morning, estimate the time you actually fell asleep the night before, if you awakened during the night, and the time you woke up in the morning. Also note how well you slept, again using a 10-point scale, with a 1 indicating that you didn't sleep a wink and a 10 being a perfect night's sleep. By reviewing the log, you can get a better sense of your sleep needs.

When we don't get enough sleep

Trying to get by on too little rest takes a psychological and physical toll. Sleepy people lack energy and motivation, have trouble concentrating, and are less creative and more irritable than their rested counterparts, researchers have found. And if they keep cutting back on sleep, they accumulate a "sleep debt." A person who runs out of credit in this sleep account can go from feeling wide awake to falling asleep in five seconds. We can pay back the sleep debt, but not minute for minute. Sleeping longer than usual on weekends and vacations can help and so can napping.

In a 1992 survey of 3,000 households, sponsored by the Better Sleep Council, 83 percent of Americans said they have fallen asleep at work or school. An alarming 1 out of 10 have nodded off while driving. According to the U.S. Department of Transportation, 200,000 sleep-related accidents each year claim more than 5,000 lives, cause hundreds of thousands of injuries, and incur billions of dollars in indirect costs. Sleep deprivation has contributed to major catastrophes, including train wrecks, mishaps in nuclear energy plants, and airplane crashes.

"Most people don't take their sleep needs or problems seriously enough," notes Thomas Roth, past president of the National Sleep Foundation and head of the division of sleep disorders medicine at Henry Ford Hospital in Detroit. "One reason is that we assume that the worst thing about not getting enough sleep is feeling drowsy the next day. That's not the case." Roth says that sleepiness can have serious long-term health implications.

An intricate connection between sleep and the immune system seems to indicate that too little sleep can affect the body as well as the mind. Sleep is believed to be a time of physical repair and rejuvenation, and people chronically deprived of adequate sleep can become more susceptible to certain illnesses. Researchers also speculate that disturbed sleep may be the reason individuals under stress—such as doctors in training or grieving widows and widowers—have lower levels of certain infection-fighting blood cells than normal, as studies have found.

If you lose an hour or two of sleep one night, you do not have to sleep an hour or two longer the next night. Nature makes up for a bad night by making the next night's sleep more efficient and restorative. During this night of recovery sleep, you spend more time in the very deep stages of sleep, even if you don't spend more time in bed.

Napping can also help and may be what people are meant to do. Researchers have found that the tendency to become drowsy in the afternoon and want to nap stems from a normal dip in body temperature that occurs about 12 hours after the midpoint of our nighttime sleep. For individuals who are not getting adequate rest at night, such as new mothers, naps can be essential for keeping energy up throughout the day. Many more people might benefit if they too could indulge in "pajamaless sleep." Among the payoffs of rest in the afternoon are increased energy, enhanced alertness, a longer attention span, improved memory, better decision-making ability, and a sunnier mood.

Getting enough sleep is especially difficult for some 40 million American adults who suffer from a chronic sleep disorder, such as persistent insomnia. An additional 20 million to 30 million people have occasional sleep difficulties, according to the National Commission on Sleep Disorders Research.

When sleep won't come

People with insomnia—a lack of sleep severe enough to interfere with daytime functioning—may toss and turn for an hour or more after going to bed, wake frequently, or not be able to sleep long enough to feel alert and energetic the next day.

Most insomnia is what doctors call transient, typically occurring before or after a major life event—such as a wedding or the start of a new job—and lasting for three or four nights. Alcohol, medications, and drugs of abuse also can disrupt sleep and create transient insomnia.

Short-term insomnia, which lasts several weeks, can occur during a period of prolonged stress, such as that brought on by a divorce or the death of a loved one. Chronic or long-term insomnia can begin at any age and persist for months or years. About one-third of those with chronic insomnia have an under-

Children's sleep problems

About 1 child out of 4 experiences some type of sleep disorder. The problems are usually temporary, or the youngsters outgrow the difficulty.

Difficulty falling asleep. Too often bedtime turns into a battle between parent and child. A pleasant, soothing sleep ritual, which may include reading and snuggling, can help avoid such showdowns and ease a child's transition from day to night.

A parent may use a neutral measure to establish bedtime, such as the clock or the end of a favorite television show, to sidestep a struggle. Parents must also remember that darkness is scary for children. A night light or soft music may reassure a child.

Nightmares are frightening dreams and are common in children, especially before age 7. The best response from a parent is reassurance and understanding. Try talking about the child's daytime worries or concerns. Frequent nightmares may indicate some serious physical or emotional stress affecting the child or the family.

Night terrors. A child experiencing a night terror awakens abruptly but not fully, usually with a scream of panic, and is so frightened that he or she may not calm down for a while. Parents should remain calm and protective while allowing the child to return to normal sleep.

Night terrors occur during the deepest stages of sleep and are not true dreams. They are con-

sidered normal in youngsters, especially between the ages of 3 and 8.

Bed-wetting. About 15 percent of all 5-year-olds and 5 percent of all 10-year-olds wet their beds. Bed-wetting can stem from various causes, including a small bladder, excessively deep sleep, increased urine output, or immature bladder muscles. Treatments include bladder control training and conditioning methods, such as using a signaling device to waken children if they begin to urinate. In some cases, an alarm clock can be set to wake the child during the night so the child can walk to the bathroom.

Sleepwalking. Between the ages of 5 and 12, from 10 percent to 15 percent of children walk in their sleep at least once. Possible causes include a still-developing central nervous system, a high fever, or extreme fatigue. Parents with a child who sleepwalks should make the home environment as safe as possible by locking windows and doors to the outside, installing protective gates at stairs, and hiding dangerous objects. Most children outgrow sleepwalking.

Sleep apnea, more common in adults, is a breathing disruption that can occur in youngsters and cause poor nighttime sleep and extreme sleepiness during the day. Removal of enlarged tonsils or adenoids, which can obstruct a child's airway during the night, can alleviate the problem in severe cases of childhood sleep apnea.

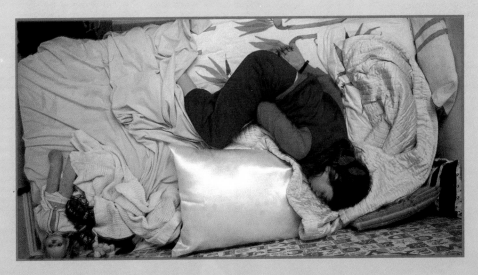

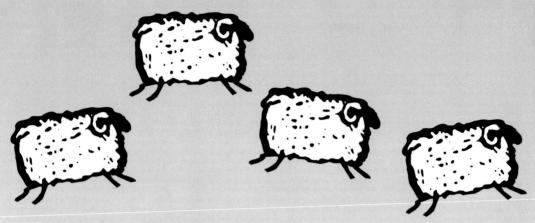

Tired of counting sheep?

You lay yourself down to sleep, tucked snugly into your bed, and wait, and wait, and wait. What can you do when the sandman doesn't show up? One of the best strategies is to use mind games that distract and relax your mind.

- Imagine yourself writing perfect numbers 6 feet high on a make-believe blackboard. Start at 100 and count backward to 0.
- Pretend you're Noah, preparing for the boarding of the ark. Think of all the types of animals you'd bring on board.
- Try to induce a feeling of warmth or heaviness in different parts of your body. Tell yourself, "My fingers are getting warmer and heavier. I can feel the sensation spreading to the palms of my hands," and so on.
- Talk to yourself, using sleepy words such as relaxed, calm, and peaceful. Say, "I am relaxed. I am falling asleep. I feel so peaceful. Soon I'll be asleep."
- In your imagination, take your favorite walk at your favorite time and place in your favorite season, either alone or with your favorite person.

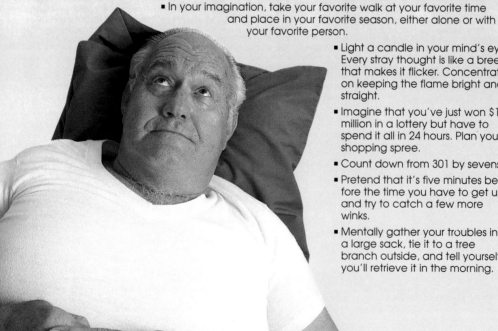

- Light a candle in your mind's eye. Every stray thought is like a breeze that makes it flicker. Concentrate on keeping the flame bright and straight.
- Imagine that you've just won $1-million in a lottery but have to spend it all in 24 hours. Plan your shopping spree.
- Count down from 301 by sevens.
- Pretend that it's five minutes before the time you have to get up, and try to catch a few more winks.
- Mentally gather your troubles into a large sack, tie it to a tree branch outside, and tell yourself you'll retrieve it in the morning.

lying mental disorder, most often depression or an anxiety disorder. These disorders affect the chemistry of the brain, which may account for the sleep problems they bring on.

Sometimes insomnia results from involuntary leg movements during the night or from a condition called restless legs, which is characterized by annoying discomfort in the lower limbs as a person is trying to fall asleep. Scientists do not know what causes these two conditions.

About 15 percent of those seeking help for chronic insomnia suffer from learned, or behavioral, insomnia. Although a life crisis may have triggered their initial sleep problems, they remain unable to sleep long after the stress eases. Each night they try harder and harder to get to sleep, but cannot. They have fallen into a habit of not being able to sleep, and the nightly anticipation of the problem only increases their anxiety and makes it more difficult to sleep.

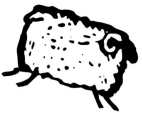

Help for insomnia

Despite the prevalence of insomnia, very few people ever seek their doctors' advice—even though treatments could help 3 out of 4 poor sleepers. "We have an array of therapies for sleep disorders that are highly effective," says psychiatrist Phil Westbrook, director of the Sleep Disorders Center at Cedars-Sinai Medical Center in Los Angeles. "And they're more likely to be behavioral than medicinal."

Sleep specialists say that the treatment of insomnia should be tailored to the individual. They point out that sleeping pills may help a specific, short-term problem, but they should be taken only under a doctor's supervision. The dangers associated with sleeping pills are numerous. See SLEEPING PILLS: SHORT-TERM GAIN on page 129.

In the long term, behavioral approaches to insomnia have proven more effective than sleeping pills. "In research studies, sleep medications seem to work better for the first few weeks," says Charles Morin, professor of psychiatry and director of the Sleep Disorders Center at Virginia Commonwealth University in Richmond. "But in follow-up studies a few months or even a year or two later, those who received nonmedical treatments do significantly better."

Long-term, nonmedicinal treatments generally involve 8 to 10 weeks of training. They seek to modify behavior through several approaches.
- *Relaxation therapy* teaches the sleeper to progressively relax each muscle, breathe deeply from the diaphragm, meditate, or go under hypnosis. Audiotapes or experienced trainers can provide instruction in these techniques.
- *Cognitive therapy* helps shift the person's mind away from the anxiety-inducing thoughts that are causing sleeplessness. For

example, people who have a difficult time turning off their racing minds may be told to read in bed until they drift into sleep. People who find themselves thinking about daytime worries may try refocusing techniques, such as memory games. See TIRED OF COUNTING SHEEP? on page 126.

- *Stimulus control therapy* helps individuals with learned insomnia unlearn the habit of sleeplessness. They must wait to go to bed until they are too tired to stay awake. If they do find themselves lying awake, they must get out of bed and find something to do until they are very sleepy. The more fatigued they become, the easier they find it to fall asleep in bed. After several weeks, they no longer associate the bed with insomnia.
- *Sleep restriction therapy* instructs insomniacs to keep a log of how much time in bed they actually spend sleeping. They are then allowed to stay in bed only that amount of time. For example, a person sleeping only four hours out of eight spent in bed must leave the bed after four hours. As a greater percentage of time is spent sleeping, more bed time is earned. Sleep restriction therapy, like stimulus control therapy, makes people so tired before they get into bed that they then fall asleep more easily.

People who are having problems falling or staying asleep at night should refrain from daytime napping, which can undermine nighttime sleep efficiency. A better alternative for people with insomnia who become tired during the day is taking a short break for relaxation exercises or meditation.

Sleep apnea and snoring

Apnea, which comes from Greek words meaning *no* and *breath*, is exactly that: the absence of breathing. People with apnea briefly stop breathing dozens or even hundreds of times during the night. As they struggle for air, they may snore extremely loudly or thrash about. Long considered a problem of older men, sleep apnea seems to be more common than thought among middle-aged men and women. In a 1993 study at the University of Wisconsin in Madison, 2 percent of the women and 4 percent of the men between ages 30 and 60 stopped breathing at least 15 times an hour during sleep.

In most cases of sleep apnea, the flow of air to the lungs is blocked by flabby throat muscles, a large tongue, or other obstruction in the airway. Obesity greatly increases the likelihood of obstructed breathing. Other causes of apnea include malfunction of respiration-control centers in the brain; disorders of the ear, nose, and throat, such as large tonsils or adenoids; and upper-airway abnormalities.

Cases of apnea range from mild to severe. How a person feels during the day is a good indicator of how serious the problem is. Apnea often causes early-morning headaches and daytime drowsiness. Severe cases can cause extreme daytime drowsiness and can lead to high blood pressure and other serious circulatory system problems. Apnea may affect as many as 10 million Americans, though most of them are unaware of the problem. "I would recommend that anyone with chronic loud snoring seek an evaluation," says Westbrook.

Treatment for apnea can include weight loss, if obesity is contributing to the problem. A mechanical breathing mask worn over the nose can also help. The mask applies continuous pressure to the airways, keeping the throat passage from closing and ensuring a steady flow of air into the lungs. In severe cases, doctors may treat apnea with surgery to enlarge the nose or throat area.

Snoring is a sound that can exasperate even the most patient of bed partners. "Snoring occurs with partial collapse of the airway during sleep," explains sleep specialist Thomas Neylan of California Pacific Medical Center in San Francisco. "While occasional mild snoring probably is not harmful, chronic snorers may suffer the same consequences as individuals with apnea, but to a lesser degree." Snoring that is accompanied by extreme daytime drowsiness may indicate sleep apnea.

To cut down on mild snoring, some simple changes can help, such as making sure the bedroom is well ventilated and using a low pillow so the snorer's neck remains straight. To keep from turning onto their backs—the position in which snoring is most likely—some snorers, or their weary partners, sew a pocket or pin a sock containing a golf or tennis ball onto the back of a pajama top. Avoiding nicotine, alcohol, and heavy meals before bedtime also may make a difference.

Other sleep problems

A few sleep problems occur only during REM sleep. The most common are nightmares, which trouble 4 percent to 5 percent of sleepers and typically begin after a major stressful life event. In most cases, occasional nightmares do not require therapy. When they occur frequently, however, they may be a sign of stress, and relaxation techniques can help.

Sleeping pills: Short-term gain

Prescription sleeping pills may alleviate a specific, short-term problem. They can speed the onset of sleep, reduce nighttime awakenings, and extend total sleep time. However, they tend to lose their effectiveness after about two weeks. The American Sleep Disorders Association recommends that sleeping pills be used in the lowest effective dose, for the shortest period of time, and only under a doctor's supervision. The dangers associated with sleeping pills include:

- Fatal overdoses, especially when combined with alcohol or other drugs that act on the central nervous system.
- Harmful interactions with other prescription medications.
- Interference with breathing.
- Impaired coordination, memory, and thinking during the daytime.
- Disruption of normal sleep stages.
- Potential damage to the kidneys, liver, and lungs.
- Difficulty awakening in the event of a nighttime crisis.
- In older people, particular sensitivity to side effects.

Over-the-counter sleeping pills also can produce disturbing side effects and should never be given to children or taken by pregnant women. Before taking these pills, be sure to consult your physician.

Source: Yudofsky, Stuart, and others. *What You Need to Know About Psychiatric Drugs*, Grove Press.

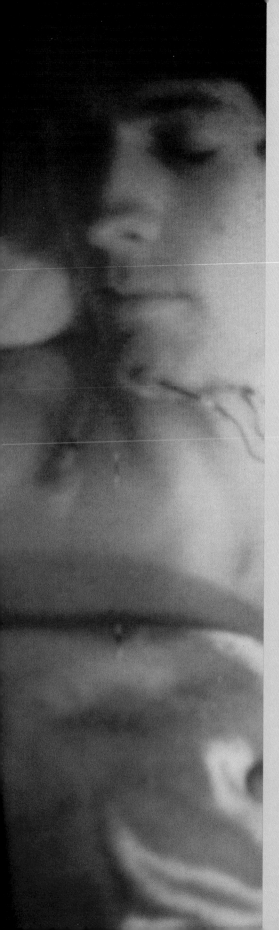

Getting a good night's sleep

What we do during the day has an enormous effect on how we sleep at night. The following recommendations can help ensure that you don't lie awake.

- **Don't drink coffee, colas, or other caffeinated beverages late in the day.** Some coffee lovers develop a tolerance for caffeine, but others do not. Caffeine can linger in the body for six to eight hours after it has been consumed.

- **Keep regular hours.** An erratic schedule makes it more difficult to fall asleep at night or wake up in the morning. Awakening at more or less the same time each day is one of the best ways to keep the body's biological clock in order.

- **Exercise regularly.** In addition to contributing to overall well-being, exercise helps relieve tension, making it easier to fall asleep quickly. A good time for a walk or workout is late afternoon or early evening, allowing the body to slow down and relax before it is time to go to bed.

- **Don't use alcohol as a sedative.** Although some people enjoy a nightcap before going to bed, alcohol can undermine the quality of sleep and lead to awakenings in the night. Even moderate drinking can interfere with the stages of deep sleep.

- **Develop a sleep ritual.** A regular routine before bedtime, such as taking a bath, reading, or listening to music, can help ease the transition from day to night. Whatever ritual you choose to unwind each night becomes a cue for your body to relax and prepare for slumber.

- **Don't bring work or worries into bed.** If you regularly curl up in bed to pay bills or catch up on work, you may associate your bed with stress rather than rest. It is best to reserve the bed for sleep only. If you find yourself fretting once you get into bed, schedule a regular time earlier in the day to think about issues in your life and work out possible solutions.

- **Create a comfortable sleep environment.** The ideal sleep setting is safe, dark, and neither too hot nor too cold. Install shades or blinds to keep out light. Use ear plugs or a machine that produces soothing sounds to ensure quiet.

- **Don't assume that more sleep is always better.** The longer people stay in bed, the shallower and more fragmented their sleep becomes. Go for quality, not quantity, and try to get as much sleep as needed to feel energetic the next day.

During the 1980's, sleep specialists identified a new and unusual problem called REM sleep behavior disorder, which occurs only during REM sleep and mostly in middle-aged or older men. For unknown reasons, possibly related to the aging brain, the major muscles of these troubled sleepers do not become paralyzed, as usually happens during dream sleep. Instead, the sleeper acts out scenes in dreams. A retired grocer, dreaming he was a football halfback, tackled his dresser so forcefully that he gashed his forehead. REM sleep behavior disorder can be treated effectively with a variety of approaches, including hypnosis, psychotherapy, and medication.

If practical strategies for getting a good night's sleep don't work, and you suspect a more serious sleep disorder, use these questions to help decide if you need professional help:

- Have you been having difficulty falling asleep?
- Do you awaken in the night and find it hard to get back to sleep?
- Do you wake in the morning not feeling rested, regardless of how long you sleep?
- Are you extremely tired during the day, and do you nod off when you don't want to?
- Do you have problems thinking, concentrating, or doing your job?
- Has a bed partner or member of your family noticed extremely loud snoring or frequent gasping for air?
- Have your sleep problems persisted for more than four to six weeks?

If you answer yes to more than one or two of these questions, you may want to seek professional help. "The best indication is the impact on your daytime functioning," says Neylan. "If you're having significant trouble at work because of fatigue, and self-help steps don't work, you definitely should see your primary-care physician or a sleep specialist."

Given that sleep is how we spend one-third of our lives, it seems that the quality of this essential activity is well worth our attention. With proper care, our time asleep can infuse our waking moments with energy and vitality.

For further reading:
Hales, Dianne. *The Complete Book of Sleep*. Addison-Wesley Publishing Company, 1981.
Hobson, J. Allan. *Sleep*. Scientific American Library, 1989.

For more information:
Information on sleep disorders and sleep treatment centers can be obtained from the American Sleep Apnea Association, P.O. Box 66, Belmont, MA 02178, and from the National Sleep Foundation, 122 S. Robertson Boulevard, 3rd Floor-HM, Los Angeles, CA 90048.

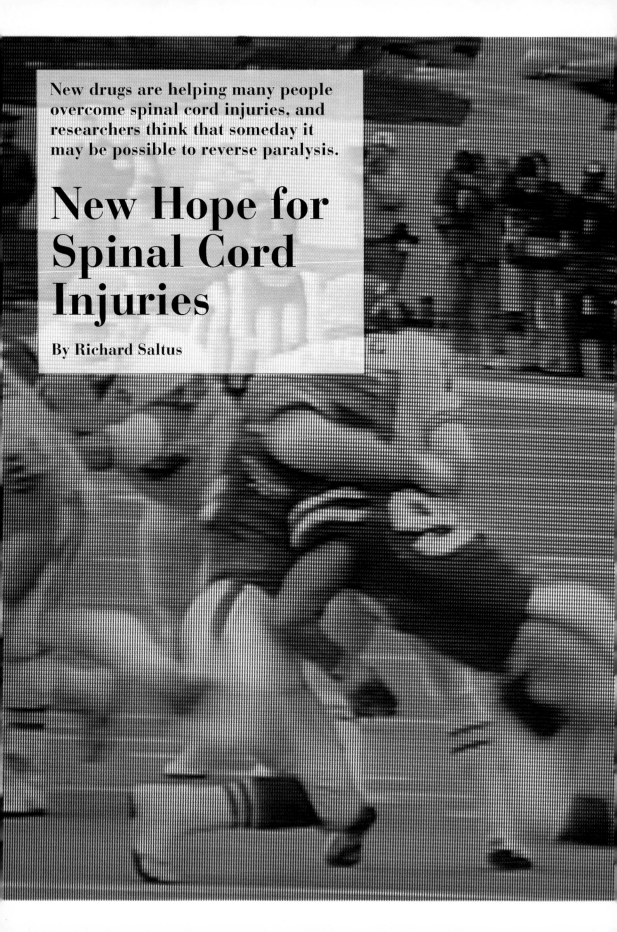

New drugs are helping many people
overcome spinal cord injuries, and
researchers think that someday it
may be possible to reverse paralysis.

New Hope for
Spinal Cord
Injuries

By Richard Saltus

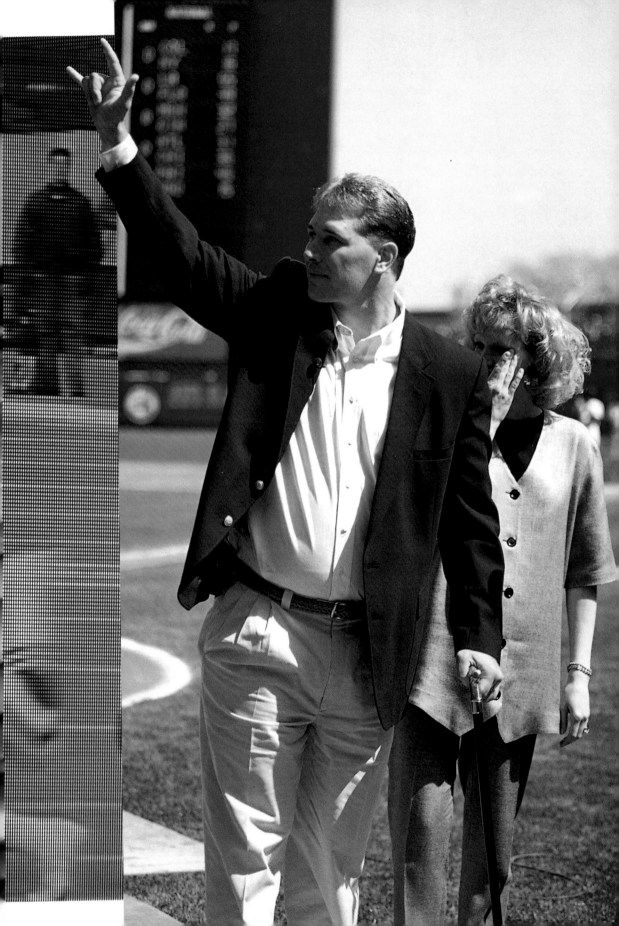

To protect the spinal cord—a vital bundle of nerve cells and nerve fibers that enables us to move and to feel—nature gave it a bony casing that can flex, turn, and roll with the punches. But there are limits to the punishment it can take. For one thing, human evolution made no provision for a violent game in which large, muscular men don hard plastic helmets and ram into one another at what can be, quite literally, breakneck speed.

So it was, on a Sunday in November 1992, for football player Dennis Byrd, a 266-pound (121-kilogram) defensive lineman for the New York Jets. In a game with the Kansas City Chiefs at Giants Stadium in New York City, Byrd hurtled at the opposing quarterback but instead slammed headfirst into a teammate. He heard a crunching sound as the impact of the collision shattered a bone in his neck. Byrd fell to the ground and was unable to move—his spinal cord had been badly damaged.

In the moment of that terrible collision on the football field, Byrd became one of an estimated 10,000 people in the United States each year who suffer injuries to the spinal cord. More than half of those people are under 30 years of age, and more than three-fourths of them are males.

Fortunately, spinal cord injuries are usually not fatal. Although as recently as the 1940's, 90 percent of people with spinal cord damage died soon after receiving the injury—usually from infections—the reverse is true today. Thanks in large part to antibiotics, about 94 percent of spinal cord injury patients now survive their first hospitalization. But they may still suffer disabling damage. An estimated 200,000 Americans are living with the consequences of spinal cord injuries. Many of them are confined to wheelchairs, partially or completely paralyzed for life. Others can walk only with the aid of crutches or leg braces.

A dramatic recovery

Byrd was fortunate. Less than five months after his catastrophic injury, aided only by a cane, he walked onto the field of base-ball's Shea Stadium, where he was cheered by New York sports fans attending the first Mets game of the season. And about a year after that, his remaining disability was relatively minor—weakness in his limbs and trunk and less endurance than he had before being injured.

Byrd was able to make such a remarkable recovery in part because the injury he suffered was not the worst that can happen to the spinal cord. But he was also helped by advances in the treatment of spinal cord injuries.

Within minutes after Byrd fell to the AstroTurf, team doctors ascertained that he had broken his neck. After placing the fallen lineman carefully onto a backboard designed to keep the spinal column straight and immobile, they sent him by ambulance to Lenox Hill Hospital in New York City. There, after evaluating

The author:

Richard Saltus is a science writer at the *Boston Globe.*

his condition, surgeons operated on Byrd for four hours. They removed chips of bone from his spinal cord and inserted metal plates and screws in his neck to shore it up and provide a scaffold for healing.

From the time he entered the hospital, Byrd was given two drugs, methylprednisolone and GM-1 ganglioside, which can limit the swelling and bleeding that often compound the damage after a spinal cord injury. Prompt treatment with those two drugs, physicians have found, can in many cases make the difference between a person's being crippled for life or regaining near-normal functioning. Researchers studying the spinal cord are even expressing guarded optimism about the possibility of one day reversing paralysis, a feat once considered impossible.

Vital and vulnerable nerves

Although it is only the thickness of an adult's little finger, the spinal cord is the most important collection of nerve tissues outside the brain, from which it extends. The spinal cord emerges from the bottom of the brain through a hole in the skull and runs for about 16 to 18 inches (41 to 46 centimeters) down the neck and the back inside the protective bony spinal column. Within the cord are more than 20 million nerve fibers, tightly packed like strands of wire in a telephone cable.

The spinal cord and the brain make up the central nervous system (CNS), the body's main "switchboard." The CNS receives sensory information from nerve cells throughout the body, analyzes the messages, and then sends instructions back to the outlying nerve cells. Those instructions control the body's internal organs and its every muscular movement.

The spinal cord ends about two-thirds of the way down the spinal column. There, the cord branches into a bundle of nerve fibers resembling a horse's tail, which in fact is its Latin name— the *cauda equina*. The cauda equina has a better ability to regain function after an injury than the spinal cord, so injuries to the lower back tend to be less devastating than ones that occur higher on the spinal column.

The cauda equina is part of the outer nerve network, called the peripheral nervous system (PNS), that ferries impulses to and from the central nervous system. The PNS includes 31 pairs of spinal nerves, each pair consisting of a sensory nerve and a motor nerve. The sensory nerves transmit information from the skin, muscles, and organs to the CNS, and the motor nerves convey the CNS's responses. For example, a sensory nerve might inform the CNS of the sensation of cold, and a motor nerve would respond with a signal to the muscles that triggers shivering. The spinal nerves are divided into groups by location: 8 pairs of cervical (neck); 12 pairs of thoracic (chest); 5 pairs of lumbar (lower back); and 5 pairs of sacral (lower end of the

Glossary

Cauda equina: A bundle of nerves that extends from the bottom of the spinal cord.

Central nervous system: The brain and spinal cord.

Paraplegia: Paralysis of the legs, lower trunk, and sometimes also the chest area.

Peripheral nervous system: The body's outer nerve network, which transmits nerve impulses to and from the central nervous system.

Spinal column: The spine or backbone, consisting of 24 interlocking bones, called vertebrae, that encase and protect the spinal cord.

Spinal cord: A collection of more than 20 million tightly packed nerve fibers that emerges from the base of the brain and extends down the back within the spinal column.

Tetraplegia: Paralysis of the arms, legs, and trunk; also called quadriplegia.

The body's main "switchboard"

The spinal cord, which consists of more than 20 million tightly packed nerves controlling all functions of the body, extends from the brain down the back. The cord is surrounded by the bony spinal column, which is made of segments called vertebrae. The spinal cord ends about two-thirds of the way down the back. From that point, a loose bundle of nerves called the cauda equina extends the rest of the way down the spinal column. The nerves extending outward from the spinal column to various parts of the body are divided into four groups: the cervical nerves, the thoracic nerves, the lumbar nerves, and the sacral nerves. Each group of nerves controls a different part of the body.

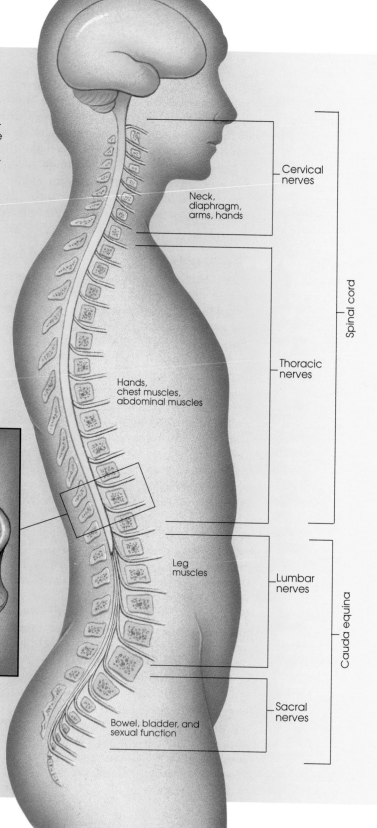

Spinal cord

Nerve fiber

Vertebra

Cervical nerves

Neck, diaphragm, arms, hands

Spinal cord

Thoracic nerves

Hands, chest muscles, abdominal muscles

Leg muscles

Lumbar nerves

Cauda equina

Bowel, bladder, and sexual function

Sacral nerves

spine). There is also one pair of coccygeal nerves at the very bottom of the spine.

The spinal column, or backbone, consisting of 24 interlocking vertebrae, is designed to protect the spinal cord and the roots of its branching nerves, including those of the cauda equina. It does that job well, but it remains vulnerable. About once an hour in the United States, someone receives an injury that twists or fractures the spinal column and damages the delicate cord. Automobile accidents are by far the most common cause of spinal cord injuries, accounting for nearly 50 percent of all spinal cord hospitalizations. The next most frequent causes of spinal cord injury are falls, which account for nearly 25 percent; shootings and other acts of violence, 15 percent; and sports injuries, particularly diving accidents, from 10 to 15 percent.

The effects of spinal cord injuries

More than half of all spinal injuries involve damage to the neck area. Another third involve the lower back, and the remainder occur in the middle of the back. The higher on the spinal cord that damage occurs, the greater is the potential loss of bodily function. All sensation and movement below the level of the injury may be lost, at least temporarily and sometimes for the rest of the person's life. Injuries to the neck area, for example, may result in tetraplegia (also called quadriplegia)—paralysis of the arms, legs, and trunk. Injuries to the back may cause paraplegia, in which the arms are spared but the legs are paralyzed. Paraplegia also involves paralysis of the lower trunk, and, if the injury is high enough on the back, the chest area as well.

The paralysis can lead to serious health problems, stemming both from the loss of CNS control over vital functions in the body and from being motionless for long periods. One of the most common complications is urinary tract infections, which develop because the individual has lost most or all control over the bladder (as well as the bowel) and must have a *catheter* (narrow tube) inserted into the bladder to allow urine to escape. The catheter can allow bacteria into the bladder, resulting in infection. The patient can also become prone to drastic swings in blood pressure caused by disruption of the nerve signals that regulate the flow of blood.

Immobility can lead to blood clots that form in the legs and migrate to the lungs, and to bedsores and other skin problems. Other complications of being confined to a bed or wheelchair include the gradual loss of bone mass, the shrinkage of muscles, and a build-up of fatty deposits in blood vessels, increasing the risk of heart attacks and strokes. Moreover, injuries or illnesses in the paralyzed areas may go undiagnosed because the person cannot feel pain or detect other warning symptoms.

These long-term effects occur despite the fact that the spinal

How spinal cord injuries occur

Automobile accidents are the greatest cause of spinal cord damage, accounting for nearly 50 percent of such injuries each year. Skiing accidents and other sports-related mishaps are responsible for 10 to 15 percent of spinal cord injuries. Other major causes of injury include falls and acts of violence.

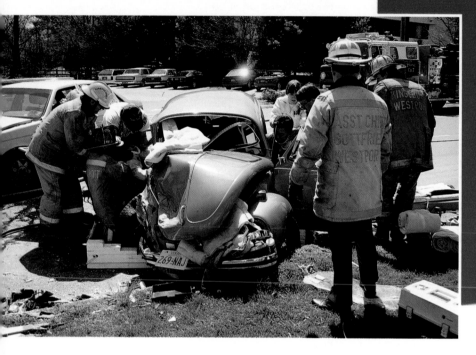

cord rarely is completely severed or even torn in an accident. In most cases, it is either crushed or bruised. Although that can be damage enough to cause lasting consequences, some of the most serious damage occurs after the initial injury. Neurologists—physicians who specialize in treating injuries and disorders of the nervous system—have learned that during the first 48 hours or so after a spinal cord injury, the body's natural responses to the injury cause the affected area of the cord to self-destruct.

During that crucial 48 hours, damaged tissues in the center of the spinal cord become inflamed and swollen. If blood vessels have been torn, *hemorrhaging* (heavy bleeding) may occur, and blood clots may form and compress the spinal cord. These effects are harmful in themselves, but they are magnified by the body's immune system, which is aroused by the injury. Scavenger cells of the immune system move into the injury site and begin cleaning up dead cells. In the process, they secrete a number of powerful chemicals that can wreak havoc on nerve tissues. In addition, dying nerve cells themselves release a number of *toxic* (poisonous) substances, including oxygen-containing molecules called free radicals, that can harm surrounding tissues.

These various events severely damage the long fibers, called

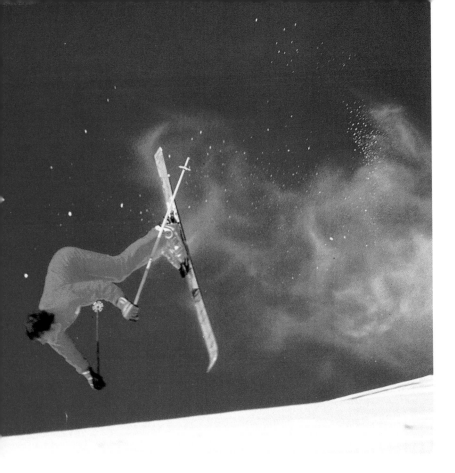

axons, that connect nerve cells to one another. The end result is a gap in the spinal cord at the site of the initial injury, bounded by scarred tissue. Because nerve impulses cannot travel across the gap, parts of the body below the injury are cut off from the brain, leaving them paralyzed.

Limiting the damage

Grim as this scenario is, researchers realized that it also offered hope for patients, if only a way could be found to stop the progressive damage. Until the 1980's, however, there were thought to be no medicines that could effectively protect the spinal cord from this assault. Then doctors began to study the effectiveness of methylprednisolone and GM-1, two drugs that showed great promise. "We now know that paralysis after spinal cord injury can be reduced by early treatment," Michael Bracken, a neurological researcher at Yale University Medical School in New Haven, Conn., announced in 1990.

In a study reported that year, Bracken and his colleagues demonstrated the protective properties of methylprednisolone, a synthetic steroid similar to cortisone. They found that people who were given high doses of methylprednisolone within eight hours after a spinal cord injury regained an average of 20 percent of lost nerve function. The drug apparently has a twofold effect. As well as reducing inflammation—and thereby warding off a response by the immune system—it attaches to free radicals and takes them out of action. By the time of Dennis Byrd's injury, doctors at many large medical centers were routinely giving methylprednisolone to patients with spinal cord injuries.

GM-1, a still-experimental drug that is undergoing clinical trials in the United States, is a chemical that occurs naturally in cell membranes of the spinal cord and brain. In 1991, physicians taking part in a small study of GM-1 at a University of Maryland medical clinic in Baltimore reported major improvements in patients given the drug right after their injury. Some of the patients, who had been immobilized by their injury, were able to walk again within a few months. Researchers theorize that GM-1 both helps halt further nerve-tissue destruction and stimulates the repair and growth of surviving nerve fibers. The drug is now being evaluated in a large-scale study at 22 medical centers in the United States and Canada.

The process of rehabilitation

Even with the help of drug therapy, however, recovery from a spinal cord injury involves months or years of rehabilitation and counseling. Dennis Byrd's regimen after his gridiron accident is typical of what many patients go through.

Byrd started on the difficult road to recovery just 10 days after his injury when he was transferred to Mount Sinai Medical Center in New York City. There, doctors and physical therapists helped Byrd through a physical training program aimed at strengthening his upper body and enhancing blood flow.

When Byrd started physical therapy, he was unable to move his arms, hands, or legs, though he retained some sensation in them. At first, therapists moved Byrd's limbs for him, but little by little he regained the ability to move them himself.

Byrd's rehabilitation began with exercise sessions on a tilt table, a board that can be rotated to various positions. Because his blood pressure was unstable and liable to plummet if he stood up, Byrd first exercised with the tilt table in a horizontal position. Over the course of weeks, the board was tilted a few degrees at a time toward the vertical, which retrained Byrd's body to maintain normal blood pressure.

When the injured athlete was ready to try standing up, he was eased into a swimming pool, which provided buoyancy for his body. In the pool, he exercised the muscles of the arms, neck, and trunk and practiced movements requiring coordination.

Other exercises were designed to improve Byrd's balance and endurance. And with the help of a device that uses electrical

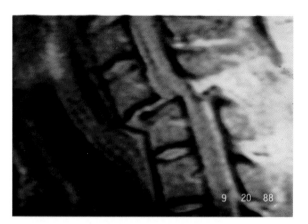

A spinal cord injury can be diagnosed with a technique called magnetic resonance imaging. In the injury above, the bony spinal column has been fractured and displaced (center of image). The spinal cord, which lies in the narrow canal just to the right of that part of the spinal column, has been compressed and damaged as a result. The body is facing left.

stimulation to trigger the contraction of muscles, he slowly regained the use of his hands.

This initial phase of Byrd's rehabilitation program lasted 11 weeks—considerably less than for many patients with spinal cord injuries. When he left the hospital at the end of that period, he was able to walk with the help of another person. And just a year after that, Byrd, though he continued with rehabilitation and would never again be able to play football, was leading a relatively normal life.

For people whose injuries cause more lasting disabilities, life can be a lot harder. Often, they try one rehabilitation program after another, seeking to regain lost function or to maintain what little they still have. Some programs are better than others, though none can offer much hope to a severely paralyzed individual.

The hope of spinal cord regeneration

Hope may be on the horizon for people disabled from spinal cord injuries. The conviction is growing among neuroscientists that it will someday be possible to use drugs to repair a badly damaged spinal cord and reverse paralysis. They have learned that nerve cells in the

From initial injury to paralysis

In the hours and days following a spinal cord injury, the body's natural responses to the injury can destroy nerve cells and the nerve fibers that extend from them. This damage may result in permanent paralysis.

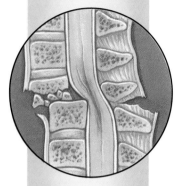

In a typical spinal injury, vertebrae in the spinal column are broken or crushed, compressing and damaging the spinal cord.

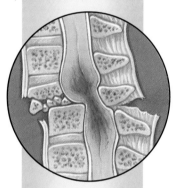

Spinal cord tissues near the site of the injury swell, become inflamed, and suffer other damaging effects. These changes lead to the death of nerve cells in the spinal cord and the disruption of nerve pathways in the damaged area.

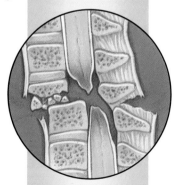

The tissue damage leaves a gap in the spinal cord, with scarred tissue at each end. Nerve connections are severed between the brain and the region below the gap. The muscles controlled by nerves at or below the gap are paralyzed.

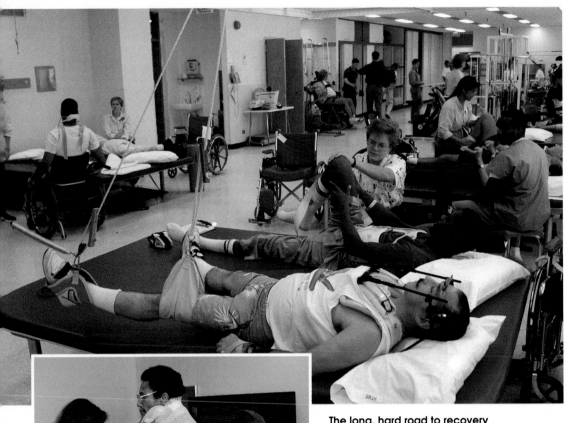

The long, hard road to recovery
People with spinal cord injuries can often be helped with physical therapy, especially if they have retained some sensation in the body areas affected by their injury. At the Rehabilitation Institute of Chicago, *above* and *left*, therapists work with patients to help them regain at least some ability to perform normal activities such as walking.

central nervous system have the capacity to *regenerate* (regrow) severed connections but are prevented from doing so by chemicals released by surrounding tissues. Some researchers think these biochemical barriers are needed to maintain a healthy CNS. If CNS nerves could easily sprout and make new connections, the nervous system might become so disorderly that it could no longer function properly.

The resistance of the CNS to regeneration was discovered in the late 1800's and early 1900's, and for decades most scientists gave up on the idea of repairing damaged spinal cords. Since the 1950's, however, scientists have again dedicated themselves to the goal of regenerating nerves in the central nervous system.

The federal government has taken an active role in this effort. Motivated in part by the large number of servicemen paralyzed by wounds in World War II (1939-1945), the government in 1950 established a research institute for neurological diseases within the National Institutes of Health. Four years later, at a meeting sponsored by the new institute, scientists asserted that regeneration of the CNS is possible, and they urged other investigators to take up the challenge. By the 1970's, researchers were learning how the CNS hinders the regrowth of CNS nerves and finding ways to counteract those natural mechanisms.

A key discovery came in 1988, when neuroscientist Martin Schwab of the University of Zurich in Switzerland, identified two chemical factors that prevent CNS nerves from regrowing. Just two years later, he showed that blocking those substances with proteins called antibodies permits severed CNS nerves in animals to regenerate for some distance.

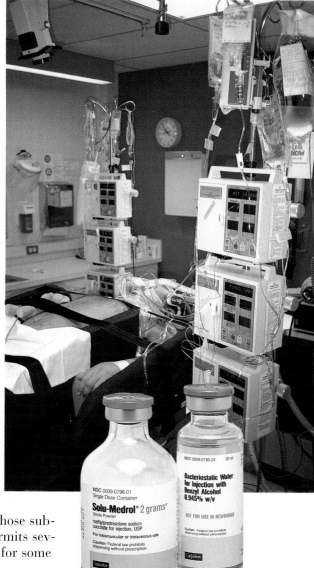

In treating spinal cord injuries, the emphasis today is on using drugs to limit the tissue damage that can lead to paralysis. Such drugs, including methylprednisolone, *above*, are given intravenously as soon as the patient enters the hospital, *top*. Researchers are now trying to develop drugs that can reverse paralysis, a goal once thought impossible.

Experiments with fetal tissue

In the 1990's, experimental attempts to regenerate the spinal cords of animals have achieved some striking results. One approach involves the implantation of fetal nerve tissue into the spinal cord. Neuroscientists consider this a promising technique because the biochemical environment in which an embryo develops encourages nerve cells to grow and interconnect. Thus, fetal tissue implanted into the scarred gap of a damaged spinal cord might stimulate nerve fibers to regrow and reestablish severed connections across the gap.

A promising series of experiments using this procedure was carried out in the early 1990's by a research team at the University of Florida in Gainesville, headed by neuroscientists Paul

J. Reier and Douglas Anderson. The investigators implanted nerve tissue from cat fetuses into the damaged spinal cords of cats. The animals regained their ability to walk, though they were less agile than before their injuries. But whether the implants actually regenerated severed nerves is unclear. It is just as possible, Reier and Anderson noted, that biochemical substances in the implanted tissue "woke up" spinal cord circuits that had survived the injury but were not functioning.

In a related approach, neuroscientist Fred Gage of the University of California at San Diego thinks that implants of cells grown in the laboratory may work just as well as fetal cells. Gage uses genetic-engineering techniques to convert rat cells into tiny "factories" producing the same substances that are in fetal tissue, including nerve growth factors—chemicals that stimulate nerves to send out new fibers.

In experimental studies with rats, Gage has implanted these genetically engineered cells into intact spinal cords and found that the cells survive, producing nerve growth factors for as long as a year. Gage says that the implanted cells stimulate an "enormously robust" sprouting of new fibers in the peripheral nerves joining the spinal cord. He is now implanting the cells into damaged rat spinal cords to see if the cords will regenerate.

Other approaches to regeneration

A research team headed by neuroscientist Richard Bunge has been tackling a different aspect of spinal cord injuries at the Miami Project to Cure Paralysis, a foundation at the University of Miami in Florida. Following spinal cord damage, surviving nerve fibers in the cord often lose their protective coating, a sheath of a fatty substance called myelin. Peripheral nerves, on the other hand, can regain their myelin coat after an injury, thanks to myelin-producing cells called Schwann cells that encapsulate these nerve fibers. Bunge thinks that Schwann cells taken from a person's own peripheral nervous system could be grown in large quantities in a laboratory dish and then used to repair a spinal cord injury. In an experiment reported in 1991, Bunge inserted plastic tubes filled with billions of Schwann cells from rats into severed rat spinal cords. He found that nerve cells in the spinal cord grew and closed the gap in the cord.

Martin Schwab, the Swiss scientist who discovered the antiregeneration substance, made news in early 1994 when he reported the results of another regeneration experiment. As in his earlier study, Schwab gave rats with spinal-cord injuries injections of an antibody that blocks the action of chemicals that ordinarily prevent nerve growth. But this time, he also injected the rats with a growth factor. With this twofold approach, Schwab and his colleagues were able to coax nerve fibers into growing across the injured area, partly repairing the damage. This experiment was one of a growing number suggesting that natural growth factors will play a very large role in future research on repairing spinal cord injuries.

All of these methods show promise, but none of them work so well that scientists think the time has come for human trials. One experimental treatment that has been tested on human subjects has become embroiled in great controversy.

That treatment was developed in the 1980's by Harry Goldsmith, a Boston University surgeon, who is still its main advocate in the United States. The procedure involves dividing and extending a blood-rich tissue in the abdomen and attaching it to the spinal cord at the injury site. Goldsmith claims that increased blood flow, together with the growth factors it secretes, appears to foster regeneration in the spinal cord.

Most other spinal cord specialists saw no persuasive evidence from animal experiments to support Goldsmith's technique. Nevertheless, Goldsmith and other surgeons at Boston University Hospital used the procedure on 26 patients with spinal cord injuries, beginning in 1992. But university officials halted the trial in the summer of 1993 after patients claimed that a recruiter for the experiment had misled them. In 1994, it was unknown whether any results from the test would be published.

Spinal cord research in the mid-1990's can be likened to the proverbial glass of water that—depending on whether you are an optimist or a pessimist—is either half full or half empty. Researchers and organizations seeking ways to regenerate damaged nerves fall more and more into the optimist camp as they emphasize the progress that has been made. The pessimists, on the other hand, point out that progress has been slow and that it's still not clear which, if any, of the many roads being explored by scientists leads in the right direction. Nonetheless, the progress is real, and investigators think that a number of approaches to repairing the spinal cord may be ready for human tests by the end of the 1990's or soon thereafter.

For more information:

The Paralyzed Veterans of America, an organization in Washington, D.C., funds a 24-hour hotline to help anyone with spinal cord injuries find support groups, rehabilitation facilities, and other types of assistance. The toll-free number is 1-800-526-3456.

The National Spinal Injury Association, an organization in Woburn, Mass., offers information on spinal cord injuries and helps victims of paralysis make contact with other paralyzed individuals who can provide emotional support. The association's toll-free number is 1-800-962-9629.

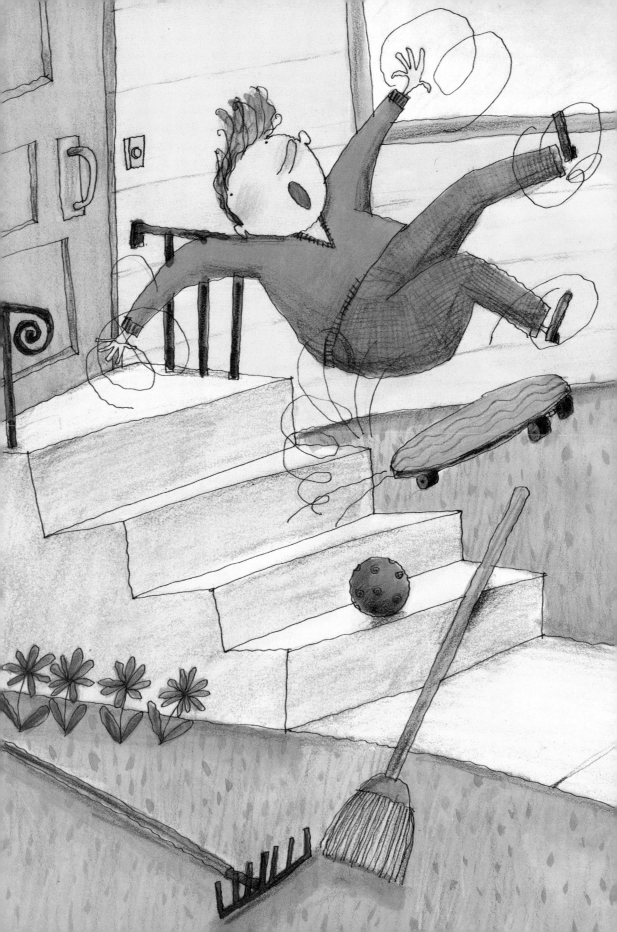

Each year, thousands of Americans die
in accidents that occur in and around
their own homes. With planning and
vigilance, most home accidents and
injuries can be prevented.

Home, Safe Home

By Michael Woods

With newspapers, talk shows, and newscasts daily barraging
audiences with stories of murder and mayhem, many Americans, naturally enough, wish to view their home as a refuge—
quiet and safe from the dangers lurking beyond their doors.
This sense of security may, however, be an illusion.

Many American homes may, in fact, be more dangerous than
the world outside, according to statistics published by the National Safety Council (NSC), a nonprofit organization dedicated
to health and safety in the home and workplace. Home accidents are the nation's fourth leading cause of death. They kill
approximately 19,500 people each year—a number greater
than the annual number of deaths resulting from all work-related accidents. The only accidents to take a greater toll involve
motor vehicles.

In terms of disabling injury—defined as physical disability
lasting 24 hours or longer—no place, according to the NSC, is
more dangerous than your own home. Approximately 6 million
injuries occurred in the home in 1992, compared with 5.8 million in public places, 3.3 million at work, and 2.2 million from
motor vehicle accidents. In the approximately 94 million houses

and apartments that Americans called home in 1992, someone suffered an accidental injury every 5 seconds, and someone died in a home accident every 27 minutes.

Home safety check

Because of the unexpected, seemingly random nature of accidents, many people regard them as uncontrollable and largely
unavoidable. Safety officials, however, say that nothing could be
further from the truth. They point out that most home accidents
are waiting to happen and can be anticipated and prevented
with simple, inexpensive measures. The NSC recommends that
people conduct a home safety check and repeat it periodically to
improve their awareness of safety hazards.

Begin your check with the entrances to your house. Make
sure that walkways are in good condition and are kept clear of
bicycles, toys, or garden tools. Make sure steps are in good repair and are fitted with a handrail. Steps and entrances should
be well lit at night.

The kitchen is the busiest room in most homes and therefore
a frequent site of accidents. Kitchens should be well lit, especially around the sink, stove, and counter tops, where knives
and other sharp tools are used. Grease and water spills on the
floor should be wiped up immediately to prevent slipping. Keep
cleaning products, disinfectants, pesticides, and alcohol in their
original, clearly labeled containers and store them either in a
locked cabinet or well out of a child's reach. If you do transfer
such products to containers with child-resistant closure (CRC)
caps, make sure you clearly note the potentially hazardous nature of the contents on the container.

A ladder, stepstool, or long-handled "grabber" should be
kept in the kitchen for reaching high shelves. A kitchen chair,
cabinet shelf, or counter top is a dangerous substitute.

Many kitchen appliances come equipped with three-pronged
plugs, requiring a grounded, electrical outlet designed to accom-
modate the third prong. To avoid fire or electric shock, do not
remove the third prong or use an adapter to force the plug into
a standard outlet. Have standard outlets replaced with grounded ones instead. Avoid trailing extension cords across counter
tops or floors, particularly in high-traffic areas. Extension cords
"hidden" under carpeting can become frayed by foot traffic
and thus pose a fire hazard. Another fire hazard is the over-
loaded "octopus" electrical outlet featuring adapters plugged
into adapters and tangles of cords.

A major offender in many American homes is the living room
home-entertainment center, where wires by the dozen interconnect television, videocassette recorder, stereo, compact disc
player, and speakers. Powering all these devices from a single
or, at best, a double outlet creates the classic accident waiting to

The author:

Michael Woods is science
editor of the *Toledo Blade*
and the author of many
articles on scientific and
medical topics.

happen. Have an electrician install additional outlets to handle appliances and home electronics. Also keep in mind that the electric circuits in most houses built before World War II (1939-1945) were not designed to carry the load of today's gadgetry.

Living room or family room fireplaces are often a potential source of house fires. Equip them with spark screens, and clean chimney flues periodically. Spark catchers installed on a chimney top can prevent fires on the roof. Many modern fireplaces consist of premade metal fireboxes called inserts. To be safe, fireplace inserts, such as wood stoves, must be properly installed and operated along guidelines supplied by the manufacturer.

In the bathroom, put abrasive strips or nonskid mats in bathtubs and showers to prevent slips. Do not store glass bottles of shampoo, lotions, or cosmetics on the bathtub rim or on a sink top, where they could fall and shatter. A night light for middle-of-the-night trips to the bathroom prevents stumbling in the dark and potentially dangerous falls.

Keep medicines in child-resistant containers and store them out of a child's reach in a high cabinet. Some safety experts recommend storing prescription drugs in the kitchen, rather than in the bathroom medicine cabinet where moisture can cause drugs to deteriorate. Do not let old prescription medicines accumulate. The Consumer Product Safety Commission (CPSC), a government agency that works to protect consumers from unsafe products, recommends flushing unused or expired medicines down the drain or toilet.

In the yard, check swing sets and other play equipment for frayed ropes, loose bolts, and other hazards. Do not disable the safety locks on power lawn mowers or lawn tractors. Make sure the grass is free of stones and other objects that could be picked up by the blades of a lawn mower and thrown into the air. When mowing the grass, keep children and pets at a safe distance. Wear eye protection and follow safety instructions when using chain saws, weed trimmers, and other power tools.

The line-up of home perils includes falls, poisonings, fires, burns, cuts, fractured bones, suffocation, gunshots, drowning, and electrocution. But most deaths and injuries result from a handful of accidents that are easily preventable.

The danger of falling

Falls are the leading cause of accidental death and serious injury in the home. They kill about 6,200 people each year and account for almost 1 out of every 3 fatal home accidents. Millions of other people are injured in falls each year. Most deaths and injuries occur when people fall down stairs, out windows, out of bed, or from ladders or roofs. But about 1 out of 4 falls occurs on a level surface, when people who are walking around the house or yard, slip, stumble, or trip over objects.

How Americans died in home accidents

- All home accidents: 19,500
- Falls: 6,200
- Poisoning: 4,500
- Fires and burns: 3,200
- Suffocation: 2,200
- Firearms: 700
- Drowning: 700
- All other home accidents: 2,200*

* Includes electrocution, explosions, and burns resulting from scalding, corrosive liquids, and steam.

Source: National Safety Council. Figures are for 1992.

Stairways are the most dangerous areas in any house. The CPSC estimates that falls down stairways account for 1.7 million serious injuries annually, more than any other kind of home injury. The American Association of Retired Persons (AARP), a nonprofit organization that addresses the needs of older people, cautions its members that "stairs are the most hazardous consumer product in the United States."

The NSC cites several ways of making stairs safer. Begin by keeping stairs clear of toys, clothing, and other objects that can trip people. Throw rugs should not be used at the very top or bottom of a stairway because they can slide and cause a fall. Worn or frayed carpeting is another potential source of falls. Stairways should have a handrail fastened securely to the wall. People who are adjusting to new bifocals should take special care because they may misjudge the location of a step.

To prevent falls in other parts of the home, make sure that throw rugs have a pad or nonskid backing. Hardware and department stores sell adhesive strips, foam rubber, and special sprays that can be applied to the back of rugs. Carpets and rugs with a short, dense pile and a pad of medium thickness provide better footing than do thick, plush carpets. Avoid polishing hardwood or tile floors with furniture waxes or dusting sprays, which can make floors very slippery. Instead, use self-polishing or nonskid floor waxes, and keep people off the floor until the

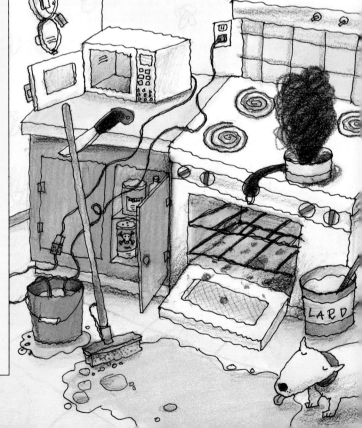

Kitchen checklist

- ☐ Mop up puddles or spills quickly to prevent slips.
- ☐ Plug major appliances, such as microwave ovens, directly into grounded outlets. Never use an extension cord.
- ☐ Check smoke alarm batteries regularly and replace them annually.
- ☐ Turn the handles of pots and pans on a hot stove inward so a child can't reach them.
- ☐ Keep used grease in an enclosed container, away from the stove top.
- ☐ Clean ovens regularly to prevent grease fires.
- ☐ Use a stepladder, never a kitchen chair, for reaching high shelves.
- ☐ Keep a chemical fire extinguisher in the kitchen.
- ☐ Store household cleaners, solvents, and alcohol in a locked cabinet in their original containers.
- ☐ Never leave knives or scissors lying on the counter in reach of a child.

Source: National Safety Council.

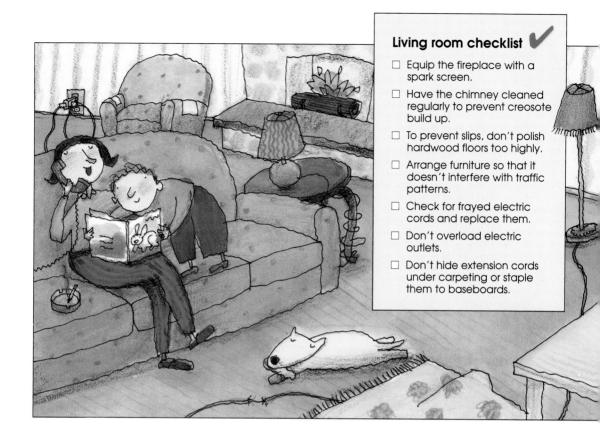

wax dries. Many falls occur when people stand on boxes, chairs, or other makeshift contraptions. It is safer to keep a stepstool or small ladder handy.

Guarding against accidental poisoning

Poisoning is the second leading cause of fatal home accidents. The National Safety Council estimates that about 4,500 fatal and 2 million nonfatal poisonings occur each year. Death rates for poisoning, unlike those for most other accidents, are increasing. They doubled between 1960 and 1990, from an average of 0.9 deaths per 100,000 people to 2.0 per 100,000. This increase is primarily due to accidental overdoses of drugs, both medications and illicit drugs.

Most fatal home poisonings—4,100 each year—involve solid and liquid substances, such as medicines, pesticides, solvents, and cleaning agents. An additional 400 deaths result from inhaling poisonous gases, especially carbon monoxide from automobile exhausts or furnaces.

Young children, who tend to "get into everything" and are unable to distinguish between food and nonfood products, are especially vulnerable to poisoning. Preventing accidental poisoning is, however, the easiest and least expensive of home safety measures.

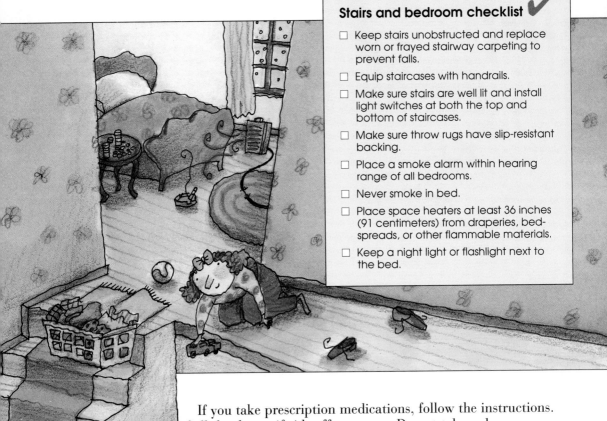

Stairs and bedroom checklist ✔

☐ Keep stairs unobstructed and replace worn or frayed stairway carpeting to prevent falls.

☐ Equip staircases with handrails.

☐ Make sure stairs are well lit and install light switches at both the top and bottom of staircases.

☐ Make sure throw rugs have slip-resistant backing.

☐ Place a smoke alarm within hearing range of all bedrooms.

☐ Never smoke in bed.

☐ Place space heaters at least 36 inches (91 centimeters) from draperies, bedspreads, or other flammable materials.

☐ Keep a night light or flashlight next to the bed.

If you take prescription medications, follow the instructions. Call the doctor if side effects occur. Do not take a drug prescribed for another person or a medicine that has expired. If you awaken during the night to take medicine, check to be sure that you have the right bottle. Store medicines, pesticides, solvents and other potentially toxic materials away from children, either locked in a cabinet or out of a child's reach. Keep these materials in their original container. If an accident does occur, you can then tell the doctor or poison control center the name of the product.

Iron tablets taken by pregnant women are the most common cause of fatal poisonings in young children and should be kept in a secure place. Children tend to imitate adults, so never drink medicine from the bottle and never tell a child that medicine is "candy."

Carbon monoxide is a colorless, tasteless, odorless gas that is extremely poisonous. It is produced when anything containing carbon—gasoline, for example—is burned without the presence of sufficient oxygen. For that reason, an automobile should never be allowed to idle in a closed garage, where carbon monoxide can accumulate. And remember that lawn mowers and garden tractors also are powered by gasoline engines and should not idle in closed areas. Furnaces that burn natural gas or oil produce carbon monoxide and should be inspected periodically for leaks.

Home fire prevention

Fires are the third leading cause of accidental death in the home. According to the National Fire Protection Association (NFPA), a nonprofit organization that works to improve fire safety, a fire strikes an American home every minute of every hour of every day. The average number of home fires per year is approximately 520,000, accounting for about 3,200 deaths and 21,500 serious injuries. About 8 out of every 10 deaths due to fire occur at home. The toll includes deaths from burns, asphyxiation or suffocation. Young children and older people are the most frequent victims of fire as they have most difficulty escaping.

Most home fires are caused by heating equipment that is improperly installed or maintained. NFPA recommends that space heaters should be placed at least 36 inches (91 centimeters) from walls, bedding, clothing, or anything else that is flammable. Check the wires of electric space heaters for deterioration, and replace frayed wires. At the start of each heating season, fireplace chimneys should be inspected for a build-up of creosote, a highly flammable, oily substance produced by tars during the burning of wood. Never burn flammable liquids, which may explode, in a fireplace. Wood or coal stoves and fireplace inserts should bear the label of a recognized testing labo-

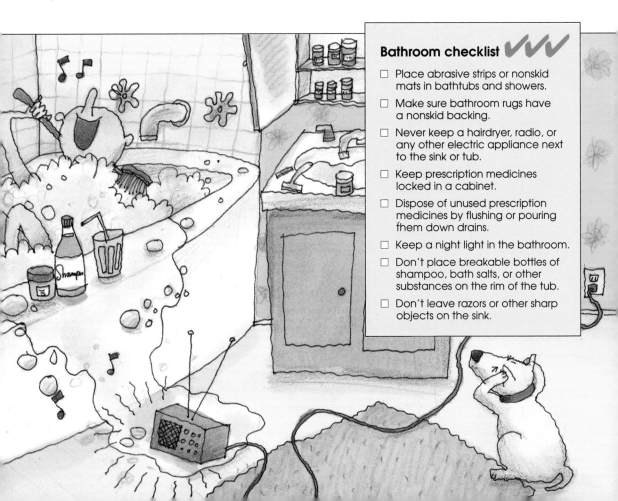

Bathroom checklist ✔✔✔

☐ Place abrasive strips or nonskid mats in bathtubs and showers.

☐ Make sure bathroom rugs have a nonskid backing.

☐ Never keep a hairdryer, radio, or any other electric appliance next to the sink or tub.

☐ Keep prescription medicines locked in a cabinet.

☐ Dispose of unused prescription medicines by flushing or pouring them down drains.

☐ Keep a night light in the bathroom.

☐ Don't place breakable bottles of shampoo, bath salts, or other substances on the rim of the tub.

☐ Don't leave razors or other sharp objects on the sink.

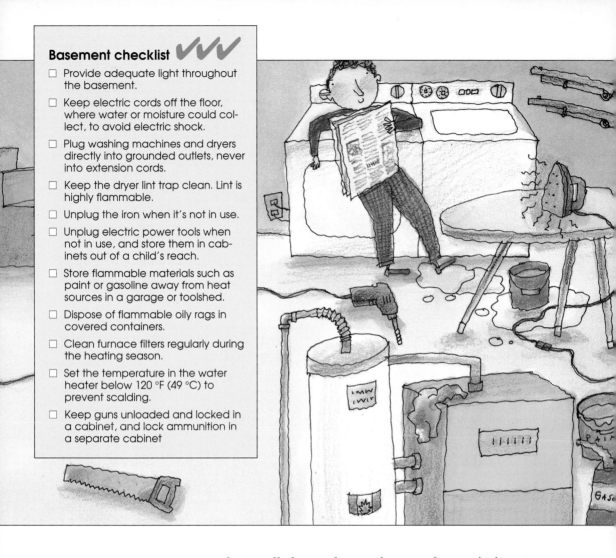

Basement checklist ✓✓✓

- ☐ Provide adequate light throughout the basement.
- ☐ Keep electric cords off the floor, where water or moisture could collect, to avoid electric shock.
- ☐ Plug washing machines and dryers directly into grounded outlets, never into extension cords.
- ☐ Keep the dryer lint trap clean. Lint is highly flammable.
- ☐ Unplug the iron when it's not in use.
- ☐ Unplug electric power tools when not in use, and store them in cabinets out of a child's reach.
- ☐ Store flammable materials such as paint or gasoline away from heat sources in a garage or toolshed.
- ☐ Dispose of flammable oily rags in covered containers.
- ☐ Clean furnace filters regularly during the heating season.
- ☐ Set the temperature in the water heater below 120 °F (49 °C) to prevent scalding.
- ☐ Keep guns unloaded and locked in a cabinet, and lock ammunition in a separate cabinet

ratory, be installed according to the manufacturer's directions, and meet all local fire codes.

Most deaths in home fires result from careless cigarette smoking. Do not smoke in bed or when drowsy. Make sure to extinguish matches and cigarette butts. Never rest a burning cigarette on the edge of a counter or table, where it could be forgotten and cause a fire. Do not flick cigarette butts into dry grass or leaves in the yard.

Most fires in the kitchen result from stoves and other cooking equipment. Always keep a fire extinguisher handy in the kitchen, and make sure that it is fully charged. (An unused fire extinguisher loses its charge over a four-year to six-year period.) Remember that throwing water on a grease fire can send the hot grease flying, possibly resulting in burns and spreading the fire beyond the confines of the pan. Instead, douse a grease fire with salt, baking soda, or a chemical fire extinguisher. Avoid cooking in garments with baggy sleeves, which can ignite or catch on the handles of hot pots and pans. Turn pot handles away from the front of the stove to prevent spills and burns.

The most important step in planning for home fire safety may be the simplest, and is certainly the least expensive: Develop a workable escape route and then test the route and teach it to your family with regular fire drills. After your family has learned the plan, continue drills twice yearly. Both the NSC and the National Fire Protection Association state that the first rule for avoiding death or injury in a fire is escape. Leave the building immediately. Call for help from a neighbor's phone. Do not go back inside.

Fire safety in the night

About one-third of fire deaths occur between midnight and 4 a.m., when the family is sound asleep. People tend to awaken to a fire disoriented by sleep, smoke, and poisonous gases, making it difficult to decide how to escape. The NFPA recommends locating two escape routes from each room, especially the bedrooms. Then if fire or smoke blocks the door, use the alternate exit, which is usually a window. Make sure that everyone is able to reach and operate locks on doors and windows. Check windows to be sure they open easily and are not painted shut. Families living in apartments should be familiar with fire exit locations. Never include an elevator in an escape plan. Not only may elevators fail during a fire, but elevator shafts draw hot air and smoke upward, much as chimneys do, making an elevator an extremely dangerous place in any fire.

Pay special attention to children in making a fire escape plan. Children may be terrified of fire fighters dressed in masks and other gear and may hide from them. Show young children pictures of fire fighters, and teach them to go to fire fighters for help. Children should know to "stop, drop, and roll" if their clothing catches fire. Instead of running, drop to the ground, cover your face with your hands, and roll to put out the fire.

Your escape plan should include an outdoor meeting spot, such as a neighbor's porch, where everyone in the family can check in. If someone is missing, tell fire fighters, but do not go back into a burning building.

Protecting bedrooms at night should be a top priority in your plan, since so many fire deaths occur from inhalation of poisonous gases when occupants are asleep. Smoke detectors can sense minute amounts of toxic gas before the odor is strong enough to awaken a person. The alarm can provide precious extra seconds to exit the house before being overcome by smoke.

NFPA recommends installing a smoke detector outside each sleeping area and on each level of your home, including the basement. If you sleep with the bedroom door closed, consider installing a smoke detector in the bedroom as well. Smoke detectors with a dead battery or no battery can do nothing to

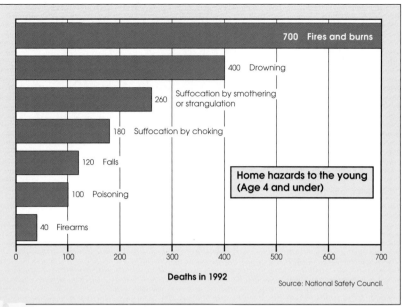

700 Fires and burns

400 Drowning

260 Suffocation by smothering or strangulation

180 Suffocation by choking

120 Falls

100 Poisoning

40 Firearms

Home hazards to the young (Age 4 and under)

0 100 200 300 400 500 600 700

Deaths in 1992

Source: National Safety Council.

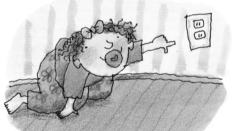

Childproofing your home

The first four years of life can be a dangerous period. It's best to begin childproofing your home before a child starts walking. Get down on your hands and knees and explore the world from your child's eye level, taking special note of what is in reach. Check stairs, kitchen, and bathrooms carefully. They are the areas of your house most dangerous to children. The greatest home hazards to the young are fires, drowning, and suffocation.

Child-safety checklist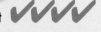

☐ Never leave any items that could cause choking, suffocation, or strangulation within a child's reach. Such items include balloons, buttons, coins, plastic bags, and small parts of toys.

☐ Never leave infants unattended on any surface above the floor.

☐ Make sure a baby's crib has slats no more than 2.75 inches (7 centimeters) apart, sides that extend at least 22 inches (56 centimeters) above the mattress, and a mattress that fits snugly.

☐ Keep cribs and chairs away from windows and install secure guards on all upper-floor windows.

☐ Strap a baby into a high chair or infant seat or onto a changing table.

☐ Install safety gates at the top and bottom of stairs.

☐ Pad sharp edges of furniture so that they cannot injure a child who runs into them.

☐ Put locks or childproof catches on cabinets or drawers where such items as cleaning supplies, medicines, alcohol, plastic wrap, matches, knives, and scissors are stored. Medicine bottles should have child-resistant caps.

☐ Keep cosmetics, shampoos, and soaps out of a child's reach.

☐ Repair peeling paint on window sills.

☐ Never leave a child unattended, even momentarily, in or near a bathtub, swimming pool, garden pool, or hot tub.

☐ Install antiscald devices on bathroom sinks and tubs, and test the water temperature before bathing a child.

☐ Cover electric outlets not in use with non-shock, childproof covers.

☐ Place light bulbs in all lamps and fixtures so that small fingers cannot touch sockets.

Sources: National Safety Council, *Parents* magazine.

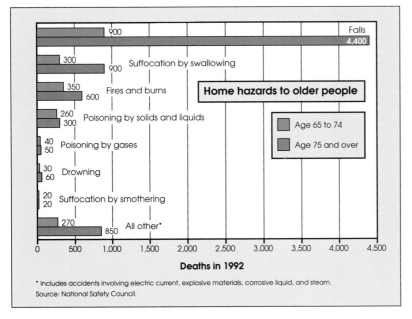

900		Falls
		4,400
300		Suffocation by swallowing
	900	
350		Fires and burns
	600	
260		Poisoning by solids and liquids
	300	
40		Poisoning by gases
50		
30		Drowning
60		
20		Suffocation by smothering
20		
270		All other*
	850	

Home hazards to older people

Age 65 to 74
Age 75 and over

0   500   1,000   1,500   2,000   2,500   3,000   3,500   4,000   4,500

Deaths in 1992

* Includes accidents involving electric current, explosive materials, corrosive liquid, and steam.
Source: National Safety Council.

Home, safe home, for the older person

The only group of Americans for whom home accidents are on the rise are those aged 65 and older. Failing eyesight and strength, along with slowed reflexes, put older people at risk of falls. And bones that have become brittle with age break easily from a fall. Moreover, some medications—or interactions among medications—can cause dizziness or disorientation, increasing the chances of a fall. Furthermore, as safety experts point out, an older person needs three times as much light as a younger person to see the same thing. All general safety measures apply to older people, but they have special safety requirements as well.

Safety checklist for older adults ✓✓✓✓

- ☐ Install handrails on all interior and exterior stairs.
- ☐ Do not place throw rugs at the top or bottom of stairs.
- ☐ Make sure all areas of the house, and particularly the stairs, are well lighted.
- ☐ Install handrails near bathtubs and toilets.
- ☐ Pad faucets in bathtubs.
- ☐ Install antiscald devices on tubs and sinks.
- ☐ Make sure that bathroom rugs have nonskid backing and that bathtubs have nonskid mats or abrasive strips.
- ☐ If there are no young children in your household, ask your pharmacist to equip medicine containers with regular caps, which are easier to open than child-resistant caps.
- ☐ Always store medicines in their original, clearly labeled containers.

Sources: National Safety Council, American Academy of Orthopedic Surgeons.

guard your family and, if they provide a false sense of security, may be worse than no detector at all. NFPA recommends testing each smoke detector once a month. Batteries should be replaced at least once a year or whenever the detector chirps. Many people change the batteries in the autumn, when setting clocks back to standard time.

Electrical system maintenance

Electricity is an important cause of both home fires and electrocution. Ideally, the electrical system in your home should comply with the current National Electrical Code, which sets standards for safe wiring. New electrical work should be done by a licensed electrician, comply with the current code, and be inspected by local building code officials. If your house has a fuse box, use only the correct size fuses. If a fuse blows out repeatedly, do not replace it with a larger fuse. Call an electrician to fix the problem. Never plug more than one large appliance into an electrical outlet. Some appliances, such as space heaters, may need their own circuit.

To avoid electrocution, do not touch electric devices when your hands are wet or when standing in water. If you feel a tingle when touching an electric device, unplug it immediately and have it repaired. The tingle means that current is leaking. Consider having ground-fault circuit interrupters (GFCIs) installed in kitchens and bathrooms. GFCIs can sense leakage of current from appliances or other equipment and instantly shut off the flow, preventing a serious shock.

Firearms in the home

Firearms are responsible for some of the most tragic home accidents, and about half of all fatal accidents involving firearms occur in or around the home. The NSC reports that approximately 700 people die in home firearms accidents annually, and for every death, there are at least 5 nonfatal injuries.

Handguns cause most firearm injuries and deaths, and children are frequent victims. Half of all children under age 16 who are injured in a handgun accident are shot in their own home. Research challenges the notion that a handgun increases personal safety. A handgun in the home triples the chances that someone will be killed there, according to an October 1993 report in *The New England Journal of Medicine*.

If you do keep a firearm, store it unloaded in a locked cabinet and keep ammunition in a separate, locked place. Always assume the gun is loaded, and never point it at anyone. If your child has toy guns, make sure they are brightly colored and look like toys. Caution a child never to point a toy gun at a stranger who, mistaking it for a real gun, may shoot in response.

Responding to a home accident

Despite all efforts at prevention, home accidents will occur, and you should be prepared to deal with them. Buy a first-aid guide, ask family members to read it, and keep it handy for quick reference. But in real emergencies, do not waste precious time. If someone is bleeding heavily, badly burned, unconscious, or suffering from other serious injuries, call for emergency help. Keep a list of emergency numbers near the kitchen phone. It should begin with the universal emergency number, 911. Children should be taught how to use the number. Some families tape a note on every phone: "For help call 911." The list also should include numbers for the police, fire department, ambulance, poison control center or hot line, pediatrician, family physician, dentist, and a reliable neighbor or friend.

One family member should know how to perform two basic first-aid procedures: cardiopulmonary resuscitation (CPR) and the Heimlich maneuver. CPR can restore breathing and heartbeat in victims of suffocation, electric shock, and such medical emergencies as heart attacks. The Heimlich maneuver can save people whose air passages are blocked by food or other objects. Local chapters of the American Red Cross, the American Heart Association, and other groups offer CPR courses.

Your home can be as safe, or as dangerous, as you choose. Prevention does work, as this century's steady decline in the number of accidental deaths proves. In 1912, when there were 21 million homes in the United States, 26,000 to 28,000 people died in home accidents. In 1992, with 94 million homes in the country, there were only 19,500 fatal home accidents. The success of home accident prevention is remarkable, but much greater progress could be made if we all were aware of the accidents waiting to happen in our own home.

For additional information

Pamphlets and fact sheets on home safety and forms for conducting home safety checkups are available from the following organizations:

National Safety Council, 1121 Spring Lake Drive, Itasca, IL 60143-3201. Toll-free telephone number: 1-800-621-7619

U. S. Consumer Product Safety Commission, Office of Information and Public Affairs, Washington, DC 20207. Toll-free telephone number: 1-800-638-2772

National Fire Protection Association, 1 Batterymarch Park, Quincy, MA 02269-9101.

American Association of Retired Persons, Consumer Affairs Section, 601 E Street, NW, Washington, DC 20049.

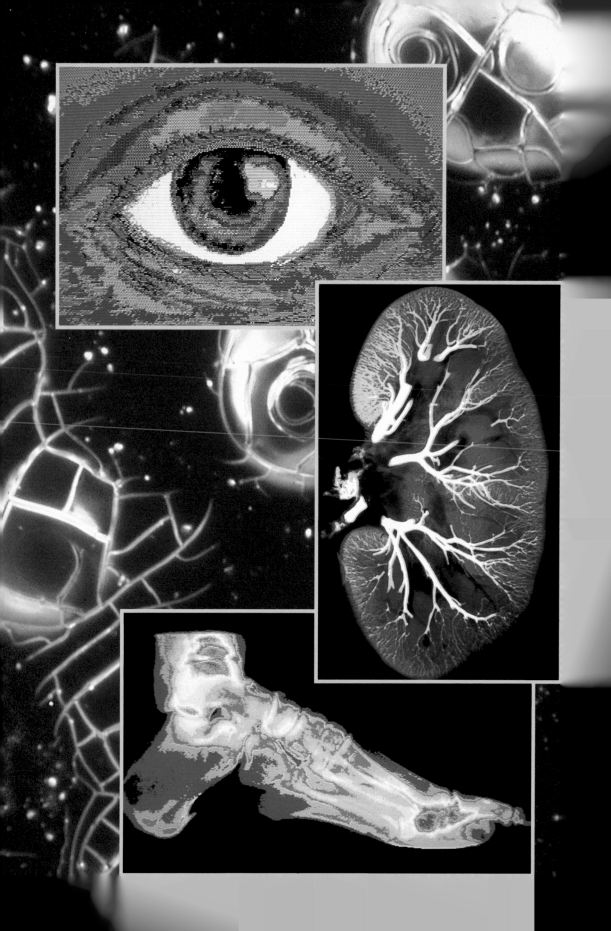

If not carefully treated, Type II diabetes can cause devastating complications. The key to preventing these complications is the close control of blood sugar levels.

Understanding Type II Diabetes

By Mark Stolar, M.D.

Ben, a 49-year-old architect, sat worriedly in the eye doctor's examining chair. Ben had never had problems with his vision. But lately, as he poured over plans and drawings, the pages seemed to blur and swim before his eyes. Ben had assumed that his deteriorating eyesight was simply an early sign of aging. But after examining Ben's eyes, his ophthalmologist had other ideas.

To Ben's surprise, she began questioning him about other symptoms. Had Ben lost weight recently, the doctor wanted to know. Yes, Ben said, he had lost some weight, even though he seemed to be eating as much as before. Did he often feel thirsty? Yes, Ben felt he needed to drink constantly. Did he need to urinate more often than he used to? To this question, too, the answer was yes.

The ophthalmologist didn't need to hear any more. She told Ben that he was probably experiencing symptoms of diabetes mellitus (commonly shortened to diabetes), a disease in which the body is unable to use sugar normally. She urged Ben to see his family physician, who would confirm the diagnosis by testing the level of sugar in Ben's bloodstream. As for his vision, the ophthalmologist said, Ben was probably suffering from a symp-

Opposite page: Type II diabetes occurs when the body cannot properly use the hormone insulin, shown greatly magnified on the right.

161

The author:

Mark Stolar is associate professor of clinical medicine at Northwestern University Medical School in Chicago.

tom of diabetes marked by changes in the lens of the eye. Fortunately for Ben, his diabetes had been diagnosed early enough that treating the disease would reverse the deterioration in his sight.

Ben is one of an estimated 13 million people in the United States who have *Type II diabetes*, the most common form of diabetes mellitus. Diabetes is one of the nation's leading causes of death, claiming more than 160,000 lives annually, according to the American Diabetes Association (ADA) in Alexandria, Va. Most of these deaths result from complications of the disease.

Diabetes patients are 2 to 4 times more likely to develop heart disease and 5 times more likely to have a stroke than members of the general population, according to the ADA. Diabetics also are nearly 20 times more likely than nondiabetics to develop kidney failure. And ADA statistics show that diabetes is the leading cause of blindness in adults aged 25 to 75 and the second leading cause of amputations, following injuries.

Doctors have no cure for diabetes, so once the disease develops, it lasts a lifetime. But the disabling and life-threatening complications of diabetes are by no means inevitable. With careful monitoring, it's possible to control the disease and prevent many problems associated with it. Moreover, by taking certain precautions, some people who might otherwise develop Type II diabetes can keep the disorder at bay.

The roles glucose and insulin play

Diabetes is a disorder of *metabolism*—the system by which living organisms use food for energy and cell growth. During digestion, the body breaks down food into simple molecules that can be transported in the bloodstream to cells throughout the body. The cells use these nutrients to build new tissues and to produce and store energy. One of the most important nutrients is *glucose*, a type of sugar. The body obtains glucose directly from sweet foods, such as honey and fruits, or indirectly by breaking down other *carbohydrates* (starches and sugars) in food. Many body cells, including nerve cells and red blood cells, depend on glucose as their exclusive energy source.

But without some mechanism to regulate the level of glucose in the bloodstream, blood sugar could reach levels *toxic* (poisonous) to body tissues. The pancreas, an organ that lies behind the stomach, orchestrates the metabolism of glucose and other nutrients. After a meal, the amount of glucose in the bloodstream rises, stimulating the pancreas to release the glucose-lowering hormone insulin. Insulin lowers glucose levels in the blood by "unlocking" special molecules called receptors on the surface of cells. This unlocking action sets off a chemical signal that enables glucose to flow into the cells. Cells use some of the glucose immediately for energy. But most of the glucose gets stored by cells in the liver and muscles and released as the body needs it.

If the insulin system fails to work properly, cells are unable to use glucose for energy or to store it for later use. Instead, the glucose builds up in the blood and eventually passes out of the body in the urine. Physicians in ancient Greece and Rome diagnosed diabetes by the sweet taste of a patient's urine. In fact, the name *diabetes mellitus* is a Latin term meaning *the spilling of something sweet.*

Types of diabetes

Diabetes is classified into two main types, which differ in how much insulin the pancreas produces and how well the body can use insulin. In Type I diabetes, the pancreas is unable to manufacture any insulin at all. Doctors refer to this form of diabetes as insulin-dependent diabetes because people with the disorder need daily doses of insulin to stay alive. The disorder is also called juvenile-onset diabetes because it typically strikes during childhood.

Type II diabetes, also called non-insulin-dependent diabetes or adult-onset diabetes, usually begins after the age of 40 and most often develops after age 55. In this form of diabetes, the pancreas usually produces insulin, but the body's cells fail to use the insulin properly. Only about a third of the people with Type II diabetes require insulin injections.

Type I diabetes is the more serious form of diabetes because of the total absence of insulin in the body. It affects 1 million to 2 million Americans. Type II diabetes, the far more common form of the disease, affects at least 90 percent of diabetes patients in the United States.

Type II diabetes develops over many years. For 10 years or more, the only symptom of the disease may be an elevated level of blood sugar, detectable only through a laboratory test. For this reason, as many as half of all Americans who have Type II diabetes are not aware of it. Experts base this estimate on two surveys conducted by the National Center for Health Statistics in the 1970's and 1980's.

Early warning signs

Although recognizing diabetes in its early stages is difficult, a number of signs can alert a person to a predisposition toward the disease. Type II diabetes tends to run in families, and studies find that one-third of patients with the disorder have a relative with the disease. And although Type II diabetes can occur in men and women of all backgrounds, it strikes at higher rates among people of African-American, Hispanic-American, or American Indian ancestry.

A disease with two faces

Doctors distinguish between two main forms of diabetes: Type I (also called insulin-dependent) and Type II (non-insulin-dependent) diabetes. Both forms involve an abnormality in the way the body uses *glucose* (a type of sugar found in food). All body cells need glucose to grow and to produce and store energy.

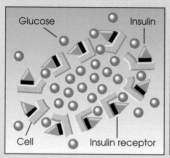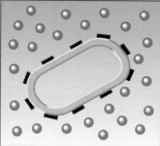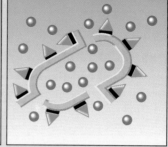

Glucose levels in the blood rise after a meal. Normally, the rising glucose levels trigger the body's production of the hormone insulin. Insulin fits into specialized molecules called insulin receptors on the surface of cells, much as a key fits into a lock. The insulin effectively unlocks a door to the cell, enabling glucose to flood into the cell.

In Type I diabetes, the body is unable to produce any insulin at all. As a result, the doors to the cell stay locked, and glucose builds up in the bloodstream.

In Type II diabetes, the body produces insulin, but the mechanism by which insulin unlocks the doors to the cell fails to work properly. Some glucose enters cells, but most of it accumulates in the blood.

For women, a mild form of diabetes that sometimes develops during pregnancy indicates an inherited tendency toward diabetes. Although blood sugar levels usually return to normal following childbirth, about 70 percent of the women who experience diabetes induced by pregnancy develop Type II diabetes later in life.

Physicians agree that factors other than heredity contribute to the onset of the disease. For instance, experts estimate that a large majority—perhaps 80 percent—of people with Type II diabetes have sedentary lifestyles, and an equal number are obese. Doctors define obesity as a body weight at least 20 percent higher than an individual's ideal body weight. Exactly why obesity increases the risk of diabetes is unclear, though researchers do know that obesity reduces insulin's effectiveness.

Symptoms of Type II diabetes become noticeable some 10 to 15 years after blood sugar levels start to rise. The most common symptoms, frequent urination and excessive thirst, develop as excess glucose draws large amounts of water into the urine. People with diabetes often experience increased hunger, weak-

Differences between Type I and Type II diabetes

Type I and Type II diabetes have similar effects on the body. But the two forms differ in their development, treatment, and cause. About 90 percent of diabetes patients in the United States have Type II diabetes.

- Type I diabetes normally strikes during childhood and generally comes on suddenly. In some cases, the patient experiences nausea, vomiting, and rapid breathing at the onset of the disease. Without immediate medical help, the patient can fall into a *coma* (state of unconsciousness), which can lead to death.

- People with Type I diabetes need daily doses of insulin supplements to survive. A low-calorie diet and exercise are also important parts of any treatment plan.

- Experts believe that Type I diabetes occurs when the body's disease-fighting immune system mistakenly attacks and destroys insulin-producing cells in the pancreas, an organ in the upper abdomen.

- Type II diabetes tends to strike adults over the age of 40. The disorder develops gradually, and noticeable symptoms may not appear for 10 to 15 years.

- Type II diabetes can usually be treated by a combination of diet, exercise, and medication that regulates blood sugar levels. Some people with the disorder require insulin injections.

- Researchers do not know what causes Type II diabetes, though about one-third of Type II diabetes patients have a relative with the disease.

ness, and sudden weight loss because the body is unable to use the calories found in glucose and because it loses large amounts of glucose in the urine. Vision may become blurred as glucose enters the lens of the eye, causing the lens to swell. Other early signs of diabetes can include tingling or pain in the legs and feet; frequent infections, especially of the gums, skin, or urinary tract; the slow healing of injuries; and dry, itchy skin. For the most part, these early signs of diabetes disappear once the patient begins to treat and control the disease.

Heading off complications

Because diabetes can go unnoticed for so long, many people fail to seek treatment soon enough to prevent complications. The earlier diabetes is detected, the easier it is to prevent, delay, or—in some cases—reverse damage caused by the disease.

To prevent the complications of diabetes, the ADA recommends that anyone over 30 who is substantially overweight or who falls into another risk group for Type II diabetes be screened at least once every three years. The main tool for diagnosing diabetes is the fasting blood sugar test. In this test, usually performed before breakfast, the patient fasts for several hours. A laboratory technician then takes a blood sample and measures the number of milligrams of glucose per deciliter (tenth of a liter) of blood (mg/dL). In a nondiabetic person, fasting blood sugar levels normally range from 70 to 110 mg/dL. Doctors diagnose diabetes if fasting blood sugar measures more than 140 mg/dL. (The typical symptoms of Type II diabetes, such as thirst and frequent urination, usually do not appear until the fasting blood sugar level exceeds 200 mg/dL.)

Doctors refer to people whose fasting blood sugar is higher than normal but lower than 140 mg/dL as having *impaired glucose tolerance* (IGT). About 30 percent of people with IGT go on to develop diabetes. Physicians recommend that people with IGT have a blood test for diabetes at least once a year.

Doctors classify the complications of diabetes according to whether the problems primarily involve small blood vessels or larger arteries. Damage to small blood vessels can affect the eyes, kidneys, nerves, and other organs. Damage to the larger arteries leads to *cardiovascular* (heart and blood vessel) disease.

About 70 percent of Type II diabetes patients develop diabetic retinopathy (*REHT uh NAHP uh thee*), an eye disease that can affect vision. Diabetic retinopathy develops when tiny blood vessels of the *retina*—the layer of light-sensitive cells at the back of the eye—leak fluid onto the retina. For most patients, vision blurs but sight is not seriously impaired. About 20 per-

Obesity reduces insulin's effectiveness on cells, raising blood sugar levels. Experts estimate that 80 percent of Type II diabetes patients are obese.

Type II diabetes: Are you at risk?

Because Type II diabetes develops gradually, it's possible to have the disease and not know it. People at risk of developing the disorder can discuss with a physician the need to have their blood sugar tested regularly. You may be at risk for Type II diabetes if you:

- Have a parent or other close relative who has had the disease.
- Are overweight.
- Are of African-American, Hispanic-American, or Native American ancestry.
- Have developed a mild form of diabetes during pregnancy.
- Are over age 40.

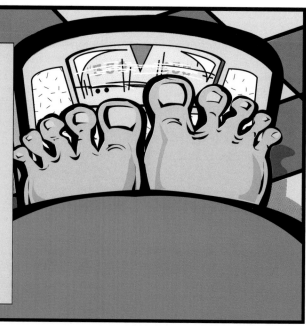

cent of retinopathy patients, however, lose some or all of their vision when repeated bleeding or scarring damage the retina.

Nearly all diabetic patients experience some decline in kidney function when high blood sugar levels cause tiny blood vessels in the kidney to swell and leak. The scarring that results can reduce the kidney's ability to filter wastes from the bloodstream. In about 15 percent of Type II diabetes patients, both kidneys gradually stop working.

Diabetic nerve damage

Another common complication of Type II diabetes is diabetic nerve damage, or *neuropathy* (*nu RAHP uh thee*). Studies show that 40 percent of patients experience some nerve damage within 25 years of being diagnosed with diabetes.

How diabetes affects nerves is not well understood, but it appears that, in many cases, high blood sugar levels damage the protective membranes that surround nerve cells. The damage most often interrupts the nerve signals that transmit sensation, causing pain or tingling, especially in the feet and legs. Eventually, nerve cells may die, causing a loss of sensation in the affected areas.

Severe cases of neuropathy involve the *autonomic nervous system*, the part of the nervous system that regulates automatic body processes such as bladder control and digestion. Damage to the nerves of the bladder can make urination difficult or reduce bladder control. Damage to the nerves of the digestive system can cause persistent diarrhea or stomach problems. Neuropathy can also affect the nerves that control sexual response, leading to a loss of sexual sensation and, in men, to impotence.

A third form of diabetic neuropathy affects a single nerve, most often in the thighs, torso, or face. Unlike the other types of neuropathy, this form usually strikes suddenly and can cause severe pain. But despite its dramatic onset, the condition usually clears up by itself within 6 to 12 months.

Consequences for the heart

People with Type II diabetes have a high risk of cardiovascular disease. In a common form of cardiovascular disease known as atherosclerosis, deposits of fat and cholesterol accumulate on the walls of arteries and clog them. When a clogged artery cuts off the flow of oxygen-rich blood to the heart, brain, or legs, the result can be a heart attack, a stroke, or *gangrene* (tissue death) in the legs or feet.

A number of factors place diabetes patients at risk for cardiovascular disease. Insulin helps cells use fat as well as glucose, and when insulin production goes awry, fats build up in the arteries. And insulin too may contribute to atherosclerosis. In

Warning signs of Type II diabetes

A number of signs can indicate the presence of Type II diabetes. Any of these symptoms should prompt a person to see a doctor.

- Frequent urination.
- Excessive thirst.
- Sudden weight loss.
- Increased hunger.
- Weakness or fatigue.
- Blurred vision.
- Tingling, pain, or numbness, especially in the legs or feet.
- Frequent infections, for example of the skin, gums, or bladder.
- Wounds or injuries that heal slowly.
- Dry, itchy skin.

1992, researchers found that when insulin accumulates in the blood, it can intensify the damaging effects of high blood sugar on arteries. Insulin can accumulate in the blood when the pancreas responds to a build-up of blood sugar by increasing its production of insulin. Smoking puts people with diabetes at even greater risk of cardiovascular disease.

The risk of infection

Perhaps the greatest day-to-day health risk for people with diabetes is infection. Damage to blood vessels slows circulation, preventing sufficient white blood cells—major players in the body's disease-fighting immune system—from reaching the infected area. High blood sugar levels also hinder the ability of white blood cells to kill invading bacteria and other microbes. And reduced blood flow hinders vital oxygen from reaching infected tissues, thereby slowing tissue healing and regrowth.

Diabetes-induced damage to nerves also increases the risk of infection in some tissues. For instance, nerve damage to the urinary tract may make a person less able to empty the bladder completely. As a result, bacteria may thrive in the bladder and other organs of the urinary tract, causing persistent infection.

Nerve damage in the legs and feet can dull sensitivity, making sores, cuts, or blisters less noticeable. Consequently, diabetes patients are at high risk for infection in their legs and feet. Such infections are particularly dangerous, because they can easily develop into gangrene. To counter the risk of infection, people with diabetes should inspect their feet daily for sores or cuts and choose comfortable shoes that fit well. They should consult their physician immediately if an area does not heal right away.

Lessening the complications

Because diabetes is a lifelong illness, treating the disease and minimizing complications require a partnership between the physician and the patient. Once the doctor has examined the patient and checked for any complications, the two set up a long-term treatment plan designed to keep the patient's blood sugar as normal as possible. This plan usually entails a combination of diet, weight control, exercise, and, for some patients, medication.

A well-planned diet is the cornerstone of diabetes care. Such a diet can help maintain normal blood sugar levels by controlling the amount of glucose and calories the patient obtains from food. A healthful diet also can help patients lose weight or keep their weight at a desirable level. And by restricting fat and cholesterol intake, it can reduce the risk of cardiovascular disease.

Experts debate the ideal diet for diabetes patients. But in guidelines issued in 1994, the ADA suggests that diabetics

Complications of Type II diabetes

If Type II diabetes is not carefully treated, the high blood sugar levels associated with the disease can damage blood vessels and other body tissues, causing a variety of complications. These complications can also occur with Type I diabetes.

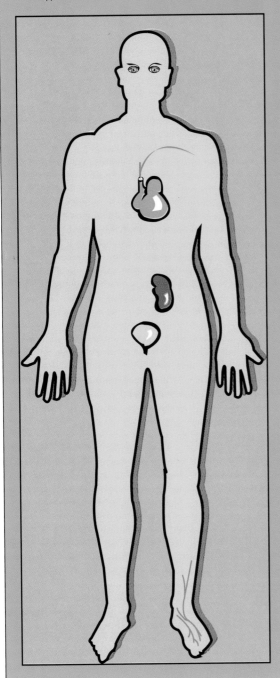

Eyes

High blood sugar can cause blood vessels of the *retina*—the layer of cells at the back of the eye—to swell and leak fluid, thereby blurring vision. In severe cases, the damage can progress to bleeding and scarring and can result in permanent blindness.

Heart and blood vessels

Diabetes can contribute to the clogging of arteries, cutting off blood flow to such organs as the heart and brain. The result can be a heart attack or stroke. Clogged arteries also increase the risk of *gangrene* (tissue death) in the feet and legs, a condition that can require amputation.

Kidneys

Elevated blood sugar can cause blood vessels of the kidney to swell and leak, reducing kidney function. In some cases, one or both kidneys may fail altogether. Diabetes also increases the susceptibility of the kidneys to infection.

Urinary and reproductive organs

Damage to nerves and blood vessels can increase the risk of infection in the bladder and other organs of the urinary tract. Women may suffer persistent vaginal infections.

Nerves

High blood sugar can damage nerve cells, causing pain, tingling, or loss of sensation. Severe nerve damage may affect such body processes as bladder control, digestion, and sexual sensation.

Legs and feet

Nerve damage in the legs and feet can dull sensitivity, making diabetes patients less likely to notice sores or cuts that may become infected. Failing to treat infections in these areas can lead to gangrene and amputation.

Treating Type II diabetes

There is no cure for diabetes. But by monitoring and regulating their blood sugar levels, Type II diabetes patients can treat the disease and reduce the likelihood—or the severity—of complications.

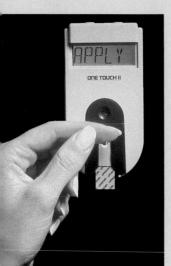

Monitoring blood sugar
Most diabetes patients need to monitor their blood sugar levels daily. To do so, the patient places a drop of blood on a strip of paper coated with a glucose-sensitive chemical, *above*. The strip changes color based on the amount of glucose in the blood. The patient then compares the color on the strip to a color chart or inserts the strip into a meter that calculates and displays the glucose level.

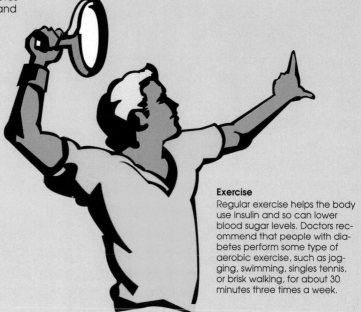

Exercise
Regular exercise helps the body use insulin and so can lower blood sugar levels. Doctors recommend that people with diabetes perform some type of aerobic exercise, such as jogging, swimming, singles tennis, or brisk walking, for about 30 minutes three times a week.

should get 10 to 20 percent of their daily calories from protein and the remaining calories from a combination of carbohydrates and fats, depending on the person's weight and other health concerns. For a patient who is not overweight, for example, up to 30 percent of calories might come from fats, whereas an overweight person—especially one with high levels of cholesterol and other fatty acids in the blood—should limit fat intake to 20 or 25 percent of calories.

The ADA also recommends that diabetes patients consume most of their fats in the form of *monounsaturated fats*, a type of fat found in such foods as olive oil, canola oil, avocados, and many nuts. In a study published in May 1994, researchers at the University of Texas Southwestern Medical Center in Dallas found that patients who ate a diet high in monounsaturated fats had lower blood levels of dangerous fats, including LDL cholesterol—the so-called bad cholesterol that increases the risk of heart disease.

Along with a well-planned diet, regular exercise helps many patients control diabetes. Exercise burns calories, making weight control easier, and it can lower fat and cholesterol levels in the blood. More important, exercise improves the effectiveness of insulin, and researchers have found that regular exercise can help lower blood sugar levels even if the exerciser does not lose weight.

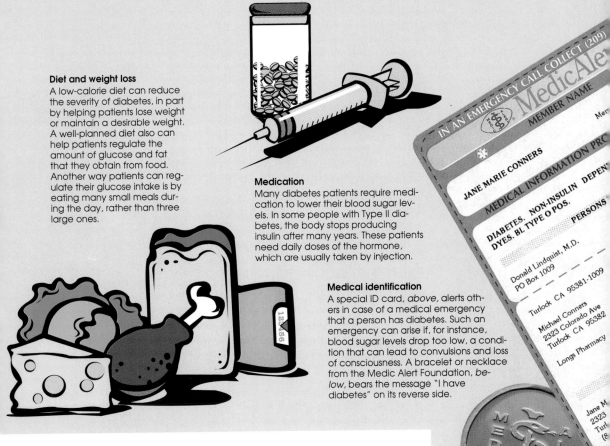

Diet and weight loss
A low-calorie diet can reduce the severity of diabetes, in part by helping patients lose weight or maintain a desirable weight. A well-planned diet also can help patients regulate the amount of glucose and fat that they obtain from food. Another way patients can regulate their glucose intake is by eating many small meals during the day, rather than three large ones.

Medication
Many diabetes patients require medication to lower their blood sugar levels. In some people with Type II diabetes, the body stops producing insulin after many years. These patients need daily doses of the hormone, which are usually taken by injection.

Medical identification
A special ID card, *above*, alerts others in case of a medical emergency that a person has diabetes. Such an emergency can arise if, for instance, blood sugar levels drop too low, a condition that can lead to convulsions and loss of consciousness. A bracelet or necklace from the Medic Alert Foundation, *below*, bears the message "I have diabetes" on its reverse side.

Medication can lower glucose levels when diet and exercise alone do not suffice. The drugs most commonly prescribed for Type II diabetes belong to a class called *sulfonylureas* (SUHL *fuh nuhl yuh REE uhs*), which facilitate the handling of insulin by the liver and muscles. These drugs also increase the amount of insulin the pancreas produces in response to meals.

Sulfonylureas effectively lower blood sugar levels for most patients. Over time, however, these drugs become less effective in stimulating the pancreas to produce insulin, and the patient needs to take larger and larger doses. Within 20 years after the patient starts using the medication, insulin production may stop altogether. In such cases, patients then require insulin injections. Doctors also may prescribe insulin injections for other patients whose pancreas does not produce enough insulin to control their diabetes.

Insulin treatment carries certain risks. Most seriously, taking too much insulin can trigger a dangerous drop in blood sugar levels, a condition doctors call *hypoglycemia*. Eating too little—especially before strenuous exercise—also can bring on hypoglycemia. A person suffering from hypoglycemia may feel weak, confused, and nauseous, and may perspire profusely. Taking some candy, juice, or other sugary food should make these symptoms disappear within 15 minutes. If not treated quickly, however, the nervous system's glucose starvation may

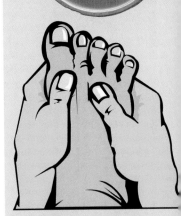

Foot care
Diabetes patients are at special risk of infection in the feet and legs. Inspecting the feet daily, bathing them in warm water, and wearing comfortable shoes can help prevent dangerous infections.

171

produce *convulsions* (muscle spasms) and loss of consciousness. A person suffering from severe hypoglycemia requires immediate medical attention.

Monitoring glucose levels

Whether people treat their diabetes through diet and exercise alone or in combination with medication, most diabetics need to monitor their blood sugar levels daily. They generally perform this task at home, using devices that measure glucose levels in a drop of blood.

Most people with diabetes check their glucose levels twice daily before meals, though doctors may ask certain patients to monitor their blood sugar more often. Unusually high or low blood sugar can harm a developing fetus, for example, so a pregnant woman may need to keep especially tight watch over her glucose levels. Patients taking insulin also may want to keep close control over their blood sugar. In 1993, a large government-sponsored study found that people with Type I diabetes who followed a regimen of "tight control" experienced reduced rates of eye, kidney, and nerve problems. The patients, all of whom required daily insulin injections, checked their blood sugar up to seven times daily and took insulin at least three times a day, adjusting the dosage as their glucose levels changed. Following a program of tight control requires close supervision by experts in diabetes treatment.

Reducing the risk of diabetes

While physicians help diabetes patients ward off the devastating complications of the disease, medical scientists are working to combat Type II diabetes on a variety of fronts. One important avenue of research involves ways in which individuals at risk for Type II diabetes can, by changing their behavior, reduce their likelihood of developing the disease. Studies suggest that regular exercise, for example, can slow or even prevent the development of Type II diabetes.

Studies are also reshaping doctors' attitudes toward diet and weight management as a way to reduce the risk of Type II diabetes. Traditionally, most doctors have counseled severely overweight diabetes patients to lose as much as 80 to 100 pounds (36 to 45 kilograms)—an extremely difficult task. Beginning in the late 1980's, researchers found that even slight weight loss can lower blood sugar levels, and the ADA's 1994 guidelines say that some patients may need to lose only 10 to 20 pounds (4.5 to 9 kilograms). Moreover, studies in the 1990's suggest that limiting calories even without weight loss may help diabetes patients control their blood sugar. Severely overweight patients who reduced their daily calorie intake to 800 calories for one week were able to stimulate insulin action and lower blood sugar levels in a 1993 study led by researchers at the University of Pittsburgh in Pennsylvania.

Possible causes

The search for a cause of Type II diabetes is another active area of investigation. Much research focuses on a protein called amylin, which the pancreas produces when it releases insulin. Studies in the late 1980's found that in people with Type II diabetes, the pancreas produces excess amylin, which accumulates in insulin-producing cells and destroys them. As a result, the pancreas eventually stops producing insulin. Scientists speculate that amylin also impairs insulin's ability to "unlock" body cells.

In April 1994, scientists at Children's Hospital in Boston announced they had discovered the mechanism by which excess amylin destroys cells in the pancreas. Meanwhile, drug treatments targeting amylin were in the works. In the early 1990's, British and American companies began conducting clinical trials on a number of drugs that prevent cells from taking up amylin.

Other scientists are searching for a genetic cause of Type II diabetes. Because the disease tends to run in families, scientists suspect that it involves defects in one or more *genes*—the components of cells that transmit hereditary information and act as the blueprints for all cell functions.

Genetics researchers are looking at stages in the glucose-delivery system that can go awry. Some patients, for instance, may have too few insulin receptors—docking sites on cell surfaces for insulin. In other cases, insulin may fail to unlock the receptors and allow glucose into cells. Or glucose may enter cells, but the cells are unable to use or store it. Researchers are investigating genes that may be involved at each of these steps.

Doctors and diabetes researchers also are working on strategies to detect diabetes in its early stages. Meanwhile, patients can take heart from the knowledge that it is possible to limit the damaging effects of Type II diabetes and to live a long and generally healthy life.

For more information:

American Diabetes Association
1660 Duke Street
Alexandria, VA 22314
(703) 549-1500 or (800) 232-3472

National Diabetes Information Clearinghouse
Box DNIC
9000 Rockville Pike
Bethesda, MD 20892
(301) 654-3327

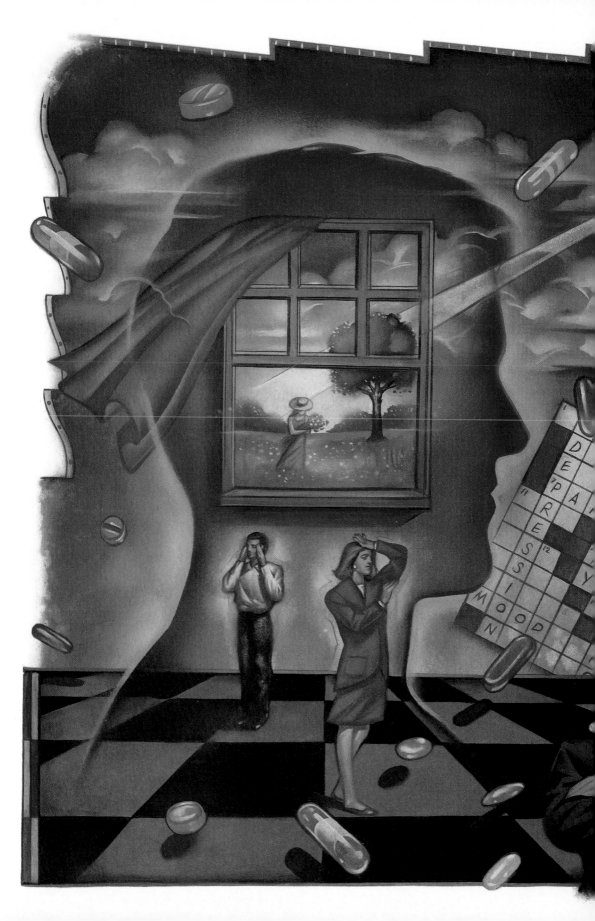

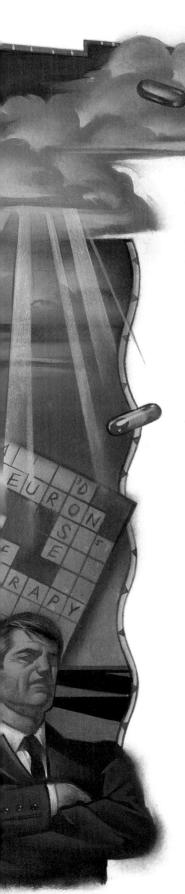

An arsenal of psychiatric drugs, which includes the widely prescribed antidepressant Prozac, can treat a range of mental disorders—disorders that affect millions of Americans.

Medicines For the Mind

By Bernard Salzman, M.D.

I met Jerry, a 45-year-old attorney, when a therapist at a local counseling center sent him to me for a psychiatric evaluation. Jerry had sought the therapist's help after he suddenly lost interest in life for no apparent reason. For nearly a month, Jerry could hardly get out of bed in the morning. He stopped enjoying his work, found it hard to think clearly, and was moody with his wife and children. At first, the therapist suspected Jerry might simply be under pressure at the office. But after two months of counseling, Jerry seemed to feel more helpless than before.

I diagnosed Jerry's problem as depression, a mental illness characterized by prolonged feelings of hopelessness or despair. I recommended that Jerry continue his treatment with the therapist, who might help him determine what had triggered his symptoms. I also prescribed for Jerry the antidepressant drug fluoxetine, better known by its trade name, Prozac.

Like many people who suffer from depression, Jerry at first resisted the idea of taking a drug to control his illness. Jerry confessed to feeling ashamed that he could not lift himself out of his low spirits. Taking medication, he felt, would be a daily reminder of his sense of failure. Jerry also worried that he would need to take the drug for the rest of his life.

The author:

Bernard Salzman is chief of the adult psychiatry unit at Bellevue Hospital Center in New York City.

Jerry seemed comforted by my assurance that only a small number of people taking antidepressant drugs must take them for more than a year. But it was only after four weeks, when his symptoms of depression were largely gone, that Jerry came to fully accept his need for the medication. The good news is that Jerry needed to take Prozac for only about six months. Today, one year later, Jerry remains free of any depressive symptoms.

Medication: Popular yet mistrusted

Jerry is one of 7 million Americans with depression who have been helped by Prozac since the drug's introduction in the United States in 1990. Partly because of its popularity, Prozac has received a great deal of publicity, though it is only one of an arsenal of drugs designed to treat a variety of mental illnesses.

Prozac's popularity notwithstanding, many people share a deeply felt mistrust of psychiatric medications. Some people worry that the drugs may change the way they feel about themselves, affecting them in ways they cannot control. Often, too, people with mental illnesses identify themselves with the disorder, saying, for example, "I am a depressed person" instead of, "I am suffering from depression." Such people may mistakenly regard a prescription for a psychiatric drug as a sign that they are to blame for their symptoms.

Experts agree, however, that people with mental illnesses are not responsible for their condition. Instead, most psychiatrists and other doctors believe that a majority of mental illnesses arise from a malfunction in the biochemistry of the brain. By correcting or compensating for that malfunction, psychiatric drugs can relieve the symptoms of the disorder without altering a patient's underlying sense of self. If used correctly and under a doctor's supervision, these drugs can restore a person's control over his or her thoughts and feelings—control that the illness had taken away.

When the blues darken into illness

All people go through times when they feel anxious, depressed, or in other ways emotionally out of whack. Usually, these feelings come in response to a particular event or situation and disappear once the situation is resolved.

Doctors distinguish between these normal episodes of psychological distress and more disturbing or persistent illnesses that can require psychiatric care. What brings on most mental illnesses is unclear, though doctors know that these disorders tend to run in families, suggesting that at least some cases are caused by one or more *genes* (components of cells that transmit inherited characteristics). Someone whose parent or grandparent has suffered from depression, for instance, has at least twice the risk

How psychiatric drugs work

Scientists believe that mental illnesses result from the abnormal operation of certain molecules that act as chemical messengers in the brain, carrying signals from one nerve cell to another. Psychiatric drugs appear to relieve the symptoms of mental illness by either increasing or decreasing the effectiveness of specific messengers, thus strengthening or weakening the signals.

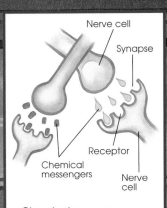

Chemical messengers carry signals between nerve cells across a gap called a synapse. Each of these chemicals binds to its own receptor, a specially configured molecule shaped to receive only one type of messenger. The messenger molecules fit into the receptors much as a key fits into a lock.

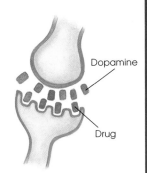

Some psychiatric drugs reduce the effectiveness of certain chemical messengers. For example, drugs designed to treat schizophrenia fit into receptors shaped to receive the brain chemical dopamine, thus reducing the amount of dopamine that binds to the receptors. Scientists believe that schizophrenia arises from either excess dopamine or overactive dopamine receptors.

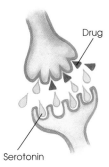

Some psychiatric drugs increase the effectiveness of chemical messengers. For instance, after a nerve cell releases the chemical messenger serotonin, the cell recaptures any serotonin remaining in the synapse. Some drugs used to treat depression block this recapture, thus increasing the amount of serotonin available to bind to receptors. Researchers believe that a shortage of serotonin may be a cause of depression.

of developing the illness as a member of the general population.

Psychiatrists classify psychiatric illnesses according to the way they affect people's emotions, thoughts, and behaviors. One group consists of the affective disorders, also called mood disorders because they involve substantial changes in mood. The most common mood disorder is depression, sometimes called clinical depression or major depression to distinguish it from ordinary sad or depressed moods.

People suffering from depression feel persistently low, unhappy, and hopeless without knowing why. They tend to feel tired all the time and to be irritable and indecisive. Often, they become flooded with feelings of worthlessness and guilt. Along with these emotional symptoms come physical changes, including an increased vulnerability to physical illness. Patients may sleep too little or too much and may lose or gain weight. Puzzlingly, depression strikes some susceptible people only once and in others recurs throughout the person's lifetime.

Bipolar disorder

Another mood disorder is bipolar disorder, also called manic depression. In bipolar disorder, patients swing between periods of depression and periods of mania, a condition marked by excessive energy, inappropriate elation, an exaggerated sense of one's abilities, irritability, and rapid speech. People in the grip of mania often act recklessly and impulsively, running up huge debts in buying sprees, for example. Once it sets in, bipolar disorder usually lasts a lifetime. Although mania most often occurs as a phase of bipolar disorder, about 10 percent of patients who experience mania have that illness alone.

Anxiety disorders

Another common group of mental illnesses are the anxiety disorders. As psychiatrists use the term, anxiety is extreme uneasiness or fear, sometimes without obvious cause, that disrupts the patient's normal life. People suffering from anxiety feel irritable and restless and have trouble concentrating. Their bodies reflect a state of anxiety with symptoms such as rapid heartbeat, excessive sweating, and tightness in the muscles. Anxiety, like depression, can strike only once or can recur throughout a lifetime, especially during periods of stress.

Severe anxiety disorders tend to last throughout life, waxing and waning over the years. In one such disorder, people experience sudden attacks of panic that can last for 10 minutes or more. Doctors sometimes refer to anxiety marked by repeated panic attacks as panic disorder.

Two other anxiety disorders are phobia and obsessive-compulsive disorder (OCD). A phobia is a persistent, excessive, and irrational fear, usually of a specific object or situation. Perhaps the most disabling phobia is agoraphobia, a fear of open spaces. In agoraphobia, every street corner or public building can seem filled with possible dangers, leading sufferers to virtually shut themselves in their homes. Another potentially serious phobia is claustrophobia, a fear of enclosed spaces such as tunnels and elevators. The most common phobia by far is the fear of flying.

In OCD, irrational thoughts and impulses intrude into a person's daily life, causing severe anxiety. Someone with OCD might spend hours each night checking and rechecking that the stove and lights are turned off, unable to banish the fear that a fire could start while the family is asleep.

The puzzle of schizophrenia

Of all the psychiatric disorders, perhaps the most devastating—and the most puzzling—is schizophrenia, another illness that usually lasts a lifetime. The main symptom of schizophrenia is repeated episodes of *psychosis* (loss of contact with reality). People with schizophrenia often hear or see imaginary voices or visions, and their thoughts and speech become disorganized and incoherent.

The cause of schizophrenia is poorly understood, though research suggests that environmental factors may help trigger the disease in genetically susceptible people. In a 1990 study of schizophrenia patients who had healthy identical twins, researchers used a scanning technique to produce images of the twins' brains. In most cases, the brains of the two siblings showed a slight difference in structure. But nobody knows with certainty whether the anatomical differences in some schizophrenics' brains are a cause or a result of the disorder.

A chance breakthrough

The modern era of psychiatric medicine began in 1950, when French biochemists developed a drug called chlorpromazine (trade name Thorazine) to reduce blood pressure and dry the mucous membranes in patients undergoing certain surgical procedures. Soon, surgeons noticed that patients who had received chlorpromazine were more tranquil following their operations than patients who had not been given the medication. That observation led to research showing that chlorpromazine could relieve symptoms of psychosis in patients with schizophrenia.

How psychiatric drugs work

Psychiatric drugs act on the vast network of nerve cells in the brain. In the early and mid-1900's, researchers discovered that these nerve cells communicate with one another through chemical messengers called neurotransmitters. After being released by a nerve cell, neurotransmitters fit into specially configured molecules known as receptors on the surface of

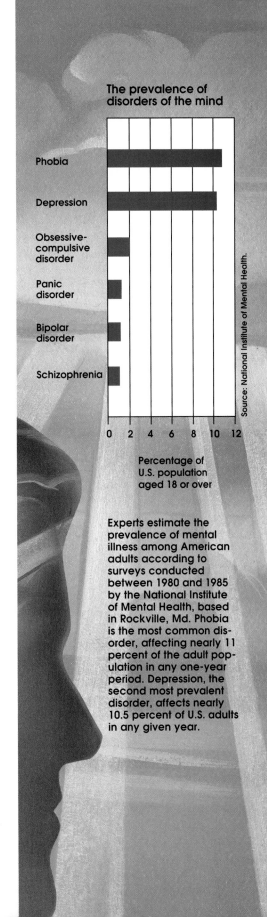

The prevalence of disorders of the mind

Phobia
Depression
Obsessive-compulsive disorder
Panic disorder
Bipolar disorder
Schizophrenia

0 2 4 6 8 10 12

Percentage of U.S. population aged 18 or over

Source: National Institute of Mental Health.

Experts estimate the prevalence of mental illness among American adults according to surveys conducted between 1980 and 1985 by the National Institute of Mental Health, based in Rockville, Md. Phobia is the most common disorder, affecting nearly 11 percent of the adult population in any one-year period. Depression, the second most prevalent disorder, affects nearly 10.5 percent of U.S. adults in any given year.

Frequently prescribed psychiatric drugs

Doctors classify psychiatric drugs according to the disorders the drugs are designed to treat and the way they work in the brain. The side effects of a medication may differ from person to person and may vary according to the dosage of the drug.

Antidepressant drugs

Antidepressant drugs are designed primarily to treat depression, though some of these drugs can also relieve the symptoms of certain other disorders. Doctors classify antidepressants into three families according to the way they work in the brain.

Tricyclics

Generic name	Trade name	Used to treat	Common side effects
Amitriptyline	Elavil, Endep, Etrafon, Limbitrol, Triavil	Depression, panic disorder, phobia. Clomipramine is also used to treat obsessive-compulsive disorder.	Drowsiness, dry mouth, sweating, constipation, blurred vision, low blood pressure, dizziness, weight gain
Clomipramine	Anafranil		
Desipramine	Norpramin		
Imipramine	Tofranil		
Nortriptyline	Aventyl, Pamelor		

Monoamine oxidase inhibitors

Generic name	Trade name	Used to treat	Common side effects
Isocarboxazid	Marplan	Depression, panic disorder, phobia.	Dizziness, drowsiness, decreased sexual function, dry mouth, rapid heartbeat, headache, trembling
Phenelzine	Nardil		
Tranylcypromine	Parnate		

Selective serotonin re-uptake inhibitors

Generic name	Trade name	Used to treat	Common side effects
Fluoxetine	Prozac	Depression, obsessive-compulsive disorder	Anxiety, headache, nausea, insomnia, dry mouth, diarrhea, decreased sexual function
Paroxetine	Paxil	Depression	Nausea, weakness, nervousness, drowsiness, sweating, decreased appetite, decreased sexual function
Sertraline	Zoloft	Depression	Nausea, diarrhea, drowsiness, sweating, dry mouth, decreased sexual function

Source: Bernard Salzman, M.D.

Mood-stabilizing drugs

Generic name	Trade name(s)	Used to treat	Common side effects
Carbamazepine	Atretol, Tegretol	Mania	Dizziness, drowsiness, clumsiness, nausea
Clonazepam	Klonopin	Anxiety, mania	Dizziness, drowsiness, clumsiness
Lithium	Cibalith-S, Eskalith, Lithobid, Lithonate	Bipolar disorder, mania	Tremors, weight gain, nausea, diarrhea, frequent urination, excessive thirst
Valproic acid	Depakene	Mania	Upset stomach, diarrhea, indigestion

Doctors typically prescribe mood-stabilizing drugs to treat mania, which generally occurs as a phase of bipolar disorder. One of these drugs, lithium, can also treat the depressive phase of this disorder.

Antianxiety drugs

Generic name	Trade name(s)	Used to treat	Common side effects
Alprazolam	Xanax	Anxiety, depression, panic disorder, phobia	Dizziness, drowsiness, clumsiness; can cause dependence. Buspirone has no significant side effects and does not cause dependence.
Buspirone	BuSpar	Anxiety	
Chlordiazepoxide	Librax, Librium	Anxiety	
Diazepam	Valium	Anxiety	
Lorazepam	Ativan	Anxiety	

Antianxiety drugs relieve the symptoms associated with prolonged or intense feelings of anxiety or stress. Some of these drugs can also be used to treat depression or specific anxiety disorders such as panic disorder.

Antipsychotic drugs

Generic name	Trade name	Used to treat	Common side effects
Chlorpromazine	Thorazine	Schizophrenia, mania	Drowsiness, low blood pressure, constipation, weight gain. All except clozapine may cause dry mouth, blurred vision, and difficulty urinating. Clozapine may cause dizziness, racing heartbeat, and watery mouth. Fluphenazine, haloperidol, and thiothixene are likely to cause tremors and other neuromuscular side effects.
Clozapine	Clozaril	Schizophrenia	
Fluphenazine	Prolixin	Schizophrenia	
Haloperidol	Haldol	Schizophrenia, mania	
Risperidone	Risperdol	Schizophrenia	
Thioridazine	Mellaril	Schizophrenia, anxiety	
Thiothixene	Navane	Schizophrenia	

Antipsychotic drugs are used mainly to treat the symptoms of psychosis (loss of contact with reality) associated with schizophrenia and, occasionally, disorders such as mania or anxiety.

neighboring nerve cells, much as a key fits into a lock. Each receptor is shaped to receive a particular type of neurotransmitter. Of the hundreds of neurotransmitters that scientists believe exist, researchers have identified at least half a dozen, each of which works on specific groups of nerve cells that regulate such activities as emotion, thinking, muscle movement, and physical sensation.

Psychiatric medications modify the activity of specific neurotransmitters, chief among them serotonin, norepinephrine, dopamine, and GABA (gamma-amino-butyric acid). These chemical messengers help regulate the limbic system, a group of brain structures that control the emotions.

Antidepressants, the largest and most diverse group of psychiatric drugs, increase the effectiveness of serotonin and, sometimes, norepinephrine. Serotonin seems to help inhibit impulsive thoughts and behaviors and to induce sleep. Norepinephrine, in contrast, causes excitement and alertness.

In depression, scientists believe, one or both of these neurotransmitters fail to lock onto receptors in sufficient numbers, and so the brain functions they control go awry. Antidepressants block the brain's mechanisms for removing certain neurotransmitters from the synapse—the gap between nerve cells—after they have been released by a cell. The brain normally clears the synapse to prevent too many neurotransmitters from binding to receptors and overstimulating them.

Antidepressants fall into three families, based on the way they keep the brain from clearing the synapse. One family, the monoamine oxidase (MAO) inhibitors, works by destroying MAO, a protein that breaks down excess serotonin and norepinephrine in the synapse. The other families block the brain's second clearing mechanism, in which releasing nerve cells recapture excess neurotransmitters from the synapse—a process known as re-uptake. Tricyclic antidepressants, sometimes called heterocyclic antidepressants, are shaped somewhat like serotonin and norepinephrine molecules and so fit into their re-uptake sites, blocking them. Selective serotonin re-uptake inhibitors (SSRI's) block the re-uptake only of serotonin.

Effects and side effects

Doctors estimate that at least 80 percent of people with depression can find relief from their symptoms through one or another of these antidepressant drugs. In addition, some antidepressants can relieve the symptoms of certain anxiety disorders as well as depression, suggesting that depression and anxiety may involve similar kinds of disorders in the brain. This agrees with studies showing that these disorders often run in the same families—a strong hint that the same defective genes may be involved in each illness.

MAO inhibitors were the first group of antidepressants to be developed. Today, doctors more often prescribe a tricyclic drug or, increasingly, Prozac—the best-known SSRI—as a first-choice therapy for depression. MAO inhibitors are reserved for patients who do not get better with one of the other drug families. In part, this is because people taking MAO inhibitors must avoid certain foods, including processed meats, certain alcoholic beverages, and most cheeses, which contain the protein-building chemical tyramine. Eating these foods while taking an MAO inhibitor can produce a dangerous build-up of norepinephrine, causing an abrupt rise in blood pressure and the possibility of a stroke.

Prozac and other SSRI's have the advantage of producing fewer side effects than other antidepressants. Psychiatric drugs can cause side effects because in modifying the actions of a neurotransmitter, they affect other targets besides those involved in emotional well-being. Also, many of these drugs act on neurotransmitters other than the ones involved in the particular mental illness. Tricyclic antidepressants, for instance, reduce levels of the neurotransmitter acetylcholine, which helps regulate body processes such as bowel function. As a result, the drugs tend to cause such side effects as constipation. Because SSRI's act only on serotonin, their side effects are usually limited.

Prozac has helped many people with depression who have failed to respond to any other antidepressant. The drug's success, along with its simplicity and ease of use—sometimes requiring only a single pill each morning—has led many people during the 1990's to believe that Prozac is a "miracle drug" that can make even healthy individuals feel happier and more alert.

Mood stabilizers

A second group of drugs are the mood stabilizers, which are used mainly to treat mania and bipolar disorder. The most important mood-stabilizing drug is lithium, in the form of lithium carbonate or lithium citrate—chemical compounds derived from the naturally occur-

Taking psychiatric drugs: Safety counts

Psychiatric medications are generally safe when taken under a doctor's supervision. But under certain conditions, taking a psychiatric drug can lead to severe complications. Observing some basic guidelines can help patients avoid these and other risks.

- Take the drug on a regular basis as prescribed by your doctor. Do not try to catch up on a missed dose by taking a double dose the next time. Doing so can dangerously raise the level of the medication in the blood.

- Tell your doctor of any illness or medical condition you may have. Some medications can cause life-threatening complications if taken by people with certain health conditions.

- Some drugs can be less effective or even dangerous when used in combination with certain other medications. Inform your doctor of any other drugs—including nonprescription products such as aspirin or vitamins—that you are taking.

- Some drugs can cause dangerous complications when combined with certain foods or with alcohol. Ask your doctor if there are any foods you should avoid while taking a drug.

- Like many medications, some psychiatric drugs can cause drowsiness, reduce mental alertness, or impair coordination. Patients taking such drugs should obtain their doctor's approval before driving or operating heavy machinery.

- If you stop taking a medication, slowly taper off the dosage according to your doctor's instructions. Discontinuing a medication abruptly can cause withdrawal symptoms, such as anxiety or sleeplessness, and can increase the likelihood that symptoms of the original illness will return.

- Tell your doctor of any side effects you experience, even mild ones.

Source: Bernard Salzman, M.D.

ring mineral lithium. Lithium is sold under a number of trade names, including Eskalith and Lithobid. Scientists do not know how lithium works, though one prominent theory is that the drug blocks a protein that helps regulate certain neurotransmitters, including serotonin and norepinephrine.

Lithium is effective in as many as 80 percent of patients who try it. But lithium takes several weeks to work, and so doctors often prescribe another drug along with lithium until the disorder is under control. Lithium also can cause some troublesome side effects, including trembling in the hands, weight gain, nausea, and frequent urination. And because lithium can affect the kidneys, some people with kidney disease are unable to take lithium.

Another problem with lithium is that when taken in large doses, the drug can build up in the blood and reach levels *toxic* (poisonous) to nerves and tissues. Without immediate medical help, the person may have seizures and eventually fall into a coma. To keep lithium at

Patients with special concerns

Certain patients have special needs when taking psychiatric medications. For example, the low body weight of children and the health problems of older adults may make them more sensitive to the effects of certain drugs. Women who are pregnant or nursing may be concerned about the possible effects of a medication on a fetus or newborn baby. Patients and their families can reduce the risk of problems by keeping these principles in mind:

Children

- Young children and adolescents may not talk readily about their feelings, making it difficult to determine whether a child's behavior is a sign of a psychiatric illness or simply the child's reaction to some event in his or her life. A qualified psychiatrist should examine the child before prescribing any medication.

- Young children may not volunteer information about any side effects they may be experiencing from a drug. Parents, teachers, and others who care for the child should watch the child carefully.

- Some medications are dangerous for children, and others can be dangerous above certain doses. Parents or other caregivers should never give a child any medication prescribed for an adult.

safe and effective levels, doctors usually perform blood tests several times a month at the start of lithium treatment and every one to three months thereafter.

For patients who cannot tolerate lithium's side effects or who do not respond to the drug, doctors can prescribe several other mood-stabilizing medications, most prominent among them carbamazepine (trade names Atretol, Tegretol). Carbamazepine works by heightening the sensitivity of receptors to the neurotransmitter GABA. Scientists believe that when GABA binds to nerve cells, it prevents those cells from releasing other neurotransmitters that would stimulate nerves in the limbic system. GABA also hinders stimulation of the nerves that control muscle movement, and carbamazepine was originally developed to prevent seizures in people with such diseases as epilepsy.

Carbamazepine and other antimanic medications relieve symptoms in about 80 percent of the people who try them. But because these drugs suppress stimulation of nerve cells, they almost always cause drowsiness. In addition, high doses of carbamazepine and some other mood stabilizers can damage certain body cells, including those of the blood and the liver. For this

Older adults

- Older people may have an underlying medical condition whose symptoms resemble those of a psychiatric illness, making diagnosis difficult. For example, many symptoms of Alzheimer's disease, such as confusion and apparent memory loss, resemble those of depression. A qualified physician should examine the patient thoroughly to rule out any underlying condition before a psychiatrist can diagnose a psychiatric disorder.

- The body of an older person may respond to a drug more rapidly or may eliminate it from the bloodstream more slowly than the body of a younger adult. Older people may therefore need a lower-than-average dosage of a drug.

- Older individuals may tend to forget that they have already taken their daily dose of a drug and so take too much of it. In addition, other medical problems in older people may mask the side effects of a psychiatric drug. The patient, family members, or friends should watch closely for any changes in the patient's health.

- Older people who take many medications may forget to inform their doctor about every drug they are taking, increasing the risk of harmful interactions between drugs. The patient or a family member should keep a list of all medications that are taken, including over-the-counter products.

Pregnant or nursing women

- Certain drugs carry a small risk of causing birth defects in a developing fetus, especially if taken during the first three months of pregnancy. Some of these drugs, moreover, can remain in the blood for up to two months after the patient stops taking them. A woman who is pregnant or plans to become pregnant should discuss these concerns with her doctor.

- Many medications can pass into a mother's breast milk and possibly affect the health of her child. A nursing mother should discuss the potential risks of any psychiatric drug with her doctor.

Source: Bernard Salzman, M.D.; National Institute of Mental Health.

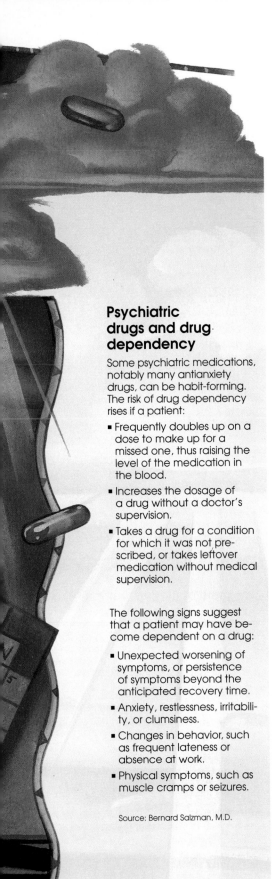

reason, patients taking these drugs, like those taking lithium, usually need periodic blood tests to monitor blood levels of the drug.

Medication for anxiety

Drug treatments for anxiety achieved a major breakthrough in the 1960's, with the development of antianxiety drugs called benzodiazepines. Like the nonlithium mood-stabilizing drugs, benzodiazepines appear to work by enhancing the sensitivity of GABA receptors.

The first benzodiazepines developed include diazepam (trade name Valium) and chlordiazepoxide (Librax, Librium). These drugs are called long-acting benzodiazepines because they can build up in the bloodstream and may have a prolonged effect. A second generation of benzodiazepines, including alprazolam (Xanax) and lorazepam (Ativan), are known as short-acting benzodiazepines because the body eliminates them from the bloodstream within hours.

Most benzodiazepines are designed mainly to treat mild to moderate anxiety, though some can also relieve symptoms of severe anxiety disorders such as panic disorder. Benzodiazepines act rapidly to relieve anxiety and nervous tension, sometimes within hours or even minutes. However, the drugs cause some drowsiness and other side effects in most patients. Short-acting benzodiazepines cause fewer side effects because they leave the body so quickly.

In addition, benzodiazepines can cause addiction if taken for more than a few weeks. The drug buspiron does not carry the risk of dependency. However, it takes two or three weeks for buspiron's effect to be felt.

Treating schizophrenia

An area of great optimism in psychiatry involves the treatment of schizophrenia. In the 1950's, when biochemists studied the effects of chlorpromazine, they discovered that the drug fits into receptors for the neurotransmitter dopamine, thus preventing dopamine from locking onto the receptors. Dopamine, which is

Psychiatric drugs and drug dependency

Some psychiatric medications, notably many antianxiety drugs, can be habit-forming. The risk of drug dependency rises if a patient:

- Frequently doubles up on a dose to make up for a missed one, thus raising the level of the medication in the blood.
- Increases the dosage of a drug without a doctor's supervision.
- Takes a drug for a condition for which it was not prescribed, or takes leftover medication without medical supervision.

The following signs suggest that a patient may have become dependent on a drug:

- Unexpected worsening of symptoms, or persistence of symptoms beyond the anticipated recovery time.
- Anxiety, restlessness, irritability, or clumsiness.
- Changes in behavior, such as frequent lateness or absence at work.
- Physical symptoms, such as muscle cramps or seizures.

Source: Bernard Salzman, M.D.

related to norepinephrine in chemical structure, appears in healthy people to play a role in stimulating the brain's reward or pleasure system. Today, most medications that treat psychosis, known as antipsychotics, work in the same way as chlorpromazine, suggesting that psychotic symptoms arise from either excess dopamine or overactive dopamine receptors.

Traditional antipsychotic drugs relieve symptoms in about 60 percent of patients. But the drugs produce numerous side effects, some of them serious. Dopamine helps regulate the nerves that control muscle movement, and so drugs that interfere with dopamine can cause neuromuscular symptoms such as tremors, muscle rigidity, and loss of facial expression. Many of these symptoms are characteristic of Parkinson's disorder, a disorder of the brain caused by a deficiency of dopamine.

Taking a drug designed to treat Parkinson's symptoms can relieve some neuromuscular side effects. But about 20 percent of patients taking antipsychotics develop a condition called tardive dyskinesia (TD), characterized by involuntary movements of the mouth, head, and body. Generally, TD disappears after patients stop taking the antipsychotic drug. Two newer antipsychotics, clozapine (trade name Clozaril) and risperidone (Risperdol), appear to be effective in many patients who do not respond to traditional antipsychotics. At the same time, these drugs produce fewer troublesome side effects.

Medication: Not for everyone

Not everyone who experiences symptoms of a mental illness needs to take medication. Some patients with anxiety or mild depression, for instance, can find relief through supportive talking therapy, in which a therapist helps the patient deal with events and relationships in the patient's life.

Even when doctors believe medication is needed to treat a disorder, they regard psychiatric drugs as more effective when used together with some other form of therapy. Over time, psychiatrists point out, living with a mental illness can change a person's behavior or thinking in potentially destructive ways. Once psychiatric drugs have relieved the symptoms of the underlying disorder, a supportive talking therapy can help the patient redirect his or her thinking in a healthy way.

For further reading:

Gorman, Jack M. *The Essential Guide to Psychiatric Drugs*. St. Martin's Press, 1990.

Salzman, Bernard. *The Handbook of Psychiatric Drugs*. Henry Holt and Company, 1991.

Yudofsky, Stuart C., and others. *What You Need to Know About Psychiatric Drugs*. Ballantine Books, 1991.

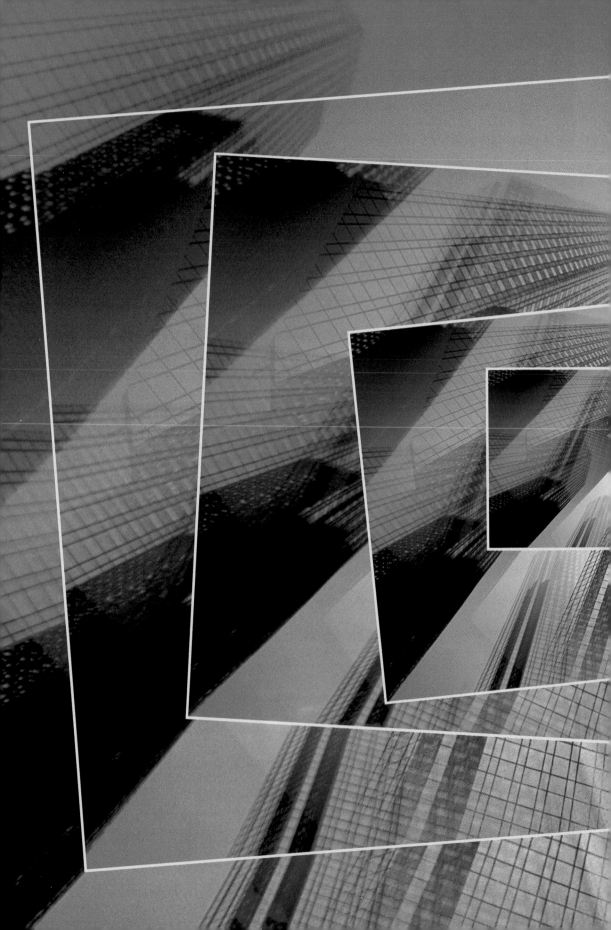

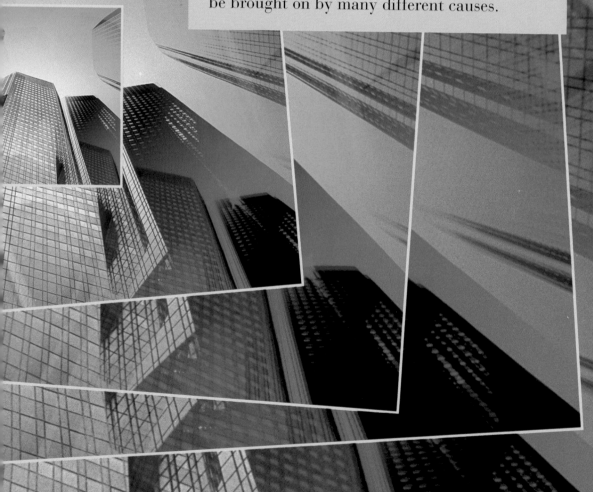

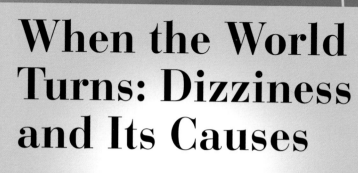

When the World Turns: Dizziness and Its Causes

By Bruce H. Dobkin, M.D.

Whether we feel just a little off-balance or as if we are spinning in space, dizziness is an unsettling sensation that can be brought on by many different causes.

The author:

Bruce H. Dobkin is a professor of neurology at the University of California at Los Angeles School of Medicine.

A young woman staggers through the doorway of a hospital emergency room. She is pale and obviously miserable. In a quavering, worried voice, she tells the attending nurse that the room is whirling and she feels nauseated. As she turns her head, her eyes jerk in the same direction. Moving her head makes her sway to the point of falling over. She says the whirling sensation, nausea, and vomiting began suddenly four hours ago.

I and my colleagues in hospitals and clinics across America see scenes like this every day. Some people report to us that the world has suddenly started to spin around them. Others describe the sensation of spinning like a top while everything else stands still. These patients suffer from an utterly disorienting and frightening form of dizziness called vertigo.

Many people have experienced far milder forms of dizziness than the whirling sensations of vertigo. Some of us may have felt momentarily light-headed or faint after standing up quickly. Perhaps a medication or bump on the head made us feel woozy. Or we may have lost our balance without experiencing any heady sensations.

Thousands of people seek medical help for dizziness each year. Although dizziness is a common complaint, its cause can be difficult to determine. Even vertigo, with its specific symptom of spinning, can be brought on by a variety of conditions.

How we keep our balance

In many cases, dizziness signals a problem within the body's intricate system for maintaining its balance. To understand what can go amiss and make us feel dizzy, it's necessary to know how the body normally maintains its balance.

Our sense of balance and of our orientation in space—leaning over to pick up a newspaper or balanced on one leg as we step off a curb—depends on information from several sources: the inner ears, eyes, and nerve endings in the muscles, tendons, and joints. The body's headquarters for receiving and coordinating this information is the brain. The brain sends back instructions that usually keep us from losing our balance.

Within the inner ear, a group of structures called the vestibular system helps steady our gaze and maintain our balance. The vestibular system, which nestles behind the eardrum, consists primarily of three fluid-filled, semicircular canals called the labyrinth. When the head bobs, turns, or tilts, fluid moves within these canals. The motion of the fluid stimulates nerves that signal the brain about changes in the position of the head. Other structures near the canals are sensitive to the pull of gravity on the body, another indication of the body's position.

The eyes send the brain messages about where our bodies are in relation to nearby and distant objects. Messages relayed by the eyes also tell the brain whether objects appear to be moving or standing still and which direction is up and which is down. The vestibular system sends back messages to the eyes to confirm that the surroundings are steady as the head moves.

Nerve endings in the muscles, and in the tendons that connect muscles to bones at the joints, signal the brain about the position of the parts of the body. These nerve endings, sometimes called position sensors, detect changes in the length and motion of muscles and in the force the muscles apply. The position sensors in the muscles and joints of the neck are especially well developed to help maintain the body's balance.

Muscles respond instantaneously and automatically to messages from the brain by adjusting the body's position to maintain its balance. When working smoothly, muscle reflexes maintain the body's balance during a simple change in position, such as taking a step, and during more complicated actions, such as hitting a tennis ball while on the run.

Two parts of the brain are involved in maintaining balance. The brain stem receives information from the labyrinths. The cerebellum coordinates the data from the vestibular system, eyes, and muscles. Because all of these systems are synchronized, the brain is able to receive data from each of them and to send appropriate messages back.

Why we feel dizzy

We feel dizzy when the brain interprets the messages it receives from the labyrinths, eyes, and muscles as contradictory. Even everyday experiences that produce a slight mismatch in messages can bring on problems. For example, when we look overhead at clouds gliding across the sky, our eyes see and report motion. But the unusual angle of the head and neck distorts the messages relayed by the vestibular system and the position sensors in the neck. As the brain momentarily struggles to correlate the conflicting signals, the body sways and starts to lose its balance. Fortunately, the brain quickly resolves the conflict.

The opposite mismatch occurs when we are in motion while our eyes relay the message that we are sitting or standing still. This mismatch can cause motion sickness in someone riding in the back seat of a car or in a boat crossing choppy water. In these situations, the vestibular system perceives small movements of the head as the car travels over bumps, depressions, and other gradations in the road or as the boat tosses in the waves. But the eyes sense little or no motion if they focus on the front seat or another part of the interior of the car or boat, which is moving along with the body.

Motion sickness often is accompanied by nausea and vomiting as the result of a misreading of messages by the vestibular system. Researchers believe that the brain triggers vomiting during motion sickness when it incorrectly interprets information from

How the body maintains its balance

The body's complex mechanism for maintaining its balance depends upon the brain's interpretation of information from the eyes, inner ears, and muscles. When functioning normally, this system operates automatically to keep us from losing our balance.

The eyes report to the brain about the body's position in relation to its surroundings. They also report on movement and direction.

The brain acts as the headquarters for the balance system, coordinating information from the eyes, inner ears, and muscles in the neck, arms, and legs. Dizziness can result when information from one of these sources contradicts the other two.

The inner ears signal the brain about the position of the head. A group of structures in the inner ear called the vestibular system detects the motion of the head as it turns, tilts, or bobs. The vestibular system also reports on changes in the pull of gravity on our bodies, another indicator of position.

Muscles, tendons, and joints in the neck and limbs signal the brain about the position of the parts of the body in relation to each other. Nerve endings in the muscles, tendons, and joints sense changes in the body's position. In response to nerve signals from the brain, the muscles quickly adjust the body's position to maintain its balance.

the vestibular system as a sign of poisoning.

Another experience that unsettles many people is looking down from a high place, such as a rooftop or the edge of a cliff. Dizziness in this case is a reaction to the labyrinths' sensitivity to the slightest motion. Our bodies naturally sway slightly, and the labyrinths report this motion to the brain. Our eyes normally adjust by focusing on a nearby object, which enables them to detect the body's sway. But when we look down from on high, our eyes focus on a distant object, and so do not readily perceive the body's sway. The signal mismatch in the brain leads to feelings of instability.

Vestibular causes

Feeling unstable while watching clouds, crossing choppy water, or looking down from a height is quite normal. But symptoms in other situations can signal a disruption in the vestibular system from injury or illness. Many people report episodes of vertigo or *disequilibrium* (loss of balance) following *whiplash*, an injury resulting from a sudden jolt that snaps the head backward and then forward. In this case, the injury usually affects the nerve endings in the labyrinth or in sprained neck muscles. But even a far milder blow to the head can injure the fragile labyrinths by shaking loose a tiny bit of debris—usually mineral grains—in the canals. The debris is heavier than the fluid, and so it exerts added pressure on the nerves. The nerves in turn send false signals to the brain, resulting in vertigo.

Many other conditions can affect the vestibular system and bring on vertigo, including ear infections caused by bacteria or viruses. Toxins released as the body breaks down alcohol or certain medications can cause a temporary malfunction of the inner ear. Migraine headaches are also associated with attacks of vertigo, though the precise mechanism is not well understood. The process of aging can hamper vestibular function. Ménière's disease, a disorder caused by increased fluid in the labyrinth, can produce repeated attacks of vertigo, ringing in the affected ear, and hearing loss.

Damage to the vestibular system also can

The vestibular system
The vestibular system is a group of structures nestled behind the eardrum in the inner ear. It plays an important role in maintaining the body's balance. Disruptions in the functioning of the vestibular system as a result of illness or injury can make us feel dizzy.

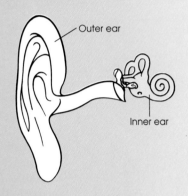

Outer ear

Inner ear

Vestibular system

Labyrinth

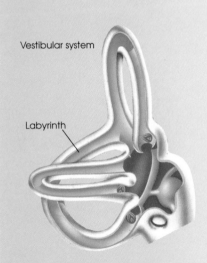

The key structures of the vestibular system are three fluid-filled, semicircular canals known as the labyrinth. When the head moves, so does the fluid in these canals. Nerve cells stimulated as a result of the fluid's motion send signals to the brain about changes in the position of the head. This information is crucial to maintaining balance.

bring on the most common type of vertigo, benign positional vertigo (BPV). People with BPV experience vertigo upon changing position. Sitting up, lying down, turning over in bed, bending over and straightening up, or looking overhead can all bring on vertigo. The sensation of spinning usually starts within 30 seconds of the position change and lasts less than one minute. Immediately repeating the motion that brought on the vertigo can usually halt an attack. But bouts of vertigo can recur daily, then stop for weeks, months, or years before another flurry of attacks begins.

An unusual pattern of involuntary, jerky movements of the eyes called nystagmus also is a characteristic of BPV. The rapid eye movements smear vision, just as rapid side-to-side turns of the head blur anyone's sight.

Although people of all ages experience BPV, it most commonly occurs after age 50 from an age-related degeneration of nerve cells in the labyrinth. BPV also can follow an acute viral infection of the labyrinth or a blow to the head.

A vestibular system injury can have lingering effects, leaving the labyrinths overly sensitive to motion so that their messages override those of the eyes and muscles. People with the condition report sensations of light-headedness, wooziness, or disequilibrium. This elusive dizziness occurs in people of all ages.

Dizziness from other causes

Dizziness doesn't always signal a problem with the body's balance system, however. Another common cause of dizziness is a reduced supply of oxygen to the brain, usually the result of a sudden dip in blood pressure. Normally, blood pressure rises when a person stands up, because the heart has to pump harder against gravity. But in some people, blood pressure fails to increase, or even falls, when they sit up or stand up. As a result, less blood and less oxygen reach the brain. The reduced supply of oxygen produces momentary light-headedness, sometimes to the point of feeling faint.

About 15 percent of people over age 70 experience this dip in blood pressure, which is known as orthostatic hypotension. The condition is also common in people who take medication for high blood pressure or other forms of heart disease. Many of these drugs partially block the mechanism that ordinarily maintains stable blood pressure.

Many people with diabetes experience disequilibrium as a result of their disease. Diabetes can cause damage to nerves in the legs. The damage dulls the signals from the nerve endings in muscles and tendons in the feet and ankles, causing feelings of imbalance when standing or walking.

Many older people have mild nerve damage that also leads to feelings of disequilibrium. When the condition is combined with poor vision and an inner ear disturbance—two other age-related problems—an older person can easily develop a fear of falling.

Vertigo also can stem from a psychological problem rather than a physical disorder. This condition is called psychogenic vertigo or dissociation. Someone with psychogenic vertigo may inadvertently bring on an attack of dizziness by *hyperventilating* (breathing unusually rapidly or deeply). The symptoms that follow include shortness of breath and a feeling of tightness in the throat or chest. The sensation of spinning can build rapidly, increasing the person's anxiety and desperate gasping for air. The symptoms result from the body's loss of carbon dioxide while hyperventilating. Breathing into a paper bag can restore carbon dioxide to the body and relieve the symptoms.

In rare cases, vertigo is the result of a more serious condition. A brain tumor, for example, can obstruct nerve connections between the brain stem and the labyrinths. Multiple sclerosis (MS), a condition in which the protective sheath around nerve fibers degenerates, can short-circuit nerve signals. In both conditions, however, other serious symptoms—such as weakness, numbness or loss of feeling in the face or limbs, loss of hearing, and double vision—may be present as well.

> ### The many causes of dizziness
> Dizziness is a symptom rather than a disorder, and it can result from a number of underlying conditions. These include:
>
> - Anxiety or depression
> - Blood pressure changes
> - Drug reactions, especially to aspirin and drugs that treat high blood pressure
> - Ear infections or inflammation, especially in the labyrinth
> - Low blood sugar
> - Ménière's disease, which involves an increase in the fluid in the inner ear
> - Motion sickness
> - Nerve damage
> - Transient ischemic attack, a brief interruption in the flow of blood to the brain
> - Tumor
> - Whiplash or other injury to the head or neck

Finally, dizziness can warn of an impending stroke if it results from a brief interruption in blood flow to the brain known as a transient ischemic attack (TIA). A TIA causes dizziness by cutting off the supply of oxygen required for the proper functioning of the brain stem, the labyrinth, and the nerve connections between the two. Other symptoms, such as slurred speech, double vision, and numbness or weakness in the arms or legs, typically accompany the dizziness.

Diagnosing dizziness

Recurrent bouts of wooziness or loss of balance should not be ignored. Anyone who experiences vertigo, disequilibrium, or light-headedness on a continuing or recurrent basis should discuss the sensation with a physician. In diagnosing the cause of dizziness, physicians are likely to ask patients for a precise description of their symptoms. This description is extremely important, even though it may be difficult for a patient to put into words.

Diagnosing dizziness

Because dizziness has many causes, a diagnostic examination encompasses a variety of tests. A test of labyrinth function, *right*, involves sending cold water into a patient's ear and then measuring the response of the eyes. Normal labyrinths produce the same response. But an injured labyrinth produces little or no response.

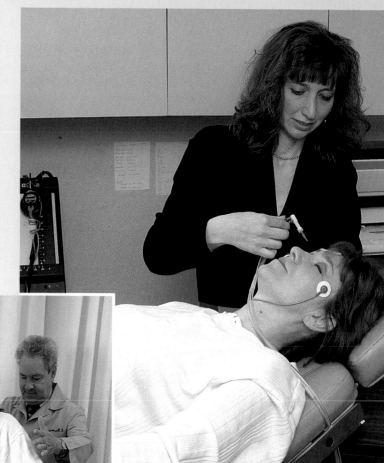

A patient wears special magnifying glasses, *below*, as a physician looks for the jerky eye motions characteristic of a common form of vertigo. Walking heel-to-toe in a straight line, first with the eyes open and then with the eyes closed, *left*, tests communication between the vestibular system and the muscles in the legs.

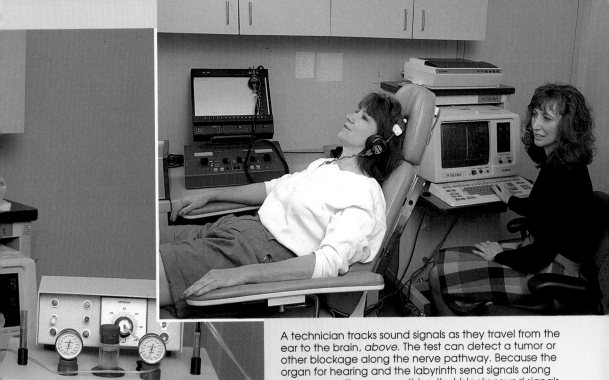

A technician tracks sound signals as they travel from the ear to the brain, *above*. The test can detect a tumor or other blockage along the nerve pathway. Because the organ for hearing and the labyrinth send signals along the same pathway, something that blocks sound signals is likely to interfere with labyrinth signals as well.

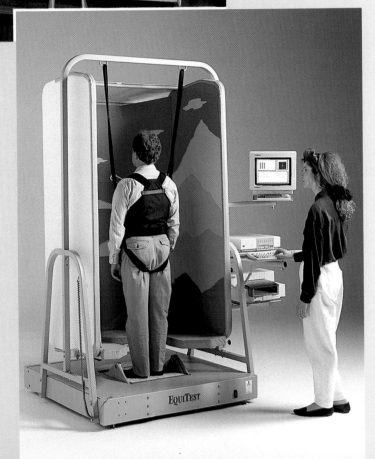

A computerized instrument tests all three components of the balance system: the eyes, inner ears, and muscles, *left*. The patient looks at surroundings that tilt back and forth while standing on a platform that also tilts. As the patient tries to maintain balance, a computer compares his responses with normal responses and prints an assessment of how well his eyes, inner ears, and muscles work together.

Treating dizziness

The treatment for dizziness depends upon its cause. In one treatment for vertigo, a therapist moves a patient's head to bring on vertigo, *right*. With repetition, this exercise may make the patient's vertigo disappear.

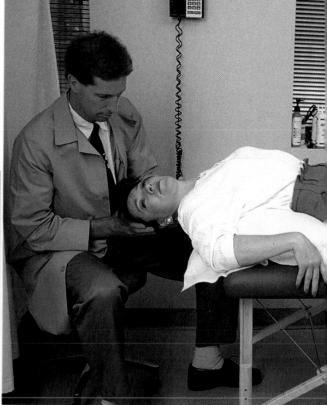

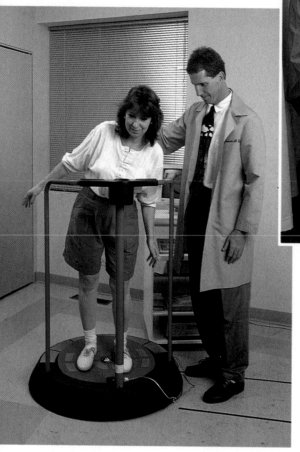

A patient who has a balance problem tries to maintain balance while standing on a platform that has areas of varying firmness. This exercise, executed with eyes open and closed, retrains nerve endings in the leg muscles that help steady a person.

The doctor may ask, for example, what occurs immediately before the onset of dizziness, such as a motion of the head, a change in body position, coughing or sneezing, or loud noises. Also of interest are any symptoms that accompany the dizziness, such as nausea and vomiting, headache, blurred or bouncing vision, hearing changes, shortness of breath, and numbness or weakness. In addition, the doctor is likely to ask about any symptoms experienced between attacks of dizziness, such as subtle sensations of disequilibrium or ringing in the ears. A medical history will cover factors that might predispose the patient to the problem, including recent viral or ear infections, head injury, diabetes, heart disease, medications the patient is taking, and a family history of equilibrium problems.

The physical examination to determine the cause of the problem encompasses a variety of tests. In an ear examination, the physician checks for fluid, an infection, or a growth, which could account for dizziness. An assessment of sensation and muscle strength in the patient's face can indicate a problem involving the vestibular nerve. Because this nerve runs alongside

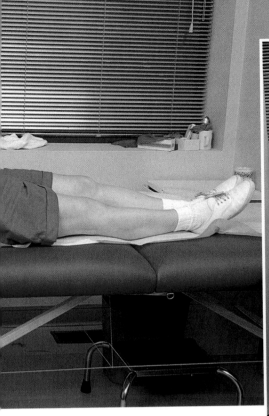

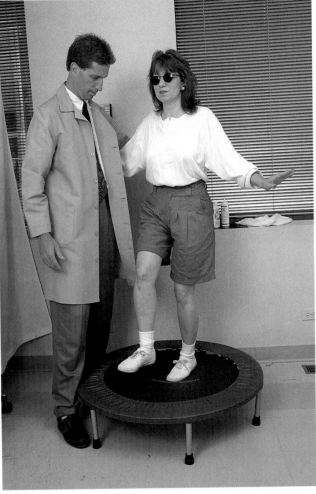

the nerve that controls facial movements and feeling, a transient ischemic attack (ministroke) or tumor involving one nerve might also involve the other. A test for hearing loss could indicate Ménière's disease or another inner ear problem. A test of eye movements can reveal the nystagmus that accompanies BPV.

A test of balance can reveal other causes of dizziness. In the test, the patient is asked to walk heel-to-toe in a straight line, first with the eyes open and then with the eyes closed. Normally, messages to the brain from the vestibular system and nerve endings in the legs compensate for the absence of visual information when the eyes are closed. But the labyrinths cannot maintain balance on their own. And so a poor performance with the eyes closed can indicate that the patient's dizziness stems from a communication problem between the vestibular system and nerves in the legs.

When benign positional vertigo is suspected, the physician looks for problems with the functioning of the labyrinth. A key indicator of labyrinth malfunction is nystagmus, so a doctor may use procedures to induce vertigo and nystagmus to confirm the diagnosis. In one such procedure, the patient is rapidly

A patient with an inner ear problem is trained to rely solely on input from her eyes and muscles in maintaining balance. As part of the training, she wears sunglasses to alter visual input and stands on a trampoline to alter input from leg muscles.

moved from a seated position on the examining table to a reclining position with the head hanging slightly over the edge. The doctor turns the head and watches the eyes for the jerky motions of nystagmus.

In another test for nystagmus, called the cold caloric test, a physician sends cool water or cool air into one ear. This stimulates the motion of the fluid in the labyrinth. The labyrinths then send conflicting messages to the brain, resulting in nystagmus and vertigo. A person without a labyrinth problem will experience the same degree of nystagmus on each side of the body. But an injured labyrinth is usually unable to respond to the test, producing little or no nystagmus on the affected side.

Blood pressure readings are important when the doctor suspects orthostatic hypotension. Blood pressure is checked while the patient is lying down as well as while standing up. The usual method of checking blood pressure—while the patient is seated—can mask the fact that a patient's blood pressure is considerably higher while lying down and dips too low upon standing.

When anxiety is the suspected cause of dizziness, the physician may ask the patient to breathe deeply for a minute or two, causing hyperventilation. If dizziness ensues, anxiety is probably the culprit that brings on the worrisome symptoms.

Other tests can rule out, or uncover, more serious disorders. Hearing tests, for example, can reveal nerve problems that affect balance. The chief organ for hearing and the labyrinth are neighbors, and each sends impulses to the brain along the same nerve. Something that obstructs the signals sent by one would likely obstruct the signals sent by the other.

A sophisticated hearing test, called the brain stem evoked potential, looks for such obstructions. In the test, a technician follows sound signals as they travel along the nerve from the inner ear to the area of the brain responsible for hearing. If there is no signal loss along the way, the pathway is probably not blocked by a tumor or another obstruction.

Other procedures look for damage within the brain stem. An imaging technique called magnetic resonance imaging (MRI) can reveal a tumor, a blood clot, or inflammation from MS that could contribute to dizziness.

Treating dizziness

The treatment for dizziness depends upon its cause. Some problems that bring on dizziness go away without treatment. For example, vertigo that results from an acute inflammation of the labyrinth, which is almost always brought on by infection, generally improves spontaneously over time. In the meantime, antihistamines can be effective in reducing inflammation brought on by a mild infection, and antibiotics can clear up a bacterial infection in the ear. A physician may prescribe tranquilizers for a patient whose bouts of dizziness stem from feelings of anxiety.

The sensation of spinning that characterizes vertigo can often be suppressed by staring at the thumb. A signal of no motion from the eyes should quickly dampen the maddening signals from a labyrinth gone awry. Ménière's disease may require surgery to drain excess fluid from the labyrinth.

Many patients suffering from dizziness benefit from a program of exercise. Movement gives nerve cells in the brain stem a chance to develop ways of compensating for the conflicting signals that a malfunctioning vestibular system is sending to the brain. People with acute vertigo, for example, should cautiously move about as soon as the sensation of spinning stops. And people experiencing vague unsteadiness because of vestibular problems should walk around rather than rest.

Physical therapists can help a patient design a program that addresses specific problems involving balance and coordination. Nerve cells in the brain stem that are activated by the vestibular system are among the most adaptable cells in our bodies.

Strangely enough, some patients with vertigo brought on by changes in position benefit from exercises designed to induce vertigo. In one exercise, the patient, who is seated, leans rapidly to one side, bringing the head to rest on a solid object such as a bed. The patient remains in this position until the vertigo ceases and then performs the same maneuver to the other side. Patients usually repeat this procedure 10 to 20 times during each of three daily sessions.

Another maneuver, performed with the assistance of a physical therapist, seems to move the mineral grain or other debris out of the canal, where it is bringing on vertigo, and to bury it in a region of the labyrinth where it can no longer cause vertigo. According to the German neurologist who developed the therapy, it cures as many as 85 percent of people with BPV.

Dizziness can be disabling, both physically and emotionally, when it interferes with work and daily life. But the disturbing sensations usually can be managed through medication, exercise, and patient education. And fortunately, bouts of dizziness often subside on their own.

For further reading:

Dizziness: Hope Through Research. National Institutes of Health Publication No. 86-76.

Watson, Mary A., and Sinclair, Helen. *Balancing Act: For People with Dizziness & Balance Disorders.* Vestibular Disorders Association, 1992.

Coping With Alzheimer's Disease

By Donna Cohen

Jean Albrecht complained of memory loss and of having difficulty finding the right word. Other people had noticed the high
school teacher's problems as well. She complimented her students on work they had not done, forgot what she had planned
to say in class, and admitted that she sometimes had difficulty
understanding what people were saying to her. Complaints
about her behavior finally led the school principal to ask for
her resignation.

Although angry at the principal's action, Albrecht realized
something was wrong and repeatedly stated that she must be
in the early stages of Alzheimer's disease. Her family and her
physician urged her to see a specialist at a local university's
memory disorders clinic.

After a series of diagnostic examinations, doctors determined
that 64-year-old Jean Albrecht indeed had Alzheimer's disease,
a disorder of unknown cause characterized by the progressive
deterioration of memory, reasoning powers, and judgment. She
and her family then met with a team of health care professionals to plan how to face the future.

Albrecht and her family are not alone. Alzheimer's disease af-

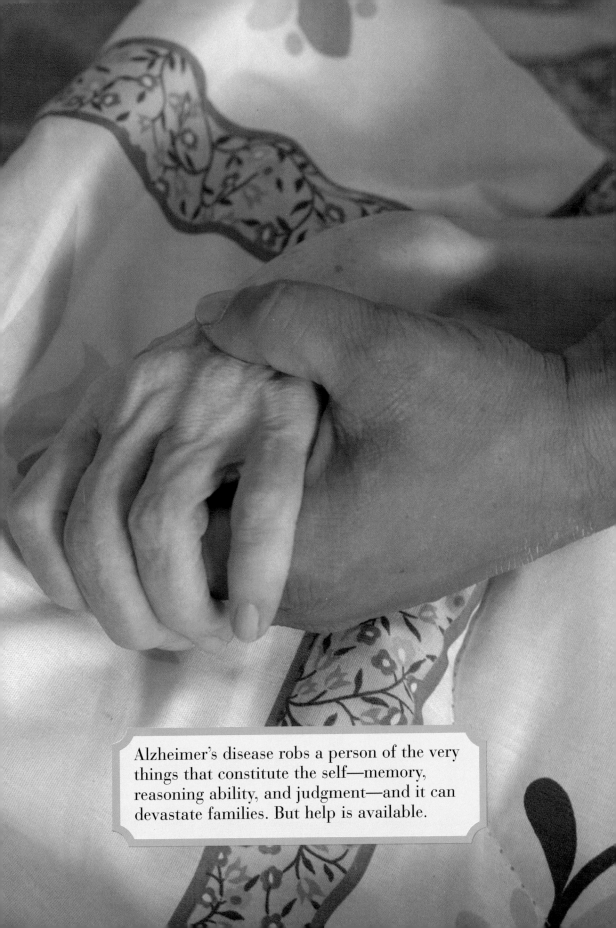

Alzheimer's disease robs a person of the very things that constitute the self—memory, reasoning ability, and judgment—and it can devastate families. But help is available.

flicts between 4 million and 6.8 million Americans, according to the Alzheimer's Disease Association in Chicago. It is the most common cause of progressive and irreversible *dementia* (mental deterioration) in the aged, but it is not the only cause. At least 50 other brain diseases can seriously impair mental abilities.

Although Albrecht received a diagnosis of Alzheimer's disease, a definitive diagnosis is possible only from an examination of the patient's brain after death. During the patient's lifetime, the diagnosis depends upon ruling out other causes of dementia.

A disease of the aged

Alzheimer's disease is primarily a disease of older people, and the number of Americans afflicted with the disease will almost certainly continue to rise. Not only are people aged 65 and older living longer than ever before, but the "oldest-old," those 85 years and older, are growing seven times faster than any other age group. This is the group at greatest risk for Alzheimer's disease. After age 85, a person has nearly a 1-in-3 chance of developing the disease, according to researchers.

Albrecht and her family, like others in their situation, had reason to fear the future. Alzheimer's disease is a long-term illness that slowly and relentlessly robs people of their mental capacities and ability to take care of themselves. On average, a person with Alzheimer's disease lives 7 years after diagnosis, but some people live on for another 20 years or more.

The course of the disease varies considerably. Some people lose their mental faculties quite rapidly. Others may show few signs of deterioration for months at a time. Different skills and abilities do not necessarily deteriorate at the same rate. Memory may decline before language skills. Motor skills may be retained longer than mental capacity, enabling the person to play tennis, for instance, but not to keep score.

In later stages of the disease, the patient's physical deterioration becomes more pronounced. For reasons not completely understood, many patients lose weight, even when eating well. They may be unable to control their bowels or bladder. Mental deterioration may progress until patients no longer recognize themselves in a mirror.

Despite important advances in our understanding of Alzheimer's disease, its cause is still unknown. Nor is there any known cure. In the absence of other treatment, families must focus on obtaining a reliable diagnosis and caring for their affected family member in the most humane way possible. My colleagues and I, who study the problems of aging, have established some clear guidelines for helping families. Much can be done to improve the well-being and quality of life of an Alzheimer's disease patient—and to assure the welfare of the rest of the family.

The author:

Donna Cohen is director of the Institute on Aging at the University of South Florida and coauthor of *The Loss of Self: A Family Resource for the Care of Alzheimer's Disease and Related Disorders.*

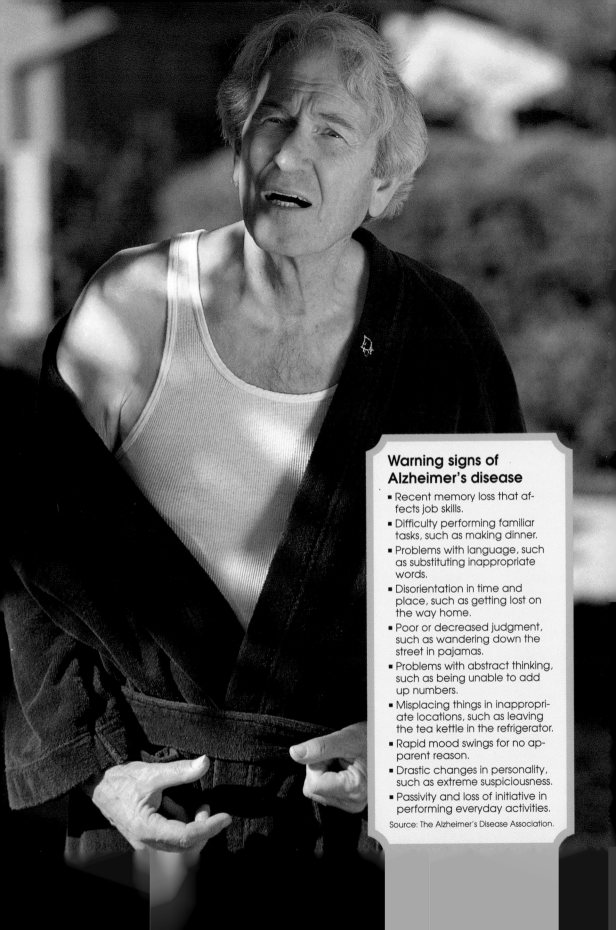

Warning signs of Alzheimer's disease

- Recent memory loss that affects job skills.
- Difficulty performing familiar tasks, such as making dinner.
- Problems with language, such as substituting inappropriate words.
- Disorientation in time and place, such as getting lost on the way home.
- Poor or decreased judgment, such as wandering down the street in pajamas.
- Problems with abstract thinking, such as being unable to add up numbers.
- Misplacing things in inappropriate locations, such as leaving the tea kettle in the refrigerator.
- Rapid mood swings for no apparent reason.
- Drastic changes in personality, such as extreme suspiciousness.
- Passivity and loss of initiative in performing everyday activities.

Source: The Alzheimer's Disease Association.

The importance of proper diagnosis

Obtaining a diagnosis depends first on recognizing the existence of a serious problem. We all have occasional memory lapses when we forget names or phone numbers or mislay keys. The problems with memory, language, or judgment experienced by someone with Alzheimer's disease are of a different order. To decide whether mental lapses require professional attention, consider the following questions. A "yes" answer to any of them indicates that a visit to a health care professional is warranted.

- Are problems with language or abstract reasoning ongoing? Everyone has trouble finding the right word at times, but people with Alzheimer's disease often demonstrate a number of ongoing language difficulties. They may forget simple words, substitute inappropriate words, or transpose words, making their sentences hard to follow. A man might say, for instance, "I used to be a boss big man, but now I'm an old, big dummy." Balancing a checkbook may thoroughly confuse someone who has had no trouble with this activity in the past, or the distinction between past and present events may become blurred.
- Do problems arise either in areas of long-time skills or in everyday activities? Calculation difficulties for a bookkeeper or an accountant, or faulty sentence structure on the part of a language instructor, suggest a serious problem. Similarly, forgetting what to do with silverware should arouse concern.
- Is behavior inappropriate or bizarre, demonstrating poor judgment? A person with Alzheimer's disease might sing a birthday song during grace at meals, wear several shirts or blouses at once, roam around outside naked, or place shoes in the refrigerator.
- Are the problems growing worse? Over time, the inability to remember familiar words or everyday activities becomes more obvious and interferes with normal functioning. Forgetfulness may also become dangerous. It is one thing to become lost while driving but another to forget what a stoplight is.
- Are there unusual changes in personality and temperament? Emotional outbursts, swearing, or aggressive or abusive behavior warrant further investigation, especially when they are out of character or unprovoked.
- Is there a loss of initiative? It is normal to tire of work or household chores, but most people regain their initiative. A person with Alzheimer's disease, on the other hand, may be passive and require prompting to engage in everyday activities.

Getting a proper diagnosis is crucial, because a number of conditions can cause symptoms resembling those of Alzheimer's disease. Next to Alzheimer's disease, stroke is the most common cause of dementia. Other disorders that can involve a deterioration of thought processes include Parkinson disease, a disorder of the brain that also reduces muscle control, and Huntington's disease, an inherited disorder of the brain and nervous system.

A number of conditions can cause less permanent memory problems in older people. Disorders that reduce blood flow, such as hardening of the arteries, also reduce the supply of oxygen that reaches the brain, which can lead to memory problems. Diabetes, poor nutrition, high blood pressure, and respiratory disorders can impair circulation and the functioning of the brain. Excessive drinking, depression, social isolation, and the use of certain drugs such as sedatives, can also cause varying degrees of confusion and memory loss.

The diagnostic evaluation for Alzheimer's disease should include a thorough physical examination. A personal and family history can reveal whether a disease that runs in the family could cause symptoms similar to those of Alzheimer's disease. A complete list of medications the person is taking provides a ba-

Ruling out other conditions

A physician reaches a diagnosis of Alzheimer's disease by ruling out other conditions that can cause the confusion, memory loss, and impaired judgment associated with the disease. To determine the extent of mental deterioration in a man suspected of having Alzheimer's, a physician gives him simple short-term memory and arithmetic tests.

Conditions whose symptoms may mimic those of Alzheimer's disease include:

- Depression
- Side effects or interactions of medications
- Poor diet or malnutrition
- Diabetes
- Infections anywhere in the body
- Heart and lung disorders that prevent sufficient oxygen from reaching the brain

- Thyroid problems
- Damage to the brain from a fall, brain tumor, or other source
- Stroke
- Heavy alcohol use
- Other diseases, including Parkinson disease and Huntington's disease

Source: Donna Cohen.

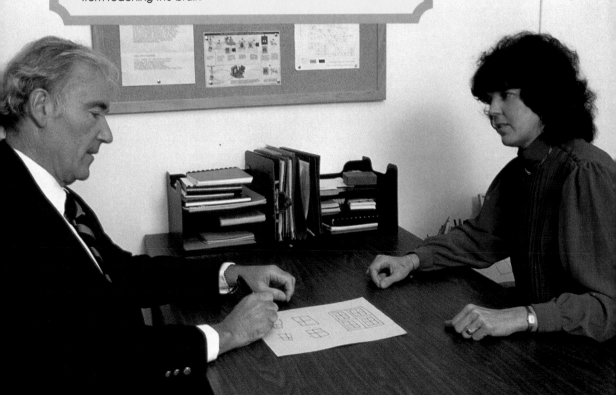

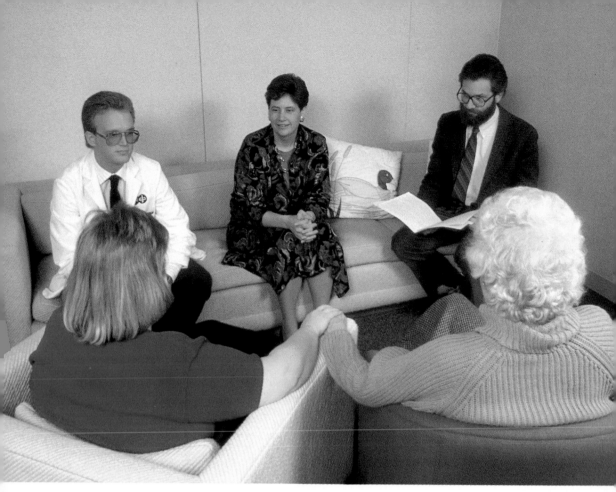

Family consultation
A patient and her family discuss the diagnosis of Alzheimer's disease with a physician, *above*. Knowing what to expect as the disease progresses enables families to plan for the future and decide how best to care for the patient. Counseling can also help the patient accept the diagnosis.

sis for determining whether side effects or drug interactions could be impairing mental function. A neurological evaluation can help rule out such disorders as Parkinson disease or Huntington's disease as the cause of the dementia. Brain scans can also help rule out various disorders of the brain.

The evaluation also should include a psychiatric examination to determine whether depression or another treatable problem may be responsible for the dementia. Other tests measure mental abilities, such as memory and arithmetic skills. A physician might ask simple questions such as "What did you eat for breakfast?" to judge short-term memory or ask the person to perform a simple calculation, such as counting backwards by sevens from 100.

Early diagnosis of a condition causing memory problems and mental confusion is important for two reasons. First, the person may have a treatable disorder that may be reversible if detected early. Second, even if the diagnosis is Alzheimer's disease, early diagnosis helps families prepare for the future while the patient is still able to participate at some level.

As much as possible, individuals with Alzheimer's should participate in decisions about their care and living arrangements.

Involvement in decision-making helps preserve the person's dignity. Discussions about long-term health care and legal control over financial resources should begin in the early stages of the illness, when the individual's mind still functions relatively well. As the disease and the impairment progress, the patient should still participate in most decisions, if only by sitting in the room during discussions.

Facing the future

Adjusting to Alzheimer's disease is deeply disturbing, not only for the patient but for everyone involved. Some families simply refuse to accept that a spouse or parent has Alzheimer's disease. Other families avoid discussing the illness out of fear of upsetting the stricken relative, precisely at a time when the person wants and needs to talk. To offer effective care, family members need to accept the diagnosis and discuss together how they are going to deal with the disease. It is also important to elicit the person's feelings about what is happening. After receiving the diagnosis, many people become angry or frustrated if the subject does not surface.

People with Alzheimer's disease usually adapt to their diminishing mental powers in six psychological stages, researchers have found. Not everyone with Alzheimer's disease experiences all the stages in the same order, but all have feelings about what is happening to them.

- Recognition and concern. The realization that something is wrong is the first stage in experiencing the disease for most people. In the early stages, many people become adept at covering up their problem, and four to six years may elapse between the initial awareness and the diagnosis.
- Denial that a problem exists commonly follows the recognition of telltale symptoms or the diagnosis of the disease. Denial can be an effective way to deal with the initial shock of bad news, if the denial does not persist. Family members should listen and offer support but also gently confront the individual with the truth. Although families may feel uncomfortable discussing something so unpleasant, this is often the stage when an individual with Alzheimer's disease most wants to talk. It's very possible that family members will have to deal with their own feelings before they can help the patient.
- Feelings of anger, sadness, and shame often follow the patient's acceptance of the diagnosis. By encouraging the expression of these emotions, family members can help the person acknowledge personal losses, identify remaining strengths, and gradually accept increasing dependency.
- Coping. During the coping phase, individuals begin to learn how to live with their impairments and develop some sense of security and involvement in their world. For example, someone

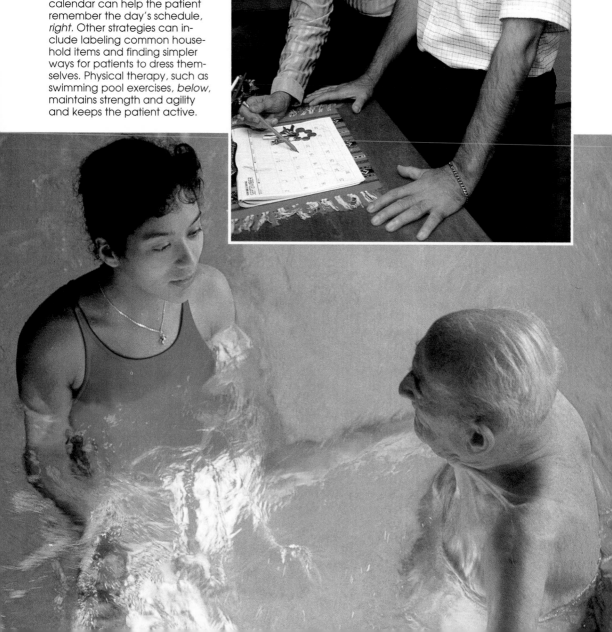

Therapy that rehabilitates

Occupational therapists help devise strategies to compensate for the patient's reduced mental capacities. Reviewing a calendar can help the patient remember the day's schedule, *right.* Other strategies can include labeling common household items and finding simpler ways for patients to dress themselves. Physical therapy, such as swimming pool exercises, *below*, maintains strength and agility and keeps the patient active.

who likes to work in the yard but has begun to get lost or confused while outside might wear a whistle to blow at such times. Neighbors or family could then come to the person's aid.

- Maturation. The maturation phase applies to Alzheimer's disease patients in advanced stages who are less able to learn coping strategies and require more care. Despite their disability and dependence on caregivers, they still need to feel emotionally connected, accepted, and safe.
- Separation from self. In the last stage of Alzheimer's disease, people lose their identities, and communication with them becomes extremely difficult if not impossible. As patients become frail, bedridden, and physically wasted, their major needs are to be kept comfortable and free of pain.

Looking for the cause

Medical researchers have not discovered the cause of Alzheimer's disease, but they have made advances in understanding how the disease interrupts normal brain functioning and causes brain cells to die. When researchers examine the brains of people who have had Alzheimer's disease, they find a loss of brain mass due to the death of brain cells. On microscopic examination, they find two major abnormalities: tangled fibers within nerve cells and dense deposits of proteins and degenerated nerve endings called plaques. Although the brains of healthy older people also have tangles and plaques, an abundance of these formations distinguishes the brains of people with Alzheimer's disease. Researchers believe that the plaques and tangles interfere with brain function, as does the death of nerve cells.

The connection between plaques and Alzheimer's disease has been known since the early 1900's. The man for whom the disease is named—German pathologist Alois Alzheimer—first described the presence of plaques in the brain of a patient who died in 1907 after suffering from severe memory loss.

A number of other brain abnormalities have been noted in patients with Alzheimer's disease since that time. These include reduced amounts of chemicals that carry messages between nerve cells; changes in brain blood flow; and a reduction in the number of connections between nerve cells.

In August 1993, scientists at Duke University in Durham, N.C., reported finding an association between Alzheimer's disease and a gene that plays a role in the transport of the fatty substance cholesterol. One variation of this gene, called the ApoE4 gene, also has been implicated in heart disease. The ApoE4 gene is rare in the healthy aged, but it has been observed in half to two-thirds of patients with Alzheimer's disease.

The fact that the disease appears to run in families increases the likelihood that at least some cases have a genetic basis. In studies of families in which the disease has affected several generations, researchers have found genetic changes known as mutations on three different *chromosomes* (structures that carry genes). The different locations of the mutations suggest that the disease has several causes.

Family coping styles

There are no simple rules about the right way to provide care for an Alzheimer's disease patient, but there are some recognized wrong ways. One of the most damaging tactics is for a family member to try to do everything alone. Unless family caregivers find others to help with certain tasks and responsibilities, they eventually burn out emotionally and may even become ill from exhaustion themselves. Nothing should prevent the caregiver from seeking the help of family, friends, clergy, and social welfare or health care professionals.

Even with help, families must bear a great burden and make serious decisions. Individual families do things differently, and a strategy that is effective in one family may be ineffective in another. Past behavior often predicts how a family will deal with a serious long-term illness. Siblings who have not had a good relationship are unlikely to cooperate in caring for the patient. After receiving the diagnosis, family members should think about how they function together before they begin to make plans and mobilize help. Caring for a patient with Alzheimer's disease creates indescribable frustration and anger, even in the most loving families. Learning as much as possible about the disease can help families prepare for the future.

Family reactions to stressful events, such as long-term illness, can be characterized under five basic headings: denying the problem, cooperating to overcome the problem, alternating leadership, fighting all the time, and breeding chaos through disorganization and hurtful behavior toward one another. Over time, most families experience a combination of these reactions.

Families in denial ignore a problem until it reaches a crisis and overwhelms them. Cooperative families communicate well and solve problems together. Families that alternate leadership do well as long as they agree about who is in charge and at which time. Some families have a long history of conflict that makes it nearly impossible for them to work together. Chaotic families are totally disorganized and often engage in fighting. At the same time, they may ignore family problems. Caring for a disabled relative creates numerous opportunities for them to attack and belittle each other—and the patient.

Whatever the family style, family members need to develop reasonable expectations about help from each other based on how the family operates. A family that encounters serious problems with denial, conflict, or anger should seek help from a trained therapist or social worker.

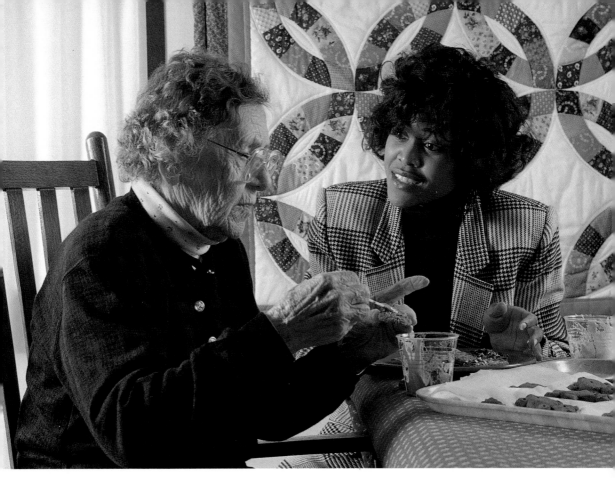

The stress of caring for someone with Alzheimer's disease affects everyone in the family, including young children. A child who does not understand the reasons for the family unhappiness may become anxious, sad, or angry. If distress is acute, a child may feel responsible for what is happening in the family. Children should have opportunities to express their feelings and ask questions, and adults should remember that children have a right to know what is happening to the family, though they do not need to know all the details. Parents can reassure the child that the family will stay together, that everyone is doing their best to deal with the situation, and that they love the child.

Even with loving attention, a child may not handle the stress in the family well. Frequent crying, difficulty sleeping or nightmares, or not wanting to play with friends are all warning signs. Other signs of a problem are new or unusual fears—of a household object, of being alone or sleeping alone, or of strangers.

Seeking outside help

Outside help for families takes many forms. Services range from health care in the home to day care, assisted-care living facilities, nurses, and nursing homes. Caregivers can learn about

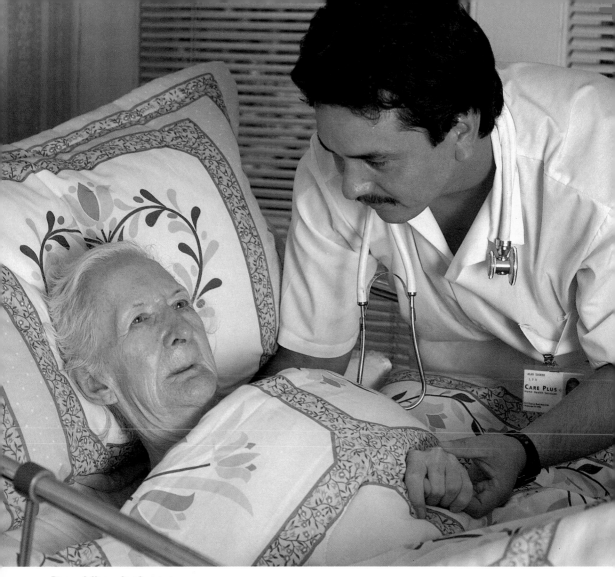

Round-the-clock care

A frail and confused patient in the final stages of Alzheimer's disease may require full-time care in a nursing home staffed by competent and caring health care workers.

available services by consulting agencies or programs on aging in their communities. Entries in the telephone book under Alzheimer's Disease Association, Area Agency on Aging, or Mayor's Office on Aging are often helpful.

At some point, families may have to consider an alternative living arrangement for the Alzheimer's disease patient. This should not be taken as a sign that the family has failed or that they do not love their relative. Assisted-living facilities and nursing homes are legitimate options when caring for the patient at home is no longer possible. Such facilities can actually improve the quality of life for the patient as well as relieve the family of an impossible responsibility. Assisted-living combines housing, health care, and support services—such as transportation to go shopping or helpers to prepare meals—for those who need some help with daily activities but do not require the skilled medical care of a nursing home.

Finding the right place usually takes time. In evaluating a facility, families should consider whether the staff genuinely cares about the patients and their quality of life. Are residents treated with care and respect? Are they given an opportunity to make choices? Does the facility protect residents' right to privacy? Are family and friends involved in planning for care as well as in implementing it? Is the facility safe? Is there a stimulating range of activities?

Some nursing homes and assisted-living programs offer a special unit devoted to meeting the needs of people with Alzheimer's disease. About 10 percent of nursing homes claim to have a special care unit. It's important to check them out, however. Many facilities advertise a special care unit but do not provide special care.

Visit as many facilities as possible and evaluate their special care units carefully. Be sure to ask questions. Is there a full-time director, and do staff have special training? Are there structured programs every day for most of the day? Are residents active? Are there family support programs or staff who do counseling? Does each resident have a personalized care plan? Is special attention given to nutrition? Spend some time at the facility and talk about your impressions with others.

Much can be done to sustain the functioning and well-being of individuals with Alzheimer's disease. Among the many challenges are remembering that the patient is first, last, and always a human being and that caregiving is an extremely difficult task, especially if the caregiver attempts to solve all problems alone. Caregivers should also bear in mind that the patient is not the only one who needs attention. There may be no more important rule in caring for someone with Alzheimer's disease than to make sure that the caregivers remain capable of doing their best for their loved one.

For further reading:

Cohen, Donna, and Eisdorfer, Carl. *The Loss of Self: A Family Resource for the Care of Alzheimer's Disease and Related Disorders.* NAL/Plume, 1987.

Goldsmith, Seth. *Choosing a Nursing Home.* Prentice-Hall, 1990.

Hoffman, Stephanie, and Platt, Constance. *Comforting the Confused— Strategies for Managing Dementia.* Springer, 1991.

For more information:

Information on Alzheimer's disease and related disorders can be obtained from the Alzheimer's Disease Association, 919 N. Michigan Ave., Chicago, IL 60611.

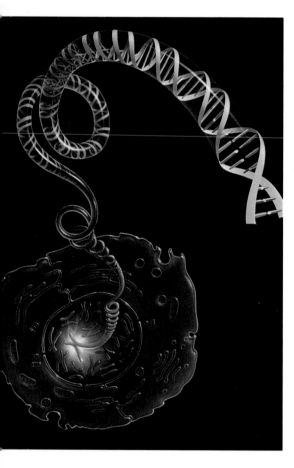

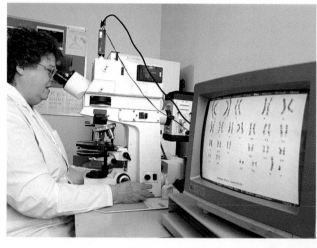

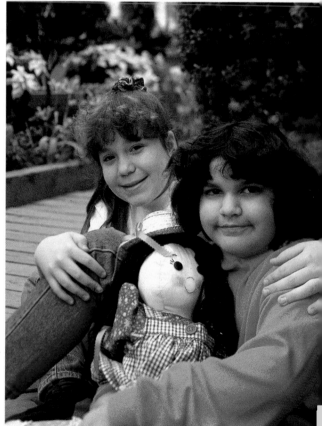

Genetic Medicine: What It's All About
by Yvonne Baskin

The one sure thing that children inherit from their parents is the genes that dictate physical characteristics. But that isn't necessarily all. Researchers are finding that the odds for good health and longevity and a predisposition to certain diseases also can be passed along in the genes. This legacy, for better or worse, was a person's lot in life—until recently.

Medicine is now in the midst of a revolution that promises to change not only the ways in which physicians heal but the very concept of health itself. This revolution was brought about by an explosion of knowledge about genes, the basic currency of heredity.

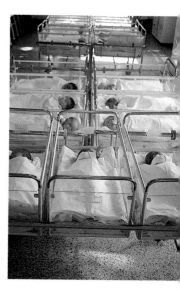

Researchers are identifying specific disease-causing genes, creating tests for those genes, and developing treatments for previously incurable ills. And the maps they are making of genes may one day give healthy people advance warning of potential genetic trouble ahead.

The promise of genetic medicine is immense, but such power also raises many ethical issues about its use. Doctors and other concerned individuals want to make sure that these issues surrounding genetics are also addressed in ways that allow the promise to be fulfilled completely.

The basis of genetics: Genes and chromosomes   **218**

How genes cause disease   **220**

Genetic medicine: The next revolution   **226**

Mapping our genes   **232**

Ethical issues   **236**

The basis of genetics:
Genes and chromosomes

Genes are the basic units of heredity. They determine the characteristics that are passed from one generation to the next. They also serve as the blueprint for all cell functions. In human beings, genes govern such traits as eye color and blood type. They ensure that body cells maintain themselves through such activities as taking in nutrients and giving off wastes. All living things—animals, plants, bacteria, viruses—possess genes.

The beginning of genetic science

People have long noted that children share many of the characteristics of their parents, and that certain diseases seem to run in families. However, not until the late 1800's did people begin to understand how biological inheritance works. In 1866, an Austrian monk named Gregor Johann Mendel published the results of records he had been keeping about his crossbreeding experiments with pea plants. After many thousands of crosses, Mendel figured out the rules by which traits such as color were passed from one generation of pea plant to the next. Central to Mendel's theory was the idea that it was not the traits that were passed on but "factors" that carried the recipes for reproducing the traits in the offspring.

Mendel's work went unnoticed for almost 40 years. Finally, in the early 1900's, scientists rediscovered his laws of heredity. In 1909, a Dutch botanist gave Mendel's hereditary factors the name *genes*, from a Greek word meaning *to give birth to*. And the science of genetics was born.

Deciphering the genetic code

Scientists gradually uncovered more secrets of genes. In 1944, they found that genes are made of a substance called DNA (deoxyribonucleic acid). DNA is a long molecule composed of four chemical subunits known as bases and written as A, C, G, and T. But researchers still did not know how genes were able to reproduce themselves. The answer lay in the structure of the DNA molecule.

In 1953, American biologist James D. Watson and British biologist Francis H. C. Crick determined that DNA takes a spiral form called a double helix. The double helix resembles a twisted ladder, with pairs of bases serving as the rungs. The two DNA strands in a double helix stick together because of chemical attractions between certain pairs of bases. The base A always pairs up with T, and C pairs up with G. Because of this structure, DNA can unzip to form two halves. And because the bases always pair

up in the same way, the unzipped strands will attract chemical bases formed in the cell to create two new double strands of DNA. Despite the amazing diversity of life, the genes in virtually all organisms are the same—a long sequence of these bases.

The next step for scientists was to work out the genetic code from the sequence of the bases in an organism's genes. Human genetic material is about 3 billion bases long. Scientists believe it contains from 50,000 to 100,000 genes.

Scientists already knew that genes somehow carry a code for making proteins, versatile molecules that perform nearly all the tasks of living cells. Some proteins break down other molecules, such as those in the food we eat. Other proteins provide structure for cells, repair cell damage, produce energy, or ferry molecules from one place to another. Scientists also knew that proteins are made up of long chains of building blocks called amino acids, of which there are 20. Through experimentation, researchers discovered that specific groups of three DNA bases, called codons, carry the code for the amino acids that make up each protein. By 1967, the genetic language had been deciphered for all 20 amino acids.

Understanding heredity

These discoveries about DNA completed one part of the story of how traits are passed from parents to children. Since around 1910, scientists had known that genes are carried on structures in the cell called chromosomes. Chromosomes reside within the *nucleus* (central compartment) of a cell. Different species have different numbers of chromosomes. Human beings have 46 chromosomes organized in 23 pairs. One chromosome in each pair is inherited from the father, the other comes from the mother.

Researchers also learned that the endless variety among individuals results in part from the fact that genes on each chromosome come in variations called alleles. For example, the gene for eye color has a number of alleles. One allele gives rise to blue eyes, whereas another leads to brown eyes.

The cells in a person's body contain the same set of 46 chromosomes, except for the sex cells involved in reproduction. In men, they are the sperm cells; in women, they are the egg cells. A sex cell has only half the total number of chromosomes.

A child is formed when an egg cell unites with a sperm cell. Each sex cell donates 23 chromosomes to the child. The egg and sperm cells do not contain exact copies of the chromosomes that the child's

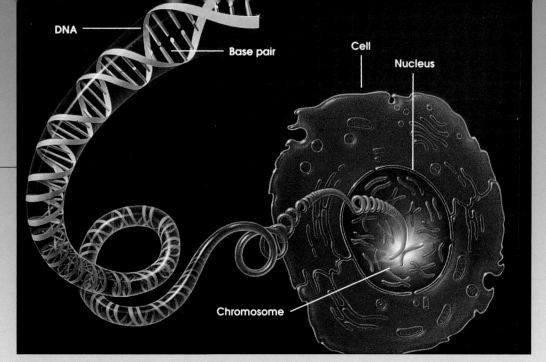

What genes are

Genes are the units of heredity. They carry instructions for all our physical characteristics and bodily functions. Genes are carried on structures called chromosomes located in the nucleus of every cell. Each chromosome contains a long strand of DNA that resembles a twisted ladder, with rungs made up of two interlocking substances called bases. A gene is a particular sequence of these base pairs.

mother and father inherited from their parents, however. During the formation of sex cells, the cells must halve the number of their chromosomes, from 46 to 23. The two chromosomes in each of the 23 pairs first line up and exchange pieces. This shuffling, called recombination, ensures that each sex cell contains a distinct set of genes. Each child, with the exception of identical twins, therefore has a unique genetic makeup.

The beginnings of genetic engineering

In the 1970's, scientists began learning how to work with genes. They discovered certain biological tools that allowed them to make changes in an organism's DNA. The ability to manipulate genes came to be called genetic engineering.

One of the most important tools the researchers found were proteins called restriction enzymes. These enzymes act as a kind of chemical scissors to cut DNA. Each restriction enzyme cuts only at a specific place on the DNA molecule.

Another important tool that scientists found was a biochemical "glue" that could link pieces of DNA together. These tools enabled scientists to cut a gene out of one piece of DNA and splice it into another. The resulting genetic material is called recombinant DNA. Working with harmless bacteria, researchers learned how to transfer a gene from one organism into another.

Bacteria provided scientists with a way to *clone*

(make copies of) genes. Because genes cannot be seen under ordinary microscopes, and a single copy is very difficult to handle or track, scientists therefore prefer to work with many copies. By 1980, they had developed two methods of cloning genes in bacteria. One method involved splicing the gene into the genetic material of viruses called phages that infect bacterial cells. Once inside the bacteria, the phages multiply rapidly, and the copy of the gene multiplies along with them. The second method involved splicing the gene into little rings of bacterial DNA called plasmids. Whenever the bacteria reproduce, so do the plasmids containing the foreign gene. After the bacteria multiply sufficiently, scientists can then recover large numbers of genes

Researchers also used recombinant-DNA techniques to induce bacteria to produce large quantities of the protein for which the spliced gene *coded* (carried the instructions). Thus, scientists learned to turn bacteria into "biological factories" for any protein they desired.

In 1983, scientists developed a third way to clone genes. The technique, called polymerase chain reaction (PCR) employs a machine containing a DNA-copying protein to make millions of copies of a gene in a matter of hours. PCR has greatly speeded up the work of geneticists.

With these discoveries, the era of genetic engineering was launched. For medical researchers, the next step was to tackle genetic diseases.

How genes cause disease

The genetic variations that make each person unique are a mixed blessing. On the one hand, they are a source of our individuality, influencing everything from our eye color to our temperament. On the other hand, they can be a source of debility and disease.

After genes were identified in the early 1900's, scientists explored the idea that mutated genes can lead to inherited disease by producing defective proteins. Sir Archibald E. Garrod, a physician in England, applied to human disease genetic principles developed in the late 1800's by the Austrian monk Gregor Johann Mendel. Garrod in 1903 outlined the foundations for what was to become modern genetic medicine. He proposed that certain rare conditions such as *albinism* (a lack of pigment in the skin and eyes) and cystinuria, which leads to kidney stones, were "inborn errors of metabolism" caused by glitches in the hereditary factors responsible for producing proteins. Today, we know that genes

How diseases are inherited
Genes pass physical traits from one generation to the next. An abnormal copy of a gene can pass on a disease. But inheriting a disease gene does not always lead to illness. A person inherits two copies of most genes, one from each parent, and these copies interact in different ways.

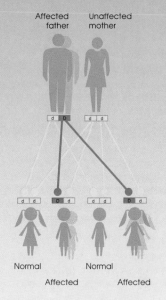

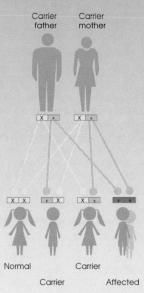

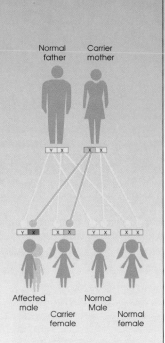

A dominant gene (D) overrides other copies of the gene (d). A child who inherits one copy of a dominant disease gene will develop the disorder. Each child has a 1 in 2 chance of inheriting the disease gene from the affected parent.

A recessive gene (x) can be masked by a normal copy of the gene (X). A child must inherit two copies of a recessive disease gene to get the disorder. When both parents carry a recessive disease gene, a child has a 1 in 4 chance of inheriting the disorder.

A sex-linked gene behaves differently in males and females. In its most common form, it acts as a dominant gene (X) in males and as a recessive gene (x) in females. A male child has a 1 in 2 chance of inheriting the disorder from a mother who carries the gene, and a female child has a 1 in 2 chance of being a carrier.

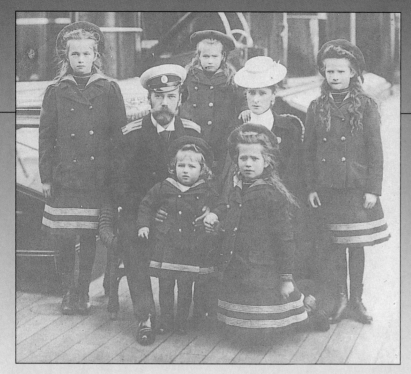

The Romanovs, who ruled Russia until 1917, carried the gene for hemophilia, a sex-linked disorder. Although only the male family members developed the bleeding disorder, female family members passed the gene to their children.

specify how to build all proteins, and faulty proteins can lead to anything from color blindness to mental deterioration and early death.

Diseases, genes, and proteins

The first to succeed in proving the link between genes and disease was American chemist Linus Pauling. In 1949, Pauling isolated the genetic cause of sickle cell anemia, a disease in which red blood cells are ineffective in carrying oxygen to the cells. In this disease, which mainly afflicts people of African ancestry, the red blood cells become misshapen and get stuck in small blood vessels, cutting off blood flow. Pauling tracked down a genetic mutation responsible for a defective version of hemoglobin, the protein in red blood cells that carries oxygen.

Since Pauling's discovery, scientists have cataloged more than 4,000 hereditary diseases and identified the defective proteins in several hundred of them. They have also learned that defective proteins can lead to disease in a variety of ways. Some proteins do essential housekeeping chores in cells, such as breaking down nutrients, clearing out wastes, and helping channel water into and out of cells. When these proteins are defective or absent, harmful chemicals can build up, cellular assembly lines can falter, and vital life processes can grind to a halt.

In a genetic disease called adenosine deaminase (ADA) deficiency, for example, a mutated gene creates a disabled form of the ADA protein. White blood cells of the body's disease-fighting immune system need ADA to do their job. When the protein is defec-tive, *toxins* (poisons) build up in the blood and eventually destroy the white blood cells, leaving the person vulnerable to infection.

Another major way that faulty proteins can lead to disease is by serving as poor *cell receptors,* molecules on the surfaces of cells that take in important biochemicals. Defective receptors can cause fatal diseases. For example, people with a genetic disorder called familial hypercholesterolemia (FH) lack key cholesterol receptors on their liver cells. These receptors normally collect cholesterol from the blood and deliver it into the liver cells for processing. The faulty receptors, however, leave the cholesterol in the blood, allowing it to accumulate on the walls of blood vessels. As a result, people with FH develop severely clogged arteries when they are children and usually suffer a fatal heart attack at a young age.

How faulty genes yield faulty proteins

Scientists now know that the defects in these proteins result from changes in the chemical subunits, or base pairs, that make up DNA. These changes, called mutations, disrupt the sequence of base pairs in a gene. Because genes carry the instructions for making a protein, mutations lead to variations in the structure or production of a protein. Many mutations are harmless. But sometimes, a mutation has very serious consequences. It can cause the cell to string together the wrong sequence of amino acids—the substances of which proteins are made. Or the mutation can cause the cell to end the assembly process before a complete protein is built, or to make

221

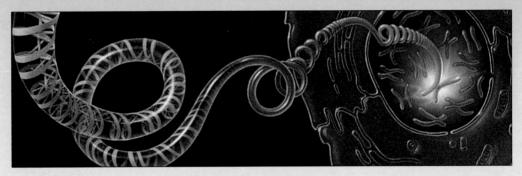

Genes and mutation

A gene can become defective as the result of a change in the sequence of its base pairs. Such a change is known as a mutation. Some mutations cause no problems, but others can lead to disease.

Environmental agents can cause mutations by reacting chemically with DNA. These agents include asbestos, tars in tobacco smoke, certain insecticides, viruses, X rays, and ultraviolet radiation from the sun. Mutations can also result from errors that occur when a cell replicates.

Normal gene   Mutated gene

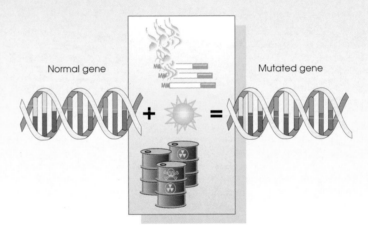

too much or too little of a protein, or to make the protein at the wrong time. Each type of error can lead to a genetic disease.

What causes mutations

There are two major causes of genetic mutations. The first occurs in the DNA-replicating or copying process that takes place whenever a cell divides. Cells are constantly dividing as our bodies grow or as our bodies replace aged or damaged cells. During DNA replication, the two strands of the DNA ladder split apart, and proteins inside the cell assemble a new half for each strand. Two copies of the original DNA molecule result, with one copy staying in the old cell and the other going to the new cell. Occasionally, a mistake occurs and the wrong base is added to one of the new DNA strands. Although there are "quality control" proteins that look out for such glitches and try to repair them, these proteins, too, can err.

The other source of genetic mutations is damage by something in the environment. Damage to DNA can be caused by chemicals in cigarette smoke, certain insecticides, viruses, and radiation such as X rays or ultraviolet light from the sun.

Mutations and genetic inheritance

However a genetic mutation arises, the consequences depend on the type of cell involved. Most of an organism's cells are *somatic* (body) cells that make up skin, muscle, bone, nerves, and various organs. Mutations in body cells can lead to a disease such as cancer. But the mutations in body cells cannot be passed on to children.

For a mutation to be inherited, it must arise in a sex cell. If a mutation occurs in a sex cell, it may become incorporated in the DNA of a sperm or egg. In this case, the mutation may cause disease in a child created from the sperm or egg. However, the mutation probably will not affect the parent, because most of the genes in a sperm or an egg are inactive until fertilization takes place.

A child will not necessarily develop a disease as the result of inheriting a harmful mutation. This is be-

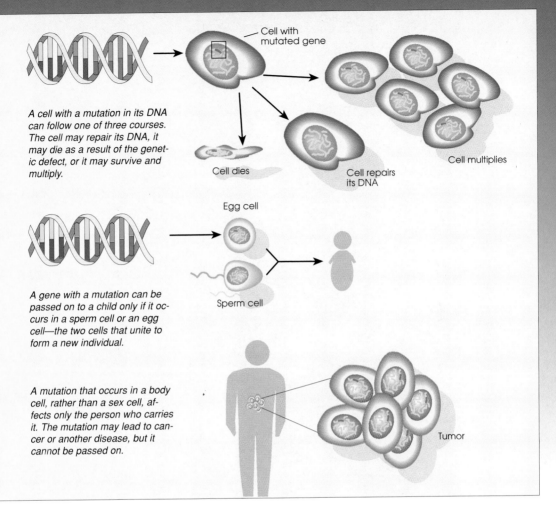

A cell with a mutation in its DNA can follow one of three courses. The cell may repair its DNA, it may die as a result of the genetic defect, or it may survive and multiply.

Cell with mutated gene

Cell dies

Cell repairs its DNA

Cell multiplies

A gene with a mutation can be passed on to a child only if it occurs in a sperm cell or an egg cell—the two cells that unite to form a new individual.

Egg cell

Sperm cell

A mutation that occurs in a body cell, rather than a sex cell, affects only the person who carries it. The mutation may lead to cancer or another disease, but it cannot be passed on.

Tumor

cause, in most cases, a child inherits two copies of a gene, one from each parent. If one copy of the gene is normal, it may produce sufficient copies of the normal protein to keep the person healthy.

Recessive and dominant diseases

Certain hereditary disorders do not develop unless a child inherits mutations in both copies of a gene. Diseases that require two flawed copies of a single gene are called recessive. Recessive genetic diseases include sickle cell anemia and cystic fibrosis (CF), characterized by abnormally thick mucus in the lungs and intestines.

Usually, a recessive disease gene is passed on to a child without consequence, because the other parent contributes a normal gene. Only when two people with the same abnormal recessive gene produce a child does the child have a possibility of inheriting the disease. Even then, the child may still inherit a normal copy of the gene if one or both parents have a normal as well as a recessive disease gene.

Rarer than recessive genetic diseases are so-

called dominant diseases. In dominant diseases, possessing a single copy of the defective gene is enough to cause illness. Huntington's disease, a fatal, progressive deterioration of the nervous system, is a dominant disease.

Sex-linked defects

A recessive disease gene can act like a dominant gene in one instance: when the recessive gene is located on the X chromosome. The X chromosome is one of two sex chromosomes that determine an individual's gender. The other is the Y chromosome. Females have two X chromosomes; males, one X and one Y.

Genetic mutations located on the X chromosome are called sex-linked defects, and the diseases they cause arise much more often in males than they do in females. Examples of sex-linked conditions include hemophilia, a disease in which the blood fails to clot, and Duchenne muscular dystrophy (DMD), a muscle disorder.

Because males have one X chromosome, a male

who inherits a defective recessive X-linked gene always gets the disease. In a female, the recessive X-linked gene is usually paired with a normal gene on the other X chromosome.

In any human female cell, however, one X chromosome is inactivated, though which X chromosome it is occurs randomly. The defective recessive gene is therefore expressed in about half of a female's cells. As a result, she may show symptoms of the disease, but they will usually be less serious than those in males.

Inheritance and environment

Some diseases may result from a combination of an inherited tendency to develop the disorder and genetic mutations caused by any number of factors in the environment. Certain cancers may be examples of such diseases.

Many people who get cancer acquire all the necessary mutations through exposure to *carcinogens* (cancer-promoting substances) in the environment, such as asbestos and radioactive materials. However, people can also be genetically *predisposed* (in-

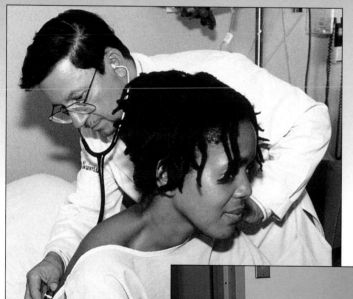

Sickle cell anemia

A doctor examines a patient who may have sickle cell anemia, a hereditary blood disease that mainly affects people of African ancestry. It results from a defect in the gene that carries the instructions for hemoglobin, the protein that transports oxygen in the blood. About 1 in 12 American blacks carries the gene, and about 1 in 600 develops the disease, in which deformed blood cells block small blood vessels, causing pain, fever, and sometimes stroke.

Cystic fibrosis

A physician tests the sweat on the arms of a youngster suspected of having cystic fibrosis (CF), a genetic disorder that involves the production of abnormally thick mucus. People with CF also have salty sweat. CF is the most common hereditary disease among whites in America. About 1 in 22 carries the gene, and 1 in 2,000 develops the disease.

How genetic defects lead to disease

Genes contain the instructions that a cell uses in the production of proteins—molecules that are essential to the cell's structure and functioning. A gene with damaged DNA may result in an abnormal protein or no protein at all. Malfunctioning proteins are the underlying cause of genetic diseases.

Normal gene

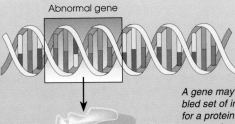

Normal protein

A normal gene produces a normal protein.

Abnormal gene

Abnormal protein

A gene may carry a garbled set of instructions for a protein. The resulting protein may not be able to carry out its usual tasks as well, or at all.

Missing gene

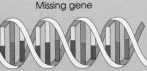

No protein

A gene may be absent entirely. If the cell is missing both copies of the gene, it cannot produce any of the protein.

Extra copies of gene

Too much protein

Extra copies of a gene may cause the cell to produce too much of the protein. The excess protein can overwhelm the cell.

clined) toward developing cancer. These people may inherit mutations in key genes, or they may be born with a heightened vulnerability to the effects of new mutations. Consequently, only one or two more mutations are needed for them to develop cancer.

Alternately, people may possess a mutated gene that is inactive. A nongenetic factor, such as a nutrient in the diet or a chemical in cigarette smoke, may activate the gene and lead to the disease. Researchers have found that certain fats, for example, may play a role in the development of colon cancer.

Cancer and genes that control cell growth

In cancer, cells grow and divide uncontrollably. Because cell growth is a complex process that involves many proteins, scientists suspect that the development of cancer requires mutations in several genes and that these mutations accumulate in a cell one by one over the course of many cell divisions.

Researchers have discovered two major classes of genes that play a role in cancer. One class regulates cell growth. Mutated versions of these genes free cells from the normal controls on cell growth and lead them to form rapidly growing masses called tumors.

The second class of genes normally stops tumors that have begun to grow by coding for the production of proteins that halt unchecked cell growth. If these tumor suppressor genes become defective as a result of a mutation, there is nothing to stop a tumor from growing.

Cancer and "quality-control" genes

Other genes can lead to cancer in an indirect way. In 1993 and 1994, researchers identified two genes involved in hereditary colon cancer. Normal versions of these genes code for some of the quality-control proteins that help guard against errors during DNA replication.

In people who inherit defective copies of these quality-control genes, errors appear in replicated DNA at a much higher rate than usual. People with mutated versions of these DNA-repair genes therefore stand a better chance of developing cancer-causing mutations in cells in their colon tissue and perhaps in other organs.

Many diseases other than cancer appear to involve genetic predispositions of some sort. Scientists in 1994 were looking for genetic components of disorders such as heart disease, *hypertension* (high blood pressure), depression, and alcoholism.

Genetic medicine:
The next revolution

The practice of medicine has undergone several revolutionary changes in the past 150 years. In the mid-1800's, the discovery of anesthetics allowed surgeons to perform longer and more complex operations. Before then, the mark of surgical skill lay in how fast a surgeon could amputate an arm or a leg. The discovery that microorganisms cause infections led to the development of antiseptic surgical practices in the late 1800's and early 1900's, which not only reduced the number of deaths from infected wounds but also ushered in an era of more sophisticated, life-saving operations.

In the 1940's and 1950's, new drugs brought about another revolution in treatment. Antibiotics routinely cured people of bacterial infections that would otherwise have killed them. Vaccines conquered viral infections ranging from polio to measles. But until the 1970's, there was no way that doctors could cure or even effectively treat many of the diseases resulting from defects in genes.

When genetic engineering techniques became available in the 1970's, the possibility of treating genetic diseases at their source took on a new reality. But first, scientists seized upon the power of recombinant-DNA technology to manufacture unlimited amounts of human proteins for use in treating disease. These genetically engineered drugs would be exactly like proteins in the human body.

Drugs from natural proteins

Most proteins are produced by the body in very small amounts and only by certain cells. But researchers developed biological factories for producing huge quantities of a particular protein. They began by creating *clones* (exact copies) of the gene responsible for directing the production of the protein. With molecules called restriction enzymes that act as biochemical scissors, the researchers cut out a particular gene from a piece of human DNA (deoxyribonucleic acid, the molecule of which genes are made). They then spliced that gene into the genetic material of a bacterium, yeast, or other fast-growing cell. When the fast-growing cell reproduced, the gene was reproduced along with it. At biotechnology companies, the cells could be grown in large vats and the desired human protein harvested.

And the harvest has proved to be a rich one. Among the genetically engineered drugs available by 1994 were: human growth hormone, a protein used to treat hereditary dwarfism in children; human insulin, a hormone used to treat diabetes; interferon, a natural substance that helps body cells ward off viruses; tissue plasminogen activator, a biochemical that breaks up the blood clots that cause heart attacks and strokes; blood-clotting factors for hemophiliacs; and erythropoietin, a protein that stimulates the production of red blood cells in anemia patients.

Human proteins have not turned out to be the wonder drugs once anticipated, however. Proteins can have multiple—even contradictory—actions in the body. And bioengineered proteins, like other drugs, can have bad side effects. For example, in some patients, treatment with human growth hormone leads to diabetes.

Another problem is that proteins are digested by stomach acids when swallowed, so they must be injected into a patient's bloodstream. However, injection is not always the best way to deliver a protein to its destination. Consequently, biotechnology companies have begun working on more effective means for administering proteins, such as pills that can survive the digestive system, aerosols that can be inhaled, or special patches to be worn on the skin.

Genetically engineered vaccines

Along with drugs, biotechnologists have been working on the development of genetically engineered vaccines. A vaccine works by stimulating the immune system to recognize a particular bacterium, virus, or other foreign invader. A conventional vaccine consists of killed or weakened microbes responsible for a particular disease, such as measles or polio. The killed or weakened organism cannot cause the disease, but when it is injected into a person, the immune system recognizes identifying proteins on the surface of the microbe and produces antibodies to immobilize and help kill it. Then, if the natural microbe invades, the immune system is primed to respond quickly, before the germ can multiply and cause disease.

Researchers are trying to develop vaccines that contain only the identifying proteins found on the surface of disease-causing organisms. A vaccine that does not contain a whole virus, for example, cannot accidentally cause a full-blown case of the disease. It might also be possible to splice genes for the identifying surface proteins of a number of viruses into the genetic material of a large, harmless virus to create one vaccine that could confer immunity against several diseases at one shot.

Moreover, genetic engineering techniques might solve the problem of creating vaccines against or-

The genetic revolution begins

During the 1970's, scientists developed the tools of genetic engineering, which enable them to manipulate individual genes. In a technique called gene splicing, they use rapidly multiplying organisms such as bacteria to churn out multiple copies of human genes and the proteins for which the genes code (carry the instructions).

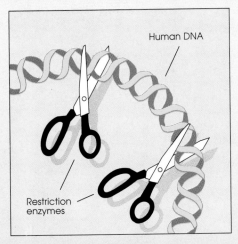

Chemical scissors called restriction enzymes are used to cut out a segment of human DNA with the desired gene.

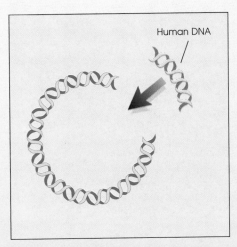

Restriction enzymes also cut open a small ring of bacterial DNA, into which the human DNA is spliced.

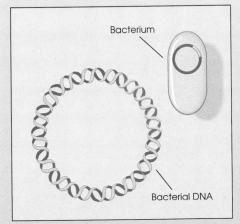

The genetically engineered rings are reinserted into bacteria. The bacteria make proteins from all the genes on the ring, including the human gene.

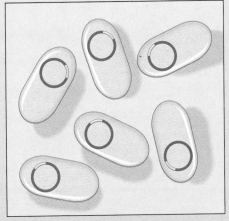

In a short time, there are millions of bacteria, each producing the human protein. Scientists can harvest the protein and give it to patients who are unable to produce the protein themselves.

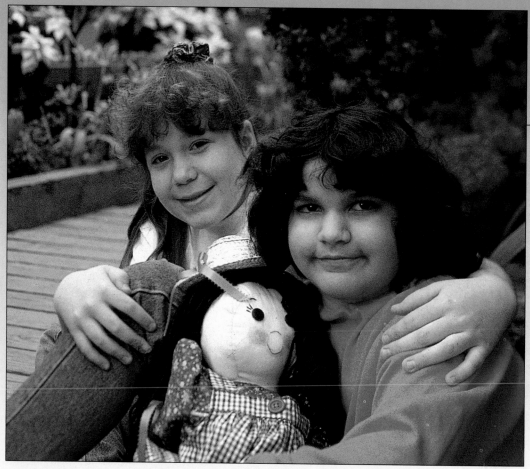

Cynthia Cutshall, left, and Ashanthi DeSilva were the first people to be treated with gene therapy in the early 1990's. Both girls received infusions of white blood cells carrying a gene that their bodies lacked. The experimental therapy treated a rare disorder of the immune system, adenosine deaminase (ADA) deficiency.

ganisms that mutate rapidly, such as the influenza virus or the virus that causes AIDS. If scientists can find a surface protein that remains the same throughout many mutations, they could clone the gene for that protein, which would always be recognized by the immune system, and create an effective, long-lasting vaccine.

Such efforts may one day provide a vaccine against certain forms of cancer. Scientists realized in the early 1990's that many cancers involve mutant forms of a gene named p53. This is a tumor suppressor gene that is responsible for directing the production of a protein that stops the uncontrolled growth of cells.

A defective p53 gene produces an abnormal protein that cannot do the job of suppressing tumor growth. Some researchers are trying to use the abnormal p53 protein as a cancer vaccine, hoping that injections of it will alert the body's defense system and "teach" it to seek out and destroy any body cells

that turn cancerous and begin making a similar mutated p53 protein.

Replacing defective genes

The development of bioengineered drugs and vaccines is one aim of genetic medicine. But a bigger quest is the treatment of genetic diseases using not the protein products of genes but the genes themselves. Gene therapy—replacing defective genes with good genes—was first undertaken in 1990.

The experiment involved a 4-year-old girl who suffered from an inherited disorder called adenosine deaminase (ADA) deficiency, in which a defective ADA protein leaves the immune system defenseless against infections. Researchers at the National Institutes of Health (NIH) in Bethesda, Md., decided to treat the girl with normal copies of the ADA gene.

From a sample of her blood, the researchers filtered out the white blood cells—the cells that normally fight infection. In the laboratory, they spliced a copy of the normal human ADA gene into the DNA of a harmless mouse virus, then infected the girl's white blood cells with the virus.

They hoped that the virus would carry the ADA gene into the DNA of some of the white blood cells, which they then returned to the girl's blood. One year later, they reported that the girl's immune system was producing ADA and fending off infection better. The therapy was a success.

The field of genetic medicine exploded after the ADA trial. By 1994, more than 50 other gene therapy trials in human beings had been approved worldwide. The experiments targeted a wide range of ills, including cystic fibrosis, heart ailments, and cancers.

Keeping gene transplants functioning

Early gene therapy researchers confronted a major problem, however. Their experiments did not provide a lasting cure. For example, the young girl who received the ADA therapy had to receive new infusions of modified white blood cells every few months as the older cells died. Scientists needed to find some way of getting the new genes into the body and of ensuring that the genes continued to function.

Scientists wondered if the solution might be found in stem cells. These are long-lived cells in bone marrow that give rise to many generations of blood cells of all types. The researchers theorized that genetically altered stem cells might supply the girl with healthy white blood cells for the rest of her life. In late 1993, doctors began treating the girl with stem cells that had been given the normal ADA gene. The therapy's outcome was not yet clear in mid-1994.

The first lasting gene therapy success was reported in April 1994. It involved a woman suffering from a genetic disorder called familial hypercholesterolemia (FH). Because of defects in both copies of a particular gene, the woman's liver cells lacked cholesterol receptors, surface proteins that remove cholesterol from the blood. The missing receptors meant that fatty deposits coated the walls of her arteries. The build-up was so severe that the woman had suffered a heart attack at age 16 and underwent coronary artery bypass surgery at 26. At age 28, already past the typical life expectancy for FH patients, the woman turned to an untried gene therapy.

Physicians at the University of Michigan in Ann Arbor removed a portion of the woman's liver in 1992. As in the ADA gene therapy, they used a harmless virus to insert normal copies of the cholesterol receptor gene into the liver cells. They then injected the altered cells through a vein that nourished the woman's liver. The researchers hoped that some of the cells would settle in the liver and begin producing the missing protein.

In 1994, two years after the surgery, the doctors reported that the woman's cholesterol levels had fallen by 20 percent and were remaining steady at that level. Scientists could not predict whether the drop was significant enough to protect the woman from further heart disease. Nevertheless, the experiment clearly marked a milestone for gene therapy. A single gene therapy operation had resulted in a seemingly permanent improvement in a patient's condition.

New gene delivery methods needed

Despite these early triumphs, researchers agree that new techniques must be developed before gene therapy becomes widespread. For example, improvement is needed in the means for delivering normal genes to a patient. In most gene therapy trials, researchers have used mouse viruses to carry copies of the human genes. The researchers first altered the DNA of the viruses so that they could not cause disease or even reproduce. However, the viruses still possessed the ability to invade cells and insert their DNA into the cell's chromosomes.

Although such viruses made the first steps in gene therapy possible, scientists do not consider them ideal gene carriers for several reasons. First, they infect only certain types of cells, and even then, they infect at a low rate. Second, they insert their genes at random in a human cell's chromosomes. However, the location of a gene is important to its proper expression, so inserted genes do not tend to work as well as naturally inherited copies. Finally, because the viruses are not selective about where they insert their DNA, they may inadvertently damage properly working genes in the cell.

Because of these problems, researchers are exploring other ways of carrying genes into cells. For example, a University of Michigan team has encased genes inside tiny balls of fat that they think might carry the genes into the cell nucleus. The genes code for a protein that stimulates the immune system to attack cancer cells. Although the therapy has not achieved a cure, the gene did enter the DNA of four of five patients treated for a deadly form of skin cancer. In one patient, the skin tumors stopped growing and several tumors disappeared.

In 1993, several research teams began to tackle cystic fibrosis (CF) using common cold viruses as gene carriers. The researchers chose cold viruses because they are naturally equipped to invade cells of the airway lining, where thick mucus builds up in CF patients and makes breathing difficult. The researchers spliced healthy versions of the CF gene into the DNA of genetically crippled cold viruses, then sprayed the viruses directly into the nasal passage and lungs of CF patients. The transferred gene has caused cells to produce a protein the patients lack, but by mid-1994, the gene had remained in place for only a few days.

Gene therapy for other diseases

Other experiments in gene therapy have been aimed not at inherited disorders but at cancer and infectious diseases such as AIDS. In these cases, the goal was not to replace a missing or defective protein but to supply more of a protein that might help stop the cancer or boost the immune system.

Researchers at the National Cancer Institute (NCI) in Bethesda, Md., were trying to provoke an immune system response that would destroy cancerous tumors. In one experiment, they removed cancer cells from a patient and added to them extra genes for a protein called tumor necrosis factor (TNF). TNF stimulates the immune system into attacking cancer cells. The researchers then injected the TNF-loaded cells back into the patient's tumor. No results from the experiment had been published by mid-1994.

Probing for defective genes

Genetic engineering techniques have also enabled medical researchers to locate disease-causing genes, develop diagnostic tests for genetic diseases, and develop genetic tests for abnormal genes in a person's DNA before they cause harm. This is accomplished using gene probes, segments of DNA that have been tagged with a radioactive compound or a special dye. The gene probes will attach to DNA at or near a defective gene.

To conduct a genetic test, doctors take a blood sample and then extract DNA from some of the cells. The DNA sample can be mixed with a chemical that causes the two strands of the molecule to "unzip," and the probe is added to the mixture. If the DNA sample contains the defective gene, the probe will attach to the DNA strand. The probes tagged with dyes or radioactivity can then be detected.

Genetic tests have been developed for a number of disorders. Disorders for which genetic tests were available by 1994 included cystic fibrosis, Duchenne muscular dystrophy, FH, hemophilia, Huntington's disease, and phenylketonuria, which causes mental retardation unless treated during infancy.

The rise of genetic screening

Many expectant parents request genetic testing for their unborn child. The doctor extracts some of the amniotic fluid from the mother's womb, then genetically analyzes cells that have flaked off from the fetus into the fluid. In 1994, about 325 genetic diseases could be detected prenatally.

Genetic testing can also be used to screen for adult carriers of genetic diseases. A carrier is a person who has one copy of a recessive disease gene. To inherit a recessive disease, a child needs to inherit two defective copies of the disease gene, one from each parent. The aim of genetic screening is to determine whether a man and a woman are both carriers for a disease and thus whether any children they had would be at risk for inheriting the disease.

Increasingly, adults are turning to genetic screening and counseling before they make decisions about childbearing, especially in families already afflicted by inherited disease. The goal of screening for these individuals is to find out whether both potential parents are carriers of the defective gene, and thus whether their children will be at risk.

One of earliest voluntary screening programs in the United States was set up to test and counsel people of eastern European Jewish ancestry who are more likely than most of the population to carry a gene for Tay-Sachs disease, a fatal disorder of the nervous system. Carrier screening for Tay-Sachs since the 1970's has reduced the incidence of that disease twentyfold.

For some genetic diseases, such as the fatal brain disorder Huntington's disease, there is no uncertainty about the fate of people who inherit the gene. But with other disorders, people who know their vulnerabilities have greater control over their fate.

For example, people born with a defective cholesterol-scavenging gene could still reduce their risk of heart disease by eating a low-fat diet, receiving regular drug treatment, and not smoking. Preventive health care and lifestyle changes could also benefit people with genes predisposing them toward such problems as diabetes, high blood pressure, and various types of cancer. With proper counseling and education, many doctors and other experts say, genetic screening may someday help prevent many of today's common health problems.

Correcting genetic abnormalities

Scientists are searching for safe, effective ways of giving patients copies of new genes that produce normal proteins. One method uses viruses to carry new genes into cells. Researchers are using this method to replace a faulty gene in white blood cells of children with an immune system disorder.

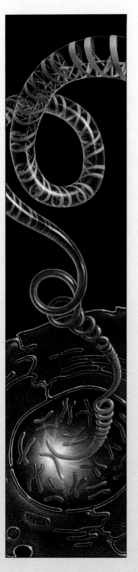

Blood is taken from the patient. The white blood cells are extracted and grown in a dish in a laboratory.

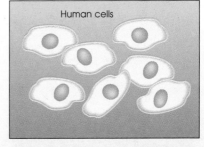

Human cells

A normal copy of the faulty gene is spliced into the DNA of a harmless virus.

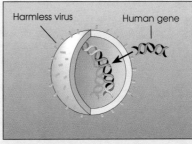

Harmless virus   Human gene

The genetically engineered viruses are mixed with the patient's white blood cells in the laboratory, and the viruses enter the cells.

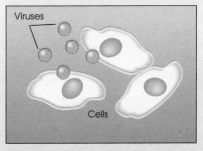

Viruses

Cells

The viruses transfer copies of the human gene into the DNA of the patient's white blood cells. These cells are then injected back into the patient, where they produce the missing immune system protein.

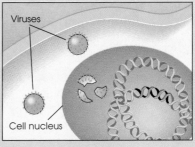

Viruses

Cell nucleus

Mapping our genes

Genetic researchers in the mid-1980's conceived a bold vision: a "map" of the human genome. Such a map would ultimately display the order of the 3 billion base pairs—chemical subunits—of DNA (deoxyribonucleic acid), the molecule of which human genes are made. Information about the order of base pairs, which scientists refer to as the DNA sequence, would be very useful to medical researchers trying to understand the mechanisms that underlie genetic diseases.

Every gene is made up of a particular DNA sequence, and this sequence *codes for* (directs the production of) a particular protein. Most genetic diseases are caused by errors in the production of proteins. These errors can result in missing proteins, malfunctioning proteins, or too many proteins. The DNA sequence of a gene indicates the chemical makeup of the protein the gene codes for, and this information, in turn, provides clues about the protein's function in the body. Learning about the role of a protein is vital to understanding how a defective version of the protein can lead to disease.

The DNA sequence of a normal gene can also help scientists hunt for defective copies of the gene in a sample of DNA. By isolating the defective genes, scientists can compare their DNA sequences with the sequence of the normal gene to learn what *mutations* (changes) have taken place in the gene. From that step, scientists can proceed to investigate how the mutations alter the structure and function of the normal protein.

Finally, a genome map could help scientists look for patterns of abnormalities among disease-causing genes. For example, in 1993, researchers isolated the gene whose defective form is responsible for Huntington's disease, an incurable disorder of the brain and nervous system. They learned that both the normal and defective versions of the gene contain a sequence of three base pairs repeated over and over, and that the versions that lead to Huntington's disease contain even more repeats than do the normal genes.

Scientists are not sure how the extra *codons* (three-base sequences) lead to illness, but the pattern has been spotted in other disease-causing genes, and some scientists now suspect that codon repetition may be a feature of many genes. A map of the human genome would help scientists test this idea by identifying other genes that have a sequence of repeated codons. The genes could then be analyzed to see whether they, too, become harmful when the number of repeated codons increases.

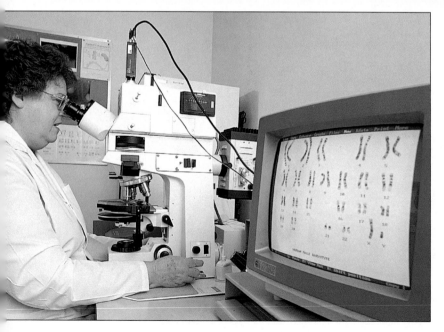

Gene detective
A medical researcher views the chromosomes from a single white blood cell, arranged with a computer according to a standard classification system. Staining with special chemicals makes banding patterns on the chromosomes visible when viewed under high-power magnification. The researcher studies these patterns for any abnormalities that could signal the presence of a genetic disease.

Spurred by the potential benefits of a human genome map, scientists acted quickly to turn the dream into a reality. In 1989, the National Research Council, an advisory body to the U.S. government, concluded that it would be possible to map the human genome in only 15 years at a cost of about $3-billion. Encouraged by this report, the NIH and the U.S. Department of Energy launched the Human Genome Project for American scientists in 1990. Since then, Japan, Russia, and the 12-nation European Community have undertaken similar projects. The worldwide mapping efforts are being coordinated by a privately funded group called the Human Genome Organization. The target date for completion of the project is the year 2005.

The first gene maps

The Human Genome Project, however, was not the first gene-mapping effort. The first gene maps, called chromosomal banding maps, were produced in the early 1970's. The human genome is not packed onto a single stand of DNA but is instead packaged on structures called chromosomes, located in the cell nucleus. Human beings have 46 chromosomes.

When cells are dividing, chromosomes are visible under the microscope. And scientists discovered that certain chemical strains create dark and light bands on chromosomes. They combined this staining technique with studies of disease-inheritance patterns in families. By studying inheritance patterns, geneticists knew that if two genes are on different chromosomes, they will be inherited independently. However, if two genes lie on the same chromosome, they may tend to be inherited together. The closer together the two genes are, the less chance that they will be separated during the formation of an egg cell or a sperm cell, when pairs of chromosomes line up and exchange pieces.

The inheritance pattern of a pair of genes therefore sheds light on whether the genes reside on the same chromosome and, if so, how far apart they are. By comparing normal banding patterns with banding patterns on chromosomes of people with an inherited disease, researchers could sometimes determine the location of abnormal or missing bands on a chromosome. But the technique of mapping genes based on inheritance patterns was time-consuming. By the mid-1970's, only about 150 human genes had been traced to specific chromosomes.

Then in 1978, biologists David Botstein of Massachusetts Institute of Technology in Cambridge and

Ronald Davis of Stanford University in California came up with an innovation in gene mapping. Along each chromosome, they identified hundreds of sites they called physical markers. These were sequences of DNA where restriction enzymes—proteins that act as chemical scissors—cut. There are many kinds of restriction enzymes, but each will make a cut only at a specific DNA sequence.

Making genetic-linkage maps

Botstein and Davis reasoned that because everyone's DNA is unique, some of the DNA cutting sites for restriction enzymes would differ from one person to another. Thus, each person's chromosomes could yield a distinctive assortment of DNA fragments when treated with restriction enzymes. Scientists further reasoned that unusual cutting sites might lie close to a defective gene. This proved to be true. An individual from a family with an inherited disorder will also inherit an unusual cutting site, or marker. Scientists searching for a disease-causing gene can now compare DNA fragments from people who have the disease with fragments from healthy people. A DNA cutting site that appears only among people with the disease can be a sign that a mutated gene is close by. Maps showing where disease-gene markers are located on chromosomes are used to make what are called genetic-linkage maps.

Sequencing the DNA in the human genome involves the creation of both genetic-linkage maps and a kind of genetic map called a physical map. While a genetic-linkage map of markers is pieced together as scientists look for particular genes, the physical map of the entire human genome involves determining the location and function of every single gene by looking at DNA. But it would be impossible to start at the beginning of a DNA strand and sequence the genes in order. There is far too much DNA for that. Instead, genetic researchers are cutting up chromosomes into ever-smaller pieces and then putting them back together in their proper order.

Making physical maps

Creating this physical map has been compared to piecing together a complicated puzzle. First, with the help of restriction enzymes, scientists cut human chromosomes into thousands of overlapping pieces. They then use the overlapping pieces to figure out the order of the pieces along the chromosomes. This is similar to cutting up two copies of a newspaper into tiny pieces of sentence fragments. If both copies were cut in the same way, it would be impossible to piece the sentences together. But if all the pieces were cut at different places, the overlapping fragments of sentences could be pieced together again.

After each successful round of DNA cutting and reassembly, the pieces of DNA are broken into smaller and smaller bits. Eventually, the pieces will consist of small segments of DNA that will be sequenced by machine.

Since 1990, geneticists have been making steady progress on both the genetic linkage and the physical maps. Researchers expected to have identified about 5,000 genetic markers along human chromosomes by the end of 1994. And in late 1993, French researchers unveiled the first rough physical map of all human chromosomes. To speed the task of detailed mapping, the researchers were using genetic engineering techniques to make copies of their DNA fragments for any scientists who wanted them.

A controversial project

Despite the advantages of a human genome map, the project has had its share of controversy. One source of concern is the project's price tag. At $3-billion, the Human Genome Project is the costliest venture ever undertaken by biologists. Many scientists oppose this move toward "big science." They fear that it will siphon funding from smaller laboratories and stifle independent research.

Proponents of the project counter that a human genome map would be a monumental scientific achievement. In addition to aiding in the treatment of disease, some biologists believe that such a map might lead to a better understanding how embryos develop, how the brain works, and why people grow up and eventually age. It may, they say, even shed light on how life itself began and evolved. The cost is negligible, proponents say, in light of the map's potential contribution to basic biological knowledge and eventual impact on medicine and human health.

Locating disease genes
A chromosome map displays the 23 pairs of chromosomes in a human cell and represents the rough location of genes or sequences of genes as bands across the chromosome. Knowing a gene's location helps gene-hunters close in on the gene itself and identify mutations that can lead to disease. An international effort to locate the 50,000 to 100,0000 genes that human chromosomes carry was underway in 1994.

Hemophilia
Blood defect making it difficult to control hemorrhaging

Neurofibromatosis, Type 2
Tumors of the auditory nerves and tissues surrounding the brain

Down Syndrome
Congenital mental deficiency condition marked by three copies of chromosome 21

Amyotrophic Lateral Sclerosis*
(Lou Gehrig's Disease)
Fatal degenerative disorder of the nervous system

ADA Immune Deficiency
Severe susceptibility to infections. First hereditary condition treated by gene therapy

Familial Hypercholesterolemia
Extremely high cholesterol

Myotonic Dystrophy
Frequent form of adult muscular dystrophy

Amyloidosis
Accumulation of a protein in the tissues

Breast Cancer*
5% to 10% of tumors in breasts

Polycystic Kidney Disease
Cysts resulting in enlarged kidneys and renal failure

Tay-Sachs Disease
Fatal hereditary disorder involving metabolism of fats

Alzheimer's Disease*
Degenerative disorder of the nervous system

Muscular Dystrophy
(Duchenne and Becker types)
Progressive deterioration of the muscles

ALD (adrenoleukodystrophy)
Nerve disease portrayed in movie *Lorenzo's Oil*

Gaucher's Disease
A chronic enzyme deficiency

Familial Colon Cancer*
One in 200 people has this gene; of those, 65% are likely to develop the disease

Retinitis Pigmentosa*
Progressive degeneration of the retina

Huntington's Disease
Degenerative disorder of the nervous system

Familial Polyposis of the Colon
Abnormal tissue growths frequently leading to cancer

Hemochromatosis
Abnormally high absorption of iron from the diet

Spinocerebellar Ataxia
Destroys nerves in the brain and spinal cord, resulting in loss of muscle control

Cystic Fibrosis
Mucus fills up the lungs, interfering with breathing

Multiple Exostoses*
A disorder of cartilage and bone

Malignant Melanoma
Tumors originating in the skin

Multiple Endocrine Neoplasia, Type 2
Tumors in endocrine glands and other tissues

Sickle Cell Anemia
Chronic inherited anemia in which red blood cells sickle, or form crescents, plugging small blood vessels

Retinoblastoma
A tumor of the eye

PKU (phenylketonuria)
An inborn error of metabolism that frequently results in mental retardation

*** Gene responsible for only some cases.**

X Y 1 2 3 4 5 6 7 8 9 10 11 12 13 14 15 16 17 18 19 20 21 22

CHROMOSOME PAIRS

Ethical issues

From the time genetic engineering techniques were developed in the 1970's, people have worried about the consequences of this new technology. At first, the concerns centered on basic safety issues. What if a harmful gene was spliced into a common organism and accidentally set loose to infect the general population? Although in 1976 the National Institutes of Health established laboratory standards for preventing the escape of microorganisms, it became clear that gene splicing was not as dangerous as had once been feared.

By the 1990's, concerns involving recombinant DNA technology had shifted to social and ethical issues. Along with the scientists who are decoding genes, many other groups, including government policymakers, insurance companies, and parents, have an interest in the discoveries. Moreover, the interests of these groups could in the future clash with the interests of society at large.

Genetic screening tests can determine if people carry genes for diseases that might endanger their children. These tests also can determine if a newborn or an unborn child has inherited the gene.

Genetic tests

Selected tests available in 1994
Adult polycystic kidney disease
Cystic fibrosis
Duchenne muscular dystrophy
Fragile X syndrome
Gaucher's disease
Hemophilia
Huntington's disease
Phenylketonuria
Retinoblastoma
Sickle cell anemia
Tay-Sachs disease

Potential future tests
Atherosclerosis
Dyslexia
Familial Alzheimer's disease
Hypertension
Manic-depressive illness
Multiple sclerosis
Rheumatoid arthritis
Schizophrenia
Type I diabetes
Ulcerative colitis

Ethics and genetic screening

Most of the potential conflicts center on genetic screening—the use of tests to determine whether people carry harmful or potentially harmful genes that have not yet manifested themselves in the form of genetic diseases. One day it may be possible for geneticists to create a complete map of a newborn's genes or to test for a host of faulty genes that may predispose the child toward developing specific illnesses later in life. Steps might then be taken to reduce the risks for this disease. Adults could also undergo genetic screening as tests for particular diseases become available.

So far genetic testing has been largely a voluntary and private decision. In an era of concern over health care costs, however, society has an interest in preventing and treating diseases with high financial and societal impacts, such as heart disease and cancer. This raises a number of difficult questions. Should government pay to provide testing, counseling, and preventive treatment for such conditions? The cost of treating a disease is usually lower if the disease is spotted early. Therefore, should testing be mandatory?

Opponents of mandatory screening say that the decision should rest with the individual. They maintain that forcing people to undergo genetic screening would be an invasion of privacy that could never be justified by a projected savings in health care costs. With genetic tests becoming increasingly available and concerns over the costs of health care continuing to be a major issue, such questions may soon rise to the forefront of public debate.

Genetic screening may also present expectant parents with difficult decisions. Scientists have learned how to detect certain genetic defects in a fetus, and this disturbs people who say the genetic makeup of a fetus should never be a factor in deciding whether to continue a pregnancy. Other people say that parents are responsible for raising a child, so they should have control over the health of the child they choose to raise.

As genetic screening becomes more widespread, people will have to weigh the personal costs and benefits of advance knowledge about their genetic heritage. Some people who undergo genetic screening may learn that they will develop a disease that has no known cure, such as Huntington's disease. Individuals would have to consider whether knowing they would develop an incurable illness would impair their ability to function and enjoy life.

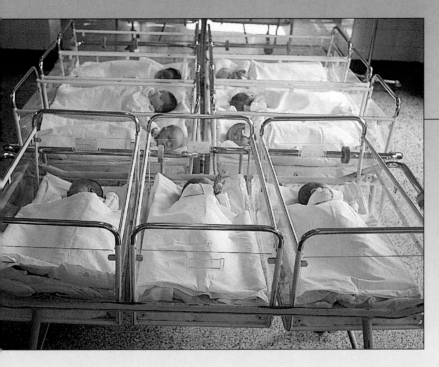

The availability of tests for more and more disease genes raises some difficult issues. Should babies be tested at birth, for example, particularly for genetic disorders for which there is no treatment?

Commercial companies are poised to offer tests for many other genetic vulnerabilities that can affect adults in the form of cancer, heart disease, kidney diseases, arthritis, and diabetes. In March 1994, however, an advisory council to the NIH asked companies to hold off making tests for genetic susceptibility to cancer widely available until certain medical, social, and legal issues can be resolved. There are questions, for example, about the accuracy of the tests. Other questions concern the age at which an individual should first be tested and who will provide counseling about the person's odds of developing the disease or about any preventive actions that the person might take.

Issues of privacy

As more and more genetic information becomes part of everyone's medical record, the pressure may increase to make some or all of this information available to health insurance and life insurance companies and even to employers. This prospect is already raising a number of ethical questions.

Since insurers base their premiums on the estimated risk of a person's developing some ailment, should insurers be allowed to reject coverage for or charge higher premiums to a person with a greater-than-average risk of heart disease, for example? And should a company be allowed to test job applicants and reject those whose genes make them more vulnerable to hazards in that particular workplace? Or could employers refuse to hire people predisposed toward heart disease, alcoholism, or mental illness? Some social observers fear the development of a "genetic underclass" of people unable to get either jobs or insurance.

Altering future generations

The area of genetics that stirs the greatest fears involves the possibility of making genetic changes that could be passed on from parents to offspring. This would require altering genes in the sex cells, the male sperm or the female egg. So far, the only human cells that have received new genes are *somatic* (body) cells, which are not involved in reproduction. In the future, however, looms the possibility of using gene therapy to permanently correct defects by making alterations to genes that will be passed from one generation to the next. While this holds the promise of ridding humanity of many terrible diseases, it also raises the specter of eugenics—the notion of improving the human species through controlled breeding. This idea gained evil notoriety in the 1930's and 1940's, when Germany's Nazi government used it to justify extreme views on "improving" the human species. Therefore, the idea of genetically altering human sex cells is very controversial.

As with all great scientific advances, the benefits of genetic medicine come at a price. The ability to repair genes carries with it the responsibility to determine when such remedies are appropriate. Ethicists say the challenge will be to improve the plight of humanity without reducing people to a DNA sequence.

The author:

Yvonne Baskin is a free-lance science writer and the author of *The Gene Doctors: Medical Genetics at the Frontier.*

Health & Medical News Update

In 40 alphabetically arranged articles, Health & Medical News Update contributors report on the year's major developments in health and medicine.

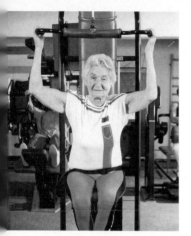

See page 240.

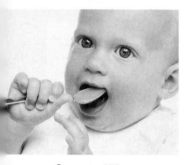

See page 273.

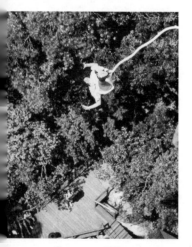

See page 295.

Aging 240
Genes and bone loss
Estrogen and Alzheimer's disease
Traffic safety

AIDS 242
AIDS research
Hemophilia and AIDS

Alcohol and Drug Abuse 246
Drug use among teens
Substance-abuse research

Allergies and Asthma 249
Asthma drugs
Treating hives

Arthritis and Connective Tissue Disorders 252
Arthritis research

Birth Control 254
Use among teen-agers
RU-486

Blood 256
Leukemia research
Thalassemia treatments
Hemophilia research

Bone Disorders 257
Genes and bone loss
Boosting bone mass

Books of Health and Medicine 259

Brain and Nervous System 261
Alzheimer's disease
Brain research

Cancer 265
Cancer research
Mammography guidelines
Close-Up:
    Prostate cancer

Child Development 271
False memories
Hyperactivity

Dentistry 275
Gum disease
New filling material

Diabetes 276
Diabetes research
Diabetes treatment

Digestive System 278
Ulcerative colitis
Cirrhosis treatment

Drugs 281
New drugs approved

Ear and Hearing 284
Tinnitus
Screening infants

Environmental Health 286
Air pollution
Questionable research
Close-Up:
    Environmental estrogens

Exercise and Fitness 290
Exercise and the heart
Preventing bone thinning

Eye and Vision 293
Nearsightedness
Cataract surgery

Genetic Medicine 297
Genes and cancer
Gene mapping

Glands and Hormones 300
Managing diabetes
Detecting thyroid cancer

Health Care Issues 302
Health care reform
Gulf War syndrome

Heart and Blood Vessels 306
Heart disease research
Treating heart disease

Infectious Diseases 310
Decline in childhood diseases
Vaccine research

Kidney 312
Diet and kidney disease
Transplants

Medical Ethics 314
Reproductive issues
Radiation experiments
Physician-assisted suicide

Mental Health 316
New drug treatments
Stress and disease
Close-Up:
    Post-traumatic stress disorder

Nutrition and Food 321
Nutrition research
Close-Up: Bovine growth hormone

Pregnancy and Childbirth 325
AIDS and pregnancy
Ultrasound screenings

Respiratory System 328
Tuberculosis
Lung cancer

Safety 330
Work-related fatalities
Infant safety
Antilock brakes

**Sexually
Transmitted Diseases** 333
Prevention program
Gonorrhea among teens
Chlamydia screening

Skin 335
Sunscreens
Psoriasis
Diet and skin cancer

Smoking 337
Health risks
Benefits of quitting
Close-Up:
    Regulating cigarettes as drugs

Stroke 342
Stroke research

Surgery 343
Breast cancer surgery
Transplants

Urology 346
Prostate cancer
Urinary tract infections

Veterinary Medicine 348
Lyme disease in dogs
Diseases from cats

Weight Control 350
Low-fat diets
Obesity and disability

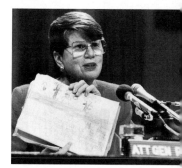

See page 302.

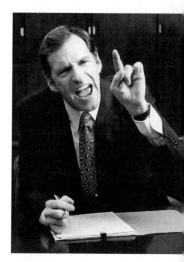

See page 308.

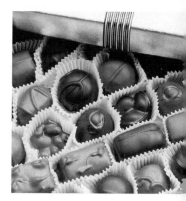

See page 321.

Genetic heritage makes some elderly women as much as four times more likely to fracture a bone than other women, according to a February 1994 study. Researchers at the Garven Institute of Medical Research in Australia showed that the strength of a woman's bones—and thus their vulnerability to fracture—is linked in part to a gene. The gene affects the activity of vitamin D within the body, and vitamin D, in turn, controls the amount of calcium absorbed by bones. Vitamin D and calcium help prevent *osteoporosis,* a condition in which bone mass diminishes, leaving the bone vulnerable to fracture.

Researchers measured the bone strength of 207 women who had reached *menopause*—the time in a woman's life when menstruation ceases. They found a strong association between low strength of bones in the spine and hip and a *mutation* (change) in the gene regulating vitamin D activity. Their findings suggest that a genetic test could identify women prone to weak bones, enabling them to receive earlier treatment with calcium, estrogen, and exercise.

Wary of CPR. Many older people, when told of their chances of surviving a heart attack, would rather not re-

Never too late
Strength training can have benefits even for people in their 80's and 90's, researchers reported in late 1993. Residents of a center for the aged in Boston increased their walking speed and their ability to climb stairs after a few weeks of lifting weights to improve strength.

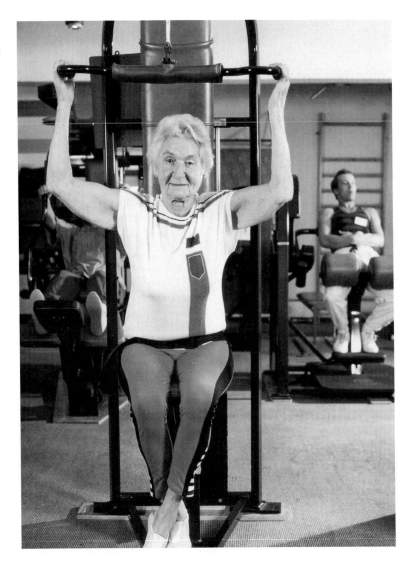

A way to drink your vitamins

Research has shown that many older people consume inadequate amounts of vitamins and minerals, either because they eat too little or because their bodies no longer absorb nutrients efficiently. Juices offer a quick, enjoyable way to add the nutritional benefits of fruits and vegetables to your diet.

Type of juice	Nutrients
Apple juice	Iron, potassium
Apricot nectar	Vitamin A, beta carotene, iron, potassium
Carrot juice	Vitamins A, C, and B_6; beta carotene; potassium; thiamine; iron; magnesium; calcium; riboflavin
Cranberry juice	Vitamin C
Grape juice	Potassium, vitamin B_6, magnesium, iron, riboflavin
Grapefruit juice	Vitamin C, folate, potassium, magnesium, thiamine
Lemonade/limeade	Vitamin C
Orange juice	Vitamin C, folate, thiamine, potassium, magnesium, niacin
Pineapple juice	Vitamins C and B_6, folate, magnesium, potassium, thiamine, iron, calcium
Prune juice	Iron, vitamins B_6 and C, potassium, niacin, riboflavin, magnesium, fiber
Tomato juice	Vitamins C, A, and B_6; folate; iron; potassium; magnesium; niacin; thiamine; fiber

Source: *Prevention Magazine's Complete Nutrition Reference Handbook.*

ceive cardiopulmonary resuscitation (CPR), especially if they are very old or chronically ill, a study reported in February 1994. Cardiopulmonary resuscitation is an emergency treatment administered to people whose breathing and heartbeat have stopped.

Researchers at a senior citizens' health care center in Denver, Colo., questioned 287 people whose average age was 77. Of this group, 41 percent said they would like to receive CPR following an acute illness. But half of them changed their minds after they were told their chances of surviving under these circumstances were very low. After learning about survival chances, only 2 of the 34 participants over age 86 said they would opt for CPR following acute illness.

Exercise can aid blood vessels.
Exercise can prevent stiffness in older people's arteries, according to a study reported in October 1993. Blood vessels must expand and contract so that blood moves through them easily. If they stiffen, as often happens with age, blood pressure is likely to rise.

Researchers at the Gerontology Research Center in Baltimore compared two groups: 146 people aged 21 to 91 who did not engage in regular aerobic exercise, and 14 men aged 54 to 75 who took part in endurance training. Arterial stiffness was about 30 percent lower in the active people than in the inactive. This suggests that regular aerobic exercise may slow age-related hardening of blood vessels and rise in blood pressure.

Bright light, good sleep. Exposure to bright light can help older people get a good night's sleep, according to an August 1993 study by researchers at Cornell University Medical College in New York City.

Sixteen people between the ages of 62 and 81 who had suffered from insomnia for at least one year were exposed to light for two hours over 12 days. Half of the participants were exposed to bright, white light and half to dim, red light. The researchers found that those exposed to the bright light showed substantial improvement (up to 90 percent) in their sleep patterns compared with the other group. Researchers believe that exposure to bright light helps reset people's internal "biological clock."

Traffic lights too brief. Don't walk, run! This, in effect, is the message older pedestrians can take from a March 1994 study by geriatrics researchers at the University of California at Los Angeles.

The researchers watched 1,200 people of all ages try to cross a busy Los Angeles intersection. All younger pedestrians got across the street before traffic signals flashed from "Walk" to "Don't Walk." But of older pedestrians, 27 percent were unable to reach the opposite curb before the signal changed. At least one-fourth of these pedestrians were stranded in traffic.

This may explain, in part, why 7,000 elderly pedestrians are killed in the United States every year. The study suggests that street crossing times should be increased, especially in areas where many older people live.

Estrogen and Alzheimer's disease. Two studies reported in December 1993 suggest that the hormone estrogen may help prevent Alzheimer's disease, a progressive deterioration of mental faculties that strikes eight times as many women as men. Women produce less and less estrogen as they age, and estrogen supplements are often prescribed to older women to prevent bone loss.

Researchers at the University of California in Los Angeles studied 253 women who were past menopause. They found that 7 percent of women who had taken estrogen supplements developed Alzheimer's disease, compared with 18 percent of the women who had not taken estrogen therapy.

In a separate study, researchers reviewed records of 2,418 women who died in southern California from 1981 to 1992. They found that those women who took estrogen supplements were 40 percent less likely to have developed Alzheimer's disease than women who had not taken the hormone. □ Rein Tideiksaar

In the Special Reports section, see COPING WITH ALZHEIMER'S DISEASE. In the Health Matters section, see WHAT YOU SHOULD KNOW ABOUT CATARACTS.

AIDS

Medical researchers worked toward a better understanding of AIDS in 1993 and 1994, but no new antiviral drugs were approved to treat AIDS, and researchers did not expect any vaccine to reach the market for at least five years. Meanwhile, the number of AIDS cases in the United States was increasing at a rate of 3 to 5 percent a year, a slower pace than the 9 percent annual growth reported as recently as 1989 by the U.S. Centers for Disease Control and Prevention (CDC) in Atlanta, Ga. At the end of 1993, the CDC had recorded a total of 361,509 cases of AIDS and 220,871 deaths due to AIDS since 1981, when the agency began tracking the disease.

In November 1993, the CDC reported that AIDS had become the leading cause of death in the United States among men aged 25 to 44. The disease ranked fourth in the causes of death among women in the same age group, surpassed only by cancer, accidents, and heart disease. For the U.S. population overall, AIDS ranked eighth among the causes of death.

The National Center for Health Statistics reported in December 1993 that an estimated 550,000 Americans are infected with the AIDS-causing HIV (human immunodeficiency virus). The actual number could lie between 300,000 and 1.02 million people. The center based its data on the National Health and Nutritional Examination Survey, an ongoing study.

Who gets AIDS. The CDC reported that homosexual and bisexual men made up the largest group with AIDS at the end of 1993 (193,162 cases). The next largest group was people who inject drugs (86,961 cases). Other groups included heterosexuals (23,038 cases) and homosexual and bisexual men who also inject drugs (23,483 cases).

AIDS and hemophilia. AIDS has reduced by 30 percent the average life span of people with hemophilia A, the most common form of the disease, according to a CDC study reported in February 1994. The researchers found that the median age at death dropped from 57 in the period 1979 to 1981 to 40 in the period 1987 to 1989. About 17,000 Americans have hemophilia A.

The blood of people with hemophilia does not clot properly, which can turn even a minor cut into a life-threatening situation. To prevent severe bleeding, people with hemophilia receive injections of a substance, derived from donated blood, that facilitates clotting. But until 1985, no screening test existed to determine whether donated blood was infected with HIV. Thus, before 1985, many people with hemophilia unknowingly became infected through contaminated blood and eventually developed AIDS.

The risk of becoming infected with HIV through a blood transfusion has been virtually eliminated by the screening of blood donations, according to the Red Cross. But because a lengthy period usually elapses between becoming infected by the virus and the onset of AIDS, the researchers said that the trend of reduced life spans will probably continue for the remainder of the 1990's.

Longer life brings other ills. Studies in 1994 showed that AIDS patients on average live about one year longer today than they did in the early years of the epidemic. Longevity varies widely, but the CDC's earlier estimate was that about half of all AIDS patients died within one year of diagnosis. The lengthened life span is largely a result of effective drug treatments for an AIDS-related respiratory illness called *Pneumocystis carinii* pneumonia (PCP), which afflicts about 80 percent of people with AIDS.

Longer life has given AIDS patients a greater risk of developing one of three cancers associated with AIDS, according to a study by Alexandra Levine, a hematologist at the University of Southern California School of Medicine in Los Angeles. Levine's study, reported in September 1993, found that about 40 percent of people infected with HIV develop severe or fatal cases of Kaposi's sarcoma, non-Hodgkin's lymphoma, or cervical carcinoma. Levine expected the incidence of these cancers to rise as survival rates for HIV-infected people

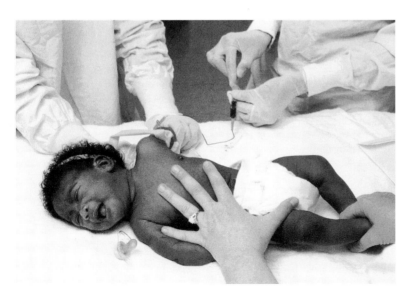

Preventing infant AIDS
An infant born to an HIV-infected mother receives an injection of AZT, a drug used to treat AIDS. Preliminary study data indicate that by taking AZT during pregnancy, an HIV-infected woman may reduce by two-thirds the chances of her baby becoming infected. Babies in the study continued to receive AZT for six weeks after birth.

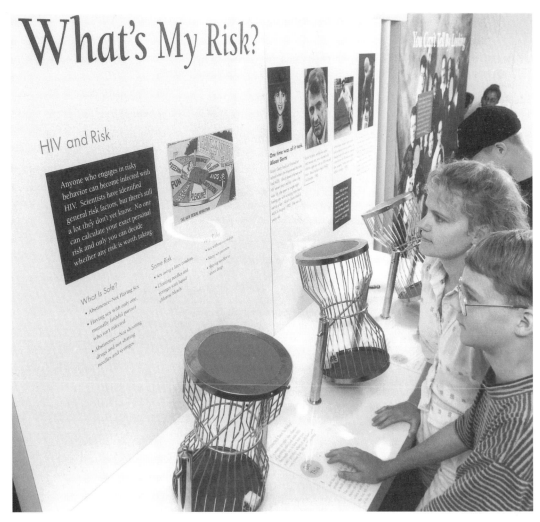

Within the image:

What's My Risk?

HIV and Risk

Anyone who engages in risky behavior can become infected with HIV. Scientists have identified general risk factors, but there's still a lot they don't yet know. No one can calculate your exact personal risk and only you can decide whether any risk is worth taking.

What Is Safe?
- Abstinence–Not Having Sex
- Having sex with only one, mutually faithful partner who isn't infected
- Abstinence—Not sharing drugs and not sharing needles and syringes.

AIDS education exhibit
Youngsters view part of an exhibit designed to educate them on a wide variety of AIDS-related issues, including the risky behaviors that can lead to AIDS. In October 1993, the exhibit began a three-year national tour of science museums across the United States.

continue to rise. Other cancers may increase as well, according to Levine, including basal cell skin cancer, which is trending upward in HIV-infected people with hemophilia.

A second study of illness in AIDS patients found that about 7 percent suffer from a deterioration of brain function known as dementia within a year after first being diagnosed with AIDS. The researchers, from Johns Hopkins University in Baltimore and other institutions, reported in November 1993 that overall, no matter how long they lived, people with AIDS had a 15 percent chance of developing dementia.

AIDS and a herpesvirus. A form of herpesvirus found in people with AIDS may speed the progression of the dis-

ease, researchers at the Medical College of Wisconsin at Milwaukee reported in March 1994. Medical researchers have observed that actively multiplying forms of the virus, human herpesvirus 6 (HHV-6), appear to cause tissue damage in infected individuals. But how the virus did so was unknown until the Wisconsin research.

The researchers detected HHV-6 mainly in disease-fighting white blood cells known as T-lymphocytes. The researchers proposed that HHV-6 may destroy these cells, further weakening the ability of the immune system to fight off the HIV infection and enabling the disease to progress more rapidly. The group of viruses known as herpesvirus cause a variety of diseases, including chickenpox and the sexually transmitted disease genital herpes.

Drug update. In December 1993, the U.S. Food and Drug Administration (FDA) approved the use of trimetrexate glucuronate for the treatment of PCP, the form of pneumonia associated with AIDS. The new medication, injected into a vein every day, is an alternative for people who experience serious side effects with previously approved PCP drugs. Researchers believe trimetrexate may be most useful for the treatment of severe cases for which other therapies have been ineffective or have caused harmful side effects.

AZT research. The use of the drug AZT (also known as zidovudine) provides only a slight delay in the progression from HIV infection to AIDS, according to a study reported in August 1993 by the CDC. Of the men in the study who developed AIDS, those taking AZT were diagnosed as having full-blown AIDS an average of 106.6 months after they tested positive for HIV. This figure compares with 97.1 months for the group not taking AZT. The results confirmed the findings of an earlier study by British and French researchers.

In another study, researchers found that AIDS patients taking AZT who experience worsening symptoms may benefit in the short term by switching to DDI, a drug also known as didanosine or dideoxyinosine. The study monitored 312 patients whose symptoms worsened after six months of taking AZT. Some of these patients were switched to DDI, while others continued to take AZT.

The DDI group experienced a 50 percent slowdown in the progression of their disease, as measured by the number of CD-4 cells in their immune system. CD-4 cells are white blood cells that HIV attacks. Although CD-4 cell counts increased in the DDI patients for about 12 weeks, the counts declined in those who kept taking AZT. Neither treatment, however, substantially prolonged life.

Another study looked at the effect of giving AZT and DDI simultaneously. Researchers at the National Cancer Institute reported in January 1994 that AIDS patients taking a combination of the two drugs had higher CD-4 counts for a longer period of time than did patients taking the two drugs alternately over a one-year period. Toxic side effects were mild and comparable, whether the drugs were administered together or separately.

Vaccine research. A number of vaccines in development in 1993 and 1994 proved to be safe and capable of making the body produce *antibodies* (infection-fighting molecules) against HIV. But long-term trials were still needed to demonstrate whether the vaccines could actually prevent HIV infection. Three studies showed that the experimental vaccines produced antibodies when injected into healthy volunteers, and the antibodies proved effective against laboratory strains of HIV. But when the experimental antibodies were tested against virus samples from AIDS patients, the antibodies did not kill HIV.

AIDS prevention. In January 1994, the CDC launched a national campaign of televised announcements aimed at men and women aged 18 to 25. The messages state that although abstinence is the only certain way to avoid sexually transmitted HIV infection, the use of latex condoms is important in protecting those who are sexually active. Kristine M. Gebbie, national AIDS policy coordinator, expressed hope that the campaign would impress upon youth that AIDS greatly affects their age group.

AIDS over 50. A study of Americans aged 50 and older found that those who were at above-average risk of contracting AIDS were only one-sixth as likely to use condoms as were comparable people in their 20's and only one-fifth as likely to have undergone an HIV test. Traits that elevated their risk included multiple sex partners or a partner with a known AIDS risk.

The study, reported in January 1994, said that 85 percent of those people at elevated risk who were sexually active never used condoms. About 10 percent of people with AIDS are 50 years of age or older, yet few AIDS prevention programs are directed at this group.   □ Richard Trubo

See also SEXUALLY TRANSMITTED DISEASES. In WORLD BOOK, see AIDS.

Alcohol and Drug Abuse

The use of drugs by American youth was on the rise in 1993 and 1994, reversing a downward trend of 14 years, according to a major annual survey by researchers at the University of Michigan in Ann Arbor. Nevertheless, drug use among youth was still well below the peak of 1979, according to Lloyd Johnston, who directed the survey of 51,000 students in the 8th, 10th, and 12th grades in more than 400 schools across the United States. In 1979, more than 54 percent of seniors said they used illegal drugs. In 1993, 31 percent said they did, up nearly 4 percent from 1992.

Marijuana use rose the most of any

drug, with 26 percent of seniors saying they smoked it, in contrast to less than 22 percent in 1992. Marijuana also gained in popularity in the lower grades, with 19 percent of the 10th-graders and 9 percent of the 8th-graders saying they had smoked it in 1993, up from 15 percent and 7 percent, respectively, in 1992. The number of 8th-graders using inhalants also rose, from 9.5 percent to 11 percent.

Although alcohol use dropped slightly, it clearly remained the favorite substance of abuse. More than half the 8th-graders in the survey said they had drunk alcoholic beverages during the year. The rate climbed to almost 70 percent among 10th-graders and 76 percent among 12th-graders.

Attitude shift. The 1993 study also found a disturbing change in attitudes toward drugs: students were less disapproving of drug use than they had been the previous year, and they were less concerned about dangerous side effects. Johnston said that attitude plays a critical role in drug use and that once perceptions soften concerning the harmfulness of drugs, an increase in their use can be expected.

Johnston's views were supported by a Health and Human Services (HHS) survey. Commenting on the survey in April 1994, HHS Secretary Donna E. Shalala expressed alarm that only 54 percent of the students surveyed believed that trying cocaine once or twice carried any risk. And 49 percent did not see that smoking a pack or more of cigarettes a day was harmful.

Racial differences in drug use. The University of Michigan study found that African-American students in all grades showed the lowest use of virtually all drugs, legal and illegal. For alcohol, the rate of heavy drinking among black seniors was 11 percent, compared with 32 percent among white seniors. Heavy drinking was defined as having five or more drinks in a row on at least one occasion.

Other studies found that tobacco use also was less prevalent among African-American youth than among white youth. For example, in March 1994, a report by U.S. Surgeon General M. Joycelyn Elders indicated that

An ancient Chinese cure for alcoholism?
A tea brewed from the kudzu vine has been used to treat alcohol abuse in China since at least 200 B.C. In November 1993, researchers from the Harvard Medical School in Boston reported that they had isolated two substances in the kudzu root that may cause alcoholics to lose their taste for liquor. The researchers injected an extract made from the root into hamsters that prefer alcohol to water. After the kudzu injection, the hamsters drank only half their usual amount of alcohol. The researchers are now trying to find out how the two substances suppress the desire to drink. They have an abundant supply of kudzu to work with. The vine grows wild in the Southern United States, climbing over everything in its path.

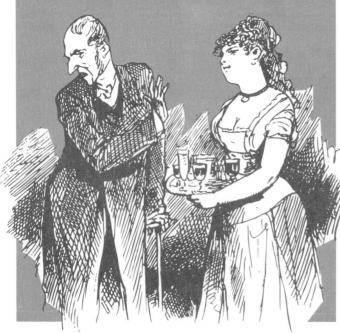

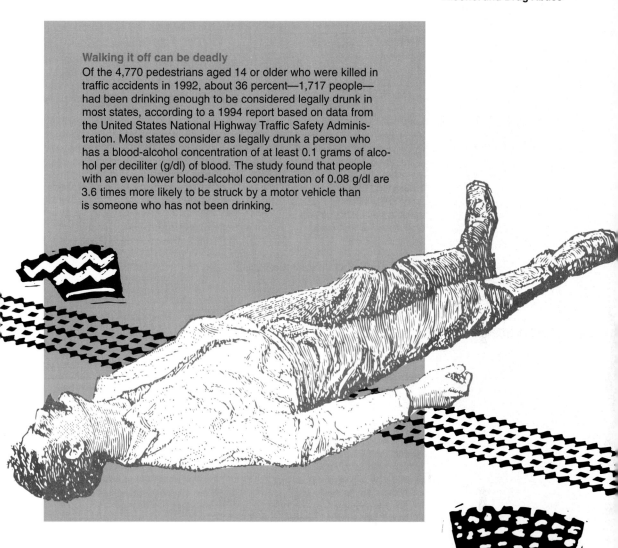

Walking it off can be deadly
Of the 4,770 pedestrians aged 14 or older who were killed in traffic accidents in 1992, about 36 percent—1,717 people—had been drinking enough to be considered legally drunk in most states, according to a 1994 report based on data from the United States National Highway Traffic Safety Administration. Most states consider as legally drunk a person who has a blood-alcohol concentration of at least 0.1 grams of alcohol per deciliter (g/dl) of blood. The study found that people with an even lower blood-alcohol concentration of 0.08 g/dl are 3.6 times more likely to be struck by a motor vehicle than is someone who has not been drinking.

smoking among African-American youth decreased from 38 percent in 1976 to 8.2 percent in 1993. Smoking among white youth, which also was at 38 percent in 1976, fell far less, to 32 percent in 1993. As for crack and cocaine, a survey by Partnership for a Drug-Free America found that 0.8 percent of African-American survey respondents reported using these substances, while 3.1 percent of white youth said they were users.

Such data prompted the U.S. Surgeon General's Office on Smoking and Health to suggest that African-American youths' behavior be studied for clues as to why their use is low. Gary Giovino, the agency's chief of epidemiology, said in March 1994 that he hoped the study would turn up

ways that would help other youths decrease their use of drugs.

The real cost of drugs. According to Daniel Melnick, a senior official at the Substance Abuse and Mental Health Services Administration, a federal agency, an increase in drug use translates to sharp increases in medical emergencies. In October 1993, he cited the latest available data for emergency treatment given to chronic drug users at hospitals or clinics. Treatment for cocaine overdoses increased 18 percent from 1991 to 119,800 cases in 1992; heroin overdoses increased 34 percent, to 48,000 cases; and adverse reactions to marijuana rose 48 percent, to 24,000 cases.

Moreover, the use of alcohol, cigarettes, and other drugs is causing more than 500,000 deaths each year, according to a study by researchers at Brandeis University in Waltham, Mass. Their study also looked at the economic cost of using drugs, as measured by drug-related medical expenses, lost income from missing work due to drugs, street crime committed for drug money, and car accidents involving a driver under the influence of drugs. In these terms, the economic cost of drugs reached a total of $238 billion in 1990 alone—$99-billion from alcohol use, $72 billion from tobacco use, and $67 billion from drug abuse.

Genetic influence in addiction.
People with a high tolerance for alcohol may be at higher risk for alcoholism than those who feel alcohol's effects readily, according to Mark Schuckit, a researcher with the Veterans Affairs Medical Center in San Diego. His study was reported in February 1994. Ten years earlier, Schuckit and his colleagues had tested 223 men, half of whom had alcoholic fathers, by giving them the equivalent of three to five drinks in 10 minutes. The researchers recorded who had the mildest and who had the strongest reactions to alcohol, as measured by brain wave and motor skills tests.

After 10 years, the scientists restudied the participants who had registered the mildest and strongest reactions. More than half of those with mild reactions and alcoholic fathers had become alcoholics, and 24 percent of those with mild reactions and nonalcoholic fathers had become alcoholic. In contrast, only 14 percent of those with strong reactions and alcoholic fathers had become alcoholic, and 9 percent of those with strong reactions and a nonalcoholic father had become alcoholic.

Genes also appear to play a role in cocaine abuse, according to a December 1993 study by pharmacologist Kenneth Blum at the University of Texas Health Science Center in San Antonio. Blum and his colleagues reported that they had found an unusual gene variant in 50.9 percent of 53 cocaine addicts they studied, but in only 16 percent of 100 nonaddicts in a control group.

The gene variant is responsible for an uncommon form of a cell *receptor* (docking site) for the brain chemical dopamine. Dopamine plays a role in creating pleasurable sensations. The researchers said that people with this gene variant have fewer dopamine receptors, and therefore their cells may not take up normal amounts of dopamine. As a result, they need greater stimulation than people ordinarily do to experience pleasure. Frequent doses of cocaine could provide that stimulation.

Drinking and driving. Alcohol-related traffic accidents in the United States claimed 17,699 lives in 1992 compared with 22,084 fatalities in 1990, a 20 percent drop, according to U.S. Department of Transportation Secretary Federico F. Peña. Citing the statistics in November 1993, Peña said the improved record resulted from a decrease in drinking and driving among younger drivers, especially teen-agers, and from tougher law enforcement.

Some states, such as California, are cracking down harder than ever on drinking and driving. In October 1993, California Governor Pete Wilson signed a law making it illegal for anyone under age 21 to drive with a blood-alcohol level at or above 0.01 grams of alcohol per deciliter (tenth of a liter) of blood (g/dL). Those caught breaking the law may have their driver's license suspended for up to one year. Before the new law was enacted, a driver between ages 18 and 21 had to have a blood-alcohol concentration of at least 0.08 g/dL or higher to be arrested for driving under the influence, and drivers aged 16 to 18 needed a level in excess of 0.05 g/dL.

The war on drugs took several interesting turns during 1993 and 1994. First, in December 1993, Surgeon General Elders stated that drug legalization should be studied as a means of reducing violence in society. She suggested that current strategies to curb drug use failed to deal effectively with violence.

Second, a major meeting took place in England in February 1994 to discuss employing global strategies in the war against drugs. The meeting also tried to unite leaders with differing views on the best way to combat drugs. One group wants increased law enforcement to stop the flow of drugs. Another group wants more education concerning the dangers of drugs and treatment for those already addicted. The meeting spotlighted the complexities of a global drug strategy, especially in view of the different approaches countries take toward drug legalization and drug abuse treatment.

Alcohol and the brain. A study reported in November suggested revising the current view of how alcohol affects brain cells. Scientists had thought that alcohol killed nerve cells in the brain. But researchers Grethe Badsberg Jenson and Bente Pakkenberg of Aarhus University in Denmark found no apparent decrease in the number of brain cells in alcoholics who had died, compared with the brains of nonalcoholics. However, the connections between brain cells appeared to be damaged.

This was good news. The fibers connecting nerve cells are capable of regrowth if alcohol consumption stops. Thus, because the brain cells themselves survive, there is hope of restoring some of an alcoholic's lost brain function. □ Gayle R. Hamilton

In WORLD BOOK, see ALCOHOLISM; DRUG ABUSE.

Allergies and Asthma

A new drug for the treatment of asthma, salmeterol, was released for use in the United States in early 1994. At the same time, researchers in Japan reported on a new class of asthma drugs that may soon be available.

Salmeterol belongs to a class of drugs called beta-2 agonist bronchodilators, which relieve asthma by decreasing the constriction of airways in the lungs. But compared with other bronchodilators, salmeterol relieves asthma symptoms for a longer time.

A clinical study of salmeterol was reported in May by asthma specialist Gilbert E. D'Alonzo and his associates at the University of Texas Health Science Center in Houston. They reported that patients using the drug experienced effective relief from asthma symptoms with minimal side effects.

Because salmeterol is longer-acting than other bronchodilators, asthma sufferers need to use it only twice a day to obtain relief from their symptoms. In fact, salmeterol cannot be used in the same way as other beta-2 agonists, which are short-acting and can be used when an asthma attack is in progress. Salmeterol is taken every 12 hours on a regular basis to prevent attacks. It may be especially useful for controlling asthma symptoms at night during sleep.

A new kind of asthma drug that works by reducing inflammation in the lungs was reported in June by scientists at the Minase Research Institute in Japan. The investigators said clinical trials of the drug, known as OKY-046, indicate that it is effective in preventing asthma symptoms. OKY-046 counteracts the production of irritating chemicals called prostaglandins and leukotrienes.

Much recent asthma research has focused on blocking the creation of these inflammatory substances in the lungs. OKY-046 is just one of a number of new drugs currently being investigated that seem to accomplish that. After further clinical tests, these drugs should start to become available for the treatment of asthma.

Corticosteroids and children. The prolonged use of inhaled corticosteroids by children to control asthma does not affect the children's growth or interfere with their bodies' production of hormones. That finding was reported in December 1993 by pediatrician Benjamin Volovitz and his colleagues at Golda Medical Center in Petah Tiqwa, Israel.

Corticosteroids are drugs that reduce inflammation in the lungs. The use of inhaled corticosteroids has become standard for the management of asthma in both children and adults. Some studies, however, have raised concerns about the effects of the drugs, suggesting that they inhibit growth and the normal production of hormones.

Volovitz and his colleagues studied

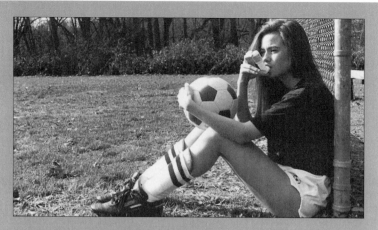

Coping with exercise-induced asthma
Up to 90 percent of people with chronic asthma, as well as some nonasthmatics, suffer asthma attacks when they exercise. Doctors say exercise-induced asthma (EIA) should not keep anyone from exercising, because a regular workout conditions and strengthens the lungs. They recommend several things that people can do to avoid or minimize EIA.

- Begin any bout of exercise with a 15-minute warm-up period to enable the lungs to adjust to the increased demand for oxygen.
- End your exercise with a 15-minute cool-down period rather than stopping abruptly.
- When exercising in cold weather, cover your nose and mouth with a scarf to warm and moisten air before it reaches the lungs.
- Follow your physician's instructions regarding the use of medications before or after exercising.
- If you experience asthma symptoms while exercising, relieve them at once with a bronchodilator. (Chromolyn and corticosteroids are not recommended because they do not immediately open blocked airways.)

Source: *FDA Consumer.*

15 asthmatic children aged 2 to 7 who used a corticosteroid called budesonide. They followed the children's progress for up to five years.

At the end of the study, the scientists found that the growth pattern of all the children—including their height, weight, and bone growth—was normal. In addition, they found that the drug had produced no effect on the functioning of the children's pituitary or adrenal glands.

These findings indicate that standard doses of inhaled corticosteroids are safe for children. The researchers pointed out, though, that precautions still need to be observed with larger doses of inhaled corticosteroid drugs or with oral corticosteroids such as prednisone.

Treating hives. A new medicated skin cream for the treatment of chronic *urticaria* (hives) was released in early 1994. The cream, which is sold under the name Zonalon, contains doxepin, a drug with an antihistamine effect. Antihistamines counteract histamine, the chemical released from certain cells of the body during an allergic attack.

Chronic urticaria is a common skin disorder characterized by itchy, raised welts. The specific cause of the condition often cannot be determined, though it is sometimes related to food allergies, heat, or exercise. Most cases of chronic urticaria are treated with oral antihistamines.

In tests, Zonalon was effective in reducing the symptoms of urticaria. Like many antihistamines, however, it can cause drowsiness.

Antihistamine-cancer link? Antihistamines may promote the growth of cancerous tumors, scientists at the University of Manitoba, in Canada, reported in May 1994. They based that finding on research with mice. The mice were given antihistamines after having tumors implanted in their bodies, and the drug apparently stimulated the cancers.

Just a few days after that report appeared, however, the U.S. Food and Drug Administration (FDA) issued a statement commenting on the study. The FDA said that neither previous clinical trials nor animal experiments with antihistamines support the findings of the Canadian researchers. The agency said antihistamines are safe for the treatment of allergies, and it urged the public not to worry about using them.

Allergies to latex are becoming a growing public health problem. The problem, and what should be done to address it, was reviewed in May 1994 by allergist Kevin J. Kelley and his associates at Children's Hospital of Wisconsin, in Milwaukee.

Latex allergies can range from simple itching, rashes, and eye irritation to fatal reactions. Until recent years, latex allergies had been a serious concern to just a few groups of people, including workers in the latex industry, patients undergoing frequent surgery, and health care workers who routinely used latex gloves.

Over the last 10 years, however, exposure of the general public to latex products has increased dramatically, in large part because of precautions that have been recommended for health care workers to prevent the spread of AIDS. Thus, say many experts, the danger of fatal reactions in people with severe, undetected latex allergies has become an international public health problem.

Kelly and his colleagues urged doctors to screen their patients for latex allergies. Although there is no skin test for sensitivity to latex that has been approved by the FDA, many allergists and immunologists have developed procedures for diagnosing latex allergies. This involves taking the patient's medical history to learn of past reactions to rubber products, such as balloons; skin tests with latex extracts; and blood tests with latex extracts.

The researchers said it is important that better methods for the detection of latex allergies be developed. In the meantime, they said, patients who suspect that they may be allergic to latex should consult their allergist or regular physician.

The use of filters to clear dust from the air in work areas could greatly reduce the incidence of asthma in aller-

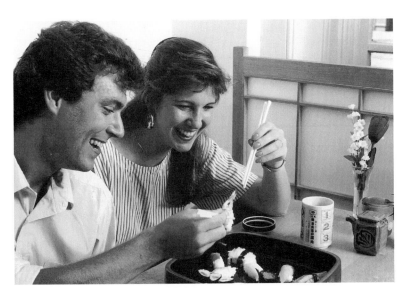

Finding may aid those with shellfish allergies
Not everyone can eat shrimp and other shellfish with abandon—some people are allergic to them. But in late 1993, scientists in the United States and India identified two molecular regions of a shellfish protein that cause allergic reactions. That finding may lead to a way of desensitizing people who are allergic to shellfish.

gic workers. That conclusion was reported in December 1993 by allergist Josep M. Antó and his colleagues in Barcelona, Spain.

Asthma can result from inhaling *allergens* (substances causing allergic reactions), such as pollen. Some allergens are encountered in the workplace and cause asthma in susceptible employees.

The Spanish investigators studied workers at a silo who were exposed to soybean dust. The researchers found that when dust levels rose, the incidence of asthmatic attacks among the employees increased. The workers suffering attacks were found to be allergic to soybean allergens.

In cooperation with the researchers, the owners of the silos installed filters in one of the silos to see if the filters would improve the workers' health. The filters greatly reduced the amount of soybean allergens in the air of that silo when soybeans were being unloaded, and allergic reactions of the employees working subsequently declined dramatically. The scientists said their finding demonstrated the need for measures to reduce dust in the soybean industry and may also be applicable to other industries in which workers are exposed to airborne allergens. □ Dominick A. Minotti

In WORLD BOOK, see ALLERGY; ASTHMA; IMMUNOLOGY.

Arthritis and Connective Tissue Disorders

Certain genes are more common in patients with either of two forms of rheumatoid arthritis (RA) than in the general population, according to research published in February 1994. RA is a type of arthritis most commonly found in women 20 to 40 years of age, in which the tissue around the joints becomes inflamed. As the disease progresses, the inflamed tissue and other substances wear away the bone and cartilage in the joint. Doctors call such progressive cases of the disease erosive RA.

Scientists have long known that RA tends to run in families, suggesting that it is inherited in at least some cases. The 1994 study advanced researchers' understanding of a possible genetic basis for the disorder. Scientists believe that RA occurs when the disease-fighting immune system mistakes the body's own tissue for a foreign substance and attacks it.

In the new research, a team from the Virginia Mason Medical Center in Seattle studied genes responsible for the body's production of *human leukocyte antigens* (HLA's), proteins on the surface of cells that alert the immune system to foreign substances in the body. The researchers looked for the prevalence of particular forms of HLA genes in 16 patients with a type of erosive RA called rheumatoid factor negative (RF-) RA. Previous research had shown that these forms were more common in patients with another type of erosive RA, rheumatoid factor positive (RF+) RA, than in the general population.

Thirteen of the 16 RF- patients, or 81 percent, had the same forms of HLA genes as are prevalent in RF+ patients. In contrast, only 17 of 39 healthy individuals studied, or 46 percent, had these forms of the genes. The researchers concluded that similar genetic mechanisms underlie the development of erosive RA in all patients, regardless of the form of the disorder.

RA relief in pregnancy. Differences in HLA types between a pregnant woman and her developing fetus may be responsible for the relief of symptoms that often occurs in women with RA during pregnancy, researchers reported in August 1993. Since the 1930's, many scientists had attributed this pregnancy-related improvement in RA to hormonal changes associated with pregnancy. But they found no evidence that hormones were indeed responsible, and the cause of the phenomenon remained a mystery.

The 1993 study grew out of speculation by J. Lee Nelson, a rheumatologist at the Fred Hutchinson Cancer Research Center in Seattle, that pregnancy might affect a woman's immune system in some way that gives rise to the temporary RA "cure." Nelson reasoned that a mother's immune system must alter during pregnancy so that it does not recognize the fetus as foreign tissue and seek to destroy it.

To test the idea, Nelson and her colleagues looked at 57 current or previous pregnancies in 41 women with RA. The women's symptoms disappeared or markedly improved in 34 of the pregnancies and did not change in 12 pregnancies. In the remaining 11 cases, the researchers could not determine whether symptoms improved during the pregnancy. The researchers based their judgments on the women's own reports, physical examinations, and medical records.

The investigators then took blood or hair samples from each mother and child. By analyzing the genetic material in the samples, they determined to what degree the child's HLA genes matched or differed from those of the mother. The researchers found that in 76 percent of the cases where the women's RA improved or disappeared during pregnancy, the mother and child had substantially different HLA types. But where RA symptoms did not improve, only 25 percent had substantially different HLA types.

Their findings suggested that the greater the degree to which the mother's and fetus's HLA types differ, the greater the degree to which the mother's immune system "turns off" to avoid attacking the fetus as foreign tissue. The turned-off immune system is also unable to attack the mother's own tissue, relieving the mother's RA.

Guarding against carpal tunnel syndrome
Carpal tunnel syndrome is a disabling disorder that affects the median nerve, one of two nerves that control movement and sensation in the hand and fingers. The syndrome occurs when the median nerve is compressed as it passes through the carpal tunnel, a narrow passage formed by the bones of the wrist and the ligament connecting them, *right*.

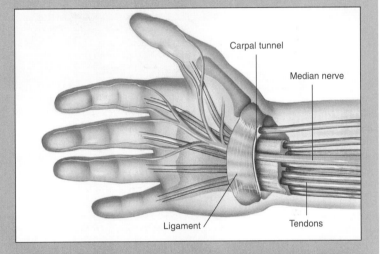

Carpal tunnel

Median nerve

Tendons

Ligament

Activities that involve repetitive wrist motions, such as typing, can produce swelling in that ligament or in the tendons that surround the median nerve, compressing the nerve. To guard against carpal tunnel syndrome while typing, experts advise holding the wrists in a neutral position so that the arm and the top of the hand form a straight line, *right*. Just as important, take a break once every 30 minutes to an hour, and use ice packs to reduce swelling at the first sign of injury.

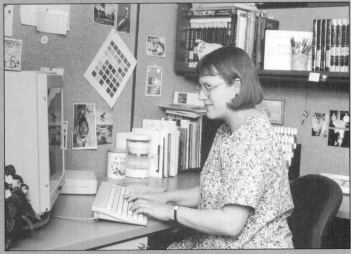

A cartilage cure for RA? In patients with rheumatoid arthritis, the immune system attacks type II collagen, a protein that helps make up the cartilage in joints. In a September 1993 study, researchers showed that giving patients oral doses of type II collagen can trick the immune system into ending its attack on its own tissues.

A team led by rheumatologists at the Harvard Medical School in Boston studied 59 volunteers with severe RA. Each day, 28 patients drank orange juice mixed with type II collagen from chickens—a substance similar to human type II collagen. The other 31 patients drank orange juice mixed with a *placebo* (substance with no active ingredients). After three months, those who received the collagen treatment showed a significant reduction in swelling and pain in their joints. In four patients, RA symptoms disappeared.

The researchers said the exact mechanism by which oral doses of collagen suppressed the body's immune reaction remained to be determined. They speculated, however, that the treatment worked because of contact between the collagen and immune cells of the stomach and intestines. Scientists believe that as a general rule the body turns off the immune system in response to proteins that pass through the intestinal tract in order to prevent food allergies. The passage of type II collagen through this tract induced a condition immu-nologists call tolerance, in which the immune response is suppressed throughout the body.

Alternative therapy for RA. A folk remedy long used by patients with rheumatoid arthritis appears to have a scientific basis, according to a report published in November 1993. A researcher at the University of Pennsylvania in Philadelphia and his colleagues studied a compound found in oils derived from the seeds of certain plants, notably borage and evening primrose. The compound, gammalinolenic acid, is converted in the body to a substance known to help reduce inflammation and to lessen the response of the immune system.

The Pennsylvania researchers gave capsules containing gammalinolenic acid in the form of borage seed oil to 19 RA patients and a placebo to 18 patients. Neither the patients nor the researchers knew which patients had received the capsules with borage seed oil. After 24 weeks, the patients taking the borage seed oil capsules showed significant improvement in their joint pain and swelling, while the patients taking the placebo experienced no relief. The finding added to a growing scientific interest in alternative medicines as a source for more effective treatments for RA and other forms of arthritis.

☐ Mark F. Gourley and John H. Klippel
In WORLD BOOK, see ARTHRITIS.

Alzheimer's Disease
See Brain and Nervous System

Birth Control

At least 70 percent of sexually active adolescents in the United States use birth control regularly, according to a study reported in June 1994 by the Alan Guttmacher Institute, a nonprofit research group. The study found that teen-agers use contraceptives about as effectively as do many adults.

For every 1,000 sexually active girls aged 15 to 19 in 1991, 208 became pregnant. This number was 18 percent lower than in 1972, when 254 out of 1,000 became pregnant. The researchers attributed this decrease to more effective use of contraception among teens. In fact, the report said, teens have prevented unwanted pregnancies more effectively than have unmarried women in their 20's.

Although teen contraceptive use is up, the report also said that more teens are engaging in premarital sex, a trend observed in other studies. The report found that over 50 percent of female adolescents and about 75 percent of males had engaged in sexual intercourse by the age of 18. In 1972, 35 percent of females and 55 percent of males had had sex by age 18.

Controversy regarding Norplant. As of August 1994, about 1,000 users of Norplant had sought to join a class-action lawsuit against the distributors of the product. The women claimed that they had experienced complications related to the removal of the contraceptive implants. Norplant con-

Method	Cost per year*	Failure rate†
Vasectomy	$34	0.2 percent
Depo-Provera injections	$198	0.3 percent
Tubal ligation	$75	0.4 percent
Norplant	$129	0.8 percent
IUD	$54	1.5 percent
Oral contraceptive	$223	3.0 percent
Condom	$62	12 percent
Diaphragm	$115	15 percent

*These estimates include physician and hospital fees in methods that require medical assistance.
†The failure rate represents the number of women who will become pregnant in a year of using the method.

Source: Wyeth-Ayerst Laboratories.

Comparing methods of birth control
Birth control methods differ in their cost and their effectivenesss, two important considerations in choosing among them. Some methods have large initial costs, but are less expensive in the long run than methods with a lower monthly or annual cost.

sists of six short, rod-shaped capsules implanted under the skin of a woman's upper arm. The capsules release low doses of a synthetic hormone that blocks ovulation.

Norplant, which first became available in 1991, provides protection against pregnancy for five years. A medical professional then removes the capsules by making a small incision and pulling them out. The lawsuit charges that some doctors have had difficulty removing the rods, causing pain, scarring, and even permanent nerve and muscle damage.

According to the distributors of Norplant, Wyeth-Ayerst Laboratories, in Radnor, Pa., most doctors have removed the rods easily and successfully. A company spokesperson said that removing the rods is a minor procedure but usually takes longer than inserting them, particularly if the capsules have not been placed properly.

In some cases, doctors have planted the rods too deeply, scar tissue has built up around the rods, or the patient has put on weight, according to Planned Parenthood of New York City. These conditions can make the rods hard to locate and remove.

In response to a separate issue, Wyeth-Ayerst said in November 1993 it would lower the cost of Norplant to public clinics in December 1995. The company had drawn criticism for the contraceptive's price of $365, when the cost of production was only about $16. In addition to the cost of the Norplant, a woman must pay about $300 in doctors' fees for the insertion and removal of the capsules. The cost of standard birth control pills, including doctor visits, runs more than $1,000 for five years.

RU-486 coming to America. In May 1994, the Population Council, a non-profit research group in New York City, announced it was undertaking studies on the safety and effectiveness of an abortion pill called mifepristone, commonly known by its trade name RU-486. The drug came on the market in 1988 but has been available only in China, France, Sweden, and the United Kingdom. The U.S. government had not approved the sale of mifepristone by August 1994, and the French manufacturer who holds the patent for the drug had refused to market it in the United States because of the controversy surrounding abortion.

Mifepristone can be used to end a pregnancy during the first three months. It works by blocking the action of progesterone, a hormone produced by the mother's body, which prepares the lining of the uterus to receive and nourish an embryo.

The French producers of RU-486 donated the U.S. patent rights to the Population Council, which will develop manufacturing and distribution plans for the drug. The group anticipates eventual approval of mifepristone by the U.S. Food and Drug Administration.   □ Mary Carvlin

In WORLD BOOK, see ABORTION; BIRTH CONTROL.

Birth Defects
See Genetics

Blood

The discovery of a protein responsible for helping blood to clot was announced in June 1994 by researchers at the University of Washington in Seattle and at two biotechnology companies. The protein, thrombopoietin, causes immature blood cells called stem cells to give rise to platelets, the blood cells that initiate clotting. The protein could be used to treat cancer patients whose ability to produce platelets has decreased as a result of chemotherapy or radiation.

A 3-year-old patient with leukemia, a cancer of the white blood cells, received a transplant of blood cells taken from the umbilical cord of an unrelated compatible donor in August 1993. Umbilical cord blood contains immature stem cells that can mature into red blood cells, white blood cells, and platelets.

Many leukemia patients rely on a transplant of bone marrow—the blood-forming tissue within large bones—from compatible donors. Such donors are usually relatives, but even a sibling has only 1 chance in 4 of providing compatible marrow. If the marrow is not compatible, the recipient's immune system will destroy the transplanted tissue. If relatives cannot provide compatible marrow, large numbers of unrelated potential donors usually must be screened.

In 1991, a team at Indiana University had shown that umbilical cord blood cells from a sibling could be transplanted to leukemia patients in place of bone marrow. The 1993 transplant, performed by pediatric surgeon Joanne Kurtzberg of Duke University Medical Center in Durham, N.C., was remarkable because the cells came from an unrelated compatible donor.

The cord blood given to the 3-year-old successfully replaced his own diseased marrow. Because cord blood produces healthy blood cells and is obtained more easily than bone marrow, which must be removed surgically from the donor, it may become an important treatment for patients who previously required transplants.

New thalassemia treatments. In September 1993, doctors reported two new treatments for thalassemia, a hereditary disease in which the body produces too little hemoglobin. Hemoglobin is the substance in red blood cells that carries oxygen to tissues throughout the body.

Until recently, the treatment for thalassemia has been lifelong transfusions of healthy red blood cells. However, patients who receive repeated transfusions of red blood cells can develop large iron deposits in the heart and other organs, which can cause severe medical problems and even death.

Researchers Christopher H. Lowrey of the Dartmouth-Hitchcock Medical

Blood shortage
Some 4 million Americans each year receive transfusions of blood collected from volunteer donors. Supplies of donated blood hit their lowest levels in years in late 1993 and early 1994. If you wish to donate blood, look in your local telephone directory under American Red Cross for the phone number and address of the center nearest you.

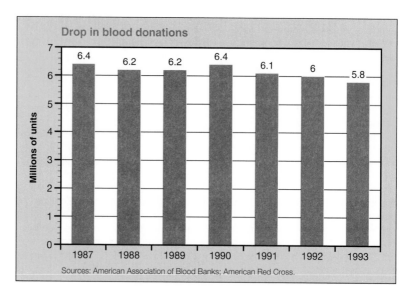

Drop in blood donations

Millions of units

1987	1988	1989	1990	1991	1992	1993
6.4	6.2	6.2	6.4	6.1	6	5.8

Sources: American Association of Blood Banks; American Red Cross.

Center in Lebanon, N.H., and Arthur W. Neinhuis of the National Institutes of Health in Bethesda, Md., reported that they successfully treated three thalassemia patients with the drug azacitidine. Azacitidine induces the body to make fetal hemoglobin rather than adult hemoglobin.

Normally, the body produces fetal hemoglobin while still in the mother's womb and at birth switches to producing adult hemoglobin. Healthy adults produce very little, if any, fetal hemoglobin. Patients with thalassemia also produce fetal hemoglobin when in the womb, but they do not make enough normal adult hemoglobin after birth. Turning on fetal hemoglobin production again after birth allows these patients to produce more red blood cells.

The patients who received azacitidine treatment no longer required transfusions of red blood cells. However, the drug does carry some risk of promoting cancer.

In another procedure, doctors in Italy transplanted bone marrow from related donors to patients who were in the early stages of thalassemia. The doctors reported good results in most patients. However, transplantation carries some risk, including death due to infection or bleeding when the patient is recovering the capacity to make blood cells. Another risk is that the transplanted cells will attack the patient's tissues. Of the 64 patients who underwent bone marrow transplants, 2 died after the procedure.

Gene therapy for hemophilia? A gene-therapy technique may offer relief to people suffering from hemophilia, according to research reported in October 1993. Hemophilia is a disorder in which the blood fails to clot normally due to a deficiency in a clotting factor, a protein that promotes clotting. As a result, patients bleed severely from even a minor injury.

A team headed by researchers Savio L. C. Woo of the Baylor College of Medicine in Houston and Kenneth M. Brinkhous of the University of North Carolina School of Medicine at Chapel Hill tested the technique on dogs bred to have a form of the disease called hemophilia B.

The researchers injected three dogs with a gene responsible for producing a clotting factor. Clotting factor IX is missing in patients with hemophilia B.

The gene was carried by a harmless virus through the dogs' bloodstream to their liver. After the virus entered the liver cells, the gene for factor IX inserted itself into the DNA (genetic material) of the cells. Afterward, the dogs' bodies began producing clotting factor IX. Although the amount of factor IX the dogs produced was 1,000 times less than normal, it was enough to improve their clotting disorders.

☐ G. David Roodman
In World Book, see Blood.

Bone Disorders

There seems to be little relation between spinal abnormalities and back pain. That conclusion was reported in July 1994 by radiologist Michael N. Brant-Zawadzki of Hoag Memorial Hospital in Newport Beach, Calif.

Brant-Zawadzki and his associates used a technique called magnetic resonance imaging to examine the spines of 98 men and women with no back pain. He found that almost two-thirds of the people had "slipped" disks or other spinal abnormalities.

Brant-Zawadzki said that although doctors find such spinal anomalies in many patients complaining of back pain, the pain may, in many instances, have nothing to do with the abnormality. He said his findings should alert physicians to be more careful about making sure that patients' symptoms are really due to whatever spinal abnormalities are identified before deciding on a treatment.

Vitamin D and bones. Vitamin D is an essential nutrient for healthy bones, enabling cells to absorb calcium. In January 1994, researchers at the Galvan Institute of Medical Research in Sydney, Australia, reported that they had found a gene that apparently plays a key role in this process. The finding suggests the possibility of a genetic test to identify individuals who are less able to incorporate vitamin D into their bone cells and who thus have a higher risk of developing *os-

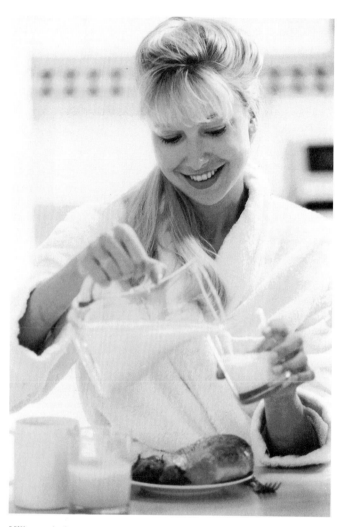

Milk can help counter bone loss from coffee

Women who drink coffee regularly can suffer significant bone loss as they age, researchers at the University of California at San Diego reported in January 1994. But their study of 980 women also revealed that drinking at least one glass of milk a day can largely counter the bone-thinning effects of coffee. The researchers cautioned, however, that a single glass of milk provides just one-third of an adult's recommended daily requirement of calcium.

teoporosis (thinning of bone tissue).

The gene carries coded information for the production of vitamin D receptors on cells. The receptors are molecular doorways through which vitamin D can enter cells.

The researchers found two forms of the gene. One form enables cells to make more efficient use of vitamin D than the other form. The investigators were uncertain why the two versions of the gene differ in their ability to help cells use vitamin D.

The scientists calculated that people with the less effective form of the gene are likely to develop osteoporosis by age 65, at least 10 years earlier than people with the other version of the gene. When they evaluated 311 middle-aged women, they found that,

indeed, women with the better-functioning gene had more bone mass than women with the other gene.

Boosting bone mass early. Doctors think people could help prevent fractures resulting from osteoporosis later in life by building up their bones while they are young. In August 1993, researchers at the Hershey Medical Center in Hershey, Pa., reported that girls taking calcium supplements were able to increase their bone mass.

Ninety-four adolescent girls participated in the study. Over an 18-month period, each girl took either two tablets of calcium citrate malate daily or a *placebo* (inactive substance). The girls taking calcium increased their intake of the nutrient from 80 percent of the recommended daily allowance to 110 percent. Those girls experienced significant gains in bone density, compared with the girls who received the placebo.

Scoliosis in boys. Scoliosis—lateral curvature of the spine—is more common in girls than boys, so screening and treatment programs for the disorder have tended to emphasize girls over boys. As a result, less is known about how scoliosis progresses in boys. A study by doctors at the Texas Scottish Rite Hospital for Crippled Children in Dallas, reported in December 1993, shed some light on this question.

The physicians evaluated the progression of scoliosis over a period of about three years in a group of 211 boys between the ages of 8 and 15. They found that one-third of the boys showed an increase of 10 degrees or more in the curvature of their spine during that time. Boys in whom the disorder began by age 10 and boys with a curvature of more than 50 degrees when first enrolled in the study fared the worst.

The investigators also noted that scoliosis often appeared in some boys at a later age than noted in girls and then progressed to a severe curvature. They concluded that boys with scoliosis should be followed carefully by a school screening program or a physician until age 18.

□ John J. Gartland

In WORLD BOOK, see BONE.

The following books on health and medicine were written for the general reader. They have been selected from books published in 1993 and 1994.

Aging. *The New Ourselves, Growing Older,* written by Paula B. Doress-Worters and Diana Laskin Siegal, in cooperation with the Boston Women's Health Book Collective, focuses on women's health from midlife to old age. The book addresses such topics as aging and well-being, reassessing body image, contraception and childbearing at midlife, sexuality, menopause, hypertension, diabetes, hysterectomy, osteoporosis, cancer, and arthritis. (Touchstone Books, 1994. 531 pp. $18.)

AIDS. *The Slow Plague: Geography of the AIDS Pandemic.* Geographer Peter Gould examines how the AIDS epidemic migrated from city to city and then spread to the areas surrounding those cities. Gould dispels the misconception that only certain minority populations are at risk of contracting AIDS. (Blackwell, 1993. 228 pp. $19.95.)

Arthritis. *Arthritis: What Exercises Work?* Dava Sobel and Arthur C. Klein examine the life-enhancing value of exercise and how it can help people who suffer from arthritis. Included is an account of how to prepare and warm up for exercising and why walking, swimming, cycling, or dancing can be beneficial for arthritis sufferers. (St. Martin's, 1993. 200 pp. $19.95.)

Breast cancer. *The Breast Cancer Handbook: Taking Control After You've Found a Lump.* Joan Swirsky, a clinical nurse specialist and a writer for *The New York Times,* and social worker Barbara Balaban give information on breast cancer diagnosis and treatment, and list questions to ask a doctor. (Harper Perennial, 1994. 232 pp. $10.)

Drugs. *Aspirin Handbook: A User's Guide to the Breakthrough Drug of the 90's.* Should you take aspirin routinely? If so, how much should you take? The authors look at the benefits and side effects of aspirin, as well as alter-natives to it. (Bantam, 1993. 243 pp. $5.99.)

The Plague Makers: How We Are Creating Catastrophic New Epidemics —and What We Must Do to Avert Them. Jeffrey A. Fisher, an anatomic and clinical pathologist, describes the threat posed by new strains of antibiotic-resistant bacteria and how the indiscriminate use of antibiotics has contributed to that threat. (Simon & Schuster, 1994. 256 pp. $23.)

General reference. *Consumer Reports Health Answer Book.* Author Jonathan Leff compiles advice from medical consultants on more than 300 frequently asked questions about such health topics as AIDS, Alzheimer's disease, anemia, weight control, and women's health. (Consumer Reports Books, 1993. 244 pp. $14.95.)

Good Operations—Bad Operations: The People's Medical Society Guide to Surgery, by Charles B. Inlander and the staff of the People's Medical Society, includes a discussion of the success and failure rates of specific operations, alternatives to surgery, controversies about surgery, and the common concerns and questions that people facing surgery have. The book also features a rating system to help weigh the advantages and disadvantages of an operation. (Viking, 1993. 430 pp. $27.50.)

Symptoms—Their Causes & Cures: How to Understand & Treat 265 Health Concerns, edited by Alice Feinstein and editors of Prevention Magazine Health Books, discusses such symptoms as aches, blisters, bloating, cold hands and feet, and headache. Symptoms are listed alphabetically. (Rodale Press, 1994. 660 pp. $29.95.)

Health care reform. *American Way of Health: How Medicine Is Changing and What It Means to You.* Janice Castro, senior health care correspondent for *Time* magazine, explains health care reform to consumers. (Little, Brown, 1994. 282 pp. $9.95.)

The Road to Reform: The Future of Health Care in America by economist Eli Ginzberg, with Miriam Ostow, cuts through the contention and confusing detail in the media to help readers understand what has gone wrong with the way health care is delivered in the United States, how it got that way, and what needs to be done. (Free Press, 1994. 216 pp. $22.95.)

Hearing loss. *When the Hearing Gets Hard: Winning the Battle Against Hearing Impairment.* Elaine Suss, novelist and poet, is one of more than 28 million Americans who have suffered severe hearing loss. She discusses the forms of hearing impairment and what can be done about this disability. (Insight Books, 1993. 282 pp. $24.50.)

Heart disease. *The Johns Hopkins Complete Guide for Preventing and Reversing Heart Disease.* Physician Peter O. Kwiterovich, Jr., discusses how to assess and reduce the risk of heart disease. Also examined are the genetic factors that contribute to heart disease, and how diet and exercise can help lower the risk of disease. (Prima, 1993. 395 pp. $12.95.)

Long-term illness. *Taking Charge: Overcoming the Challenges of Long Term Illness* by Irene Pollin, with Susan K. Golant. After Pollin's son and daughter died, she founded a medical-crisis counseling service to provide therapy for chronically ill patients, their families, and caregivers. Pollin draws on her own personal and professional experience as she discusses eight

commonly shared fears and coping strategies among the chronically ill—including the fear of dependency, abandonment, isolation, and death. (Times Books, 1994. 262 pp. $29.)

Medicine and society. *Silent Travelers: Germs, Genes, and the Immigrant Menace.* Alan M. Kraut, professor of history at American University in Washington, D.C., shows how fears of ethnic differences and of disease were often linked and how earlier generations coped with those fears. For example, the Irish were blamed for a cholera epidemic in New York City in 1832; Chinese immigrants, for an outbreak of bubonic plague in San Francisco in 1900; and Haitians, for the spread of AIDS in the 1980's. (Basic Books, 1994. 369 pp. $25.)

Your Complete Medical Record. The People's Medical Society staff describes how people can obtain and maintain their own medical records. Because most people's records are scattered among various health care agencies, private practitioners, and specialists, it can be difficult to assemble all of the records in one place. This book informs people about state laws regarding access to medical records. Also provided are blank forms for tracking family and personal medical history, and for recording laboratory results and visits to practitioners. (People's Medical Society, 1993. 208 pp. $12.95.)

Noteworthy new titles
Your Complete Medical Record tells how to obtain your records; *Arthritis: What Exercises Work?* advises people with arthritis; *The Thyroid Book* discusses thyroid disorders; *When the Hearing Gets Hard* helps people cope with hearing loss; *The Breast Cancer Handbook* advises women on managing their care; *Aspirin Handbook* explains what aspirin can do; *The Johns Hopkins Complete Guide for Preventing and Reversing Heart Disease* tells how to reduce your risk.

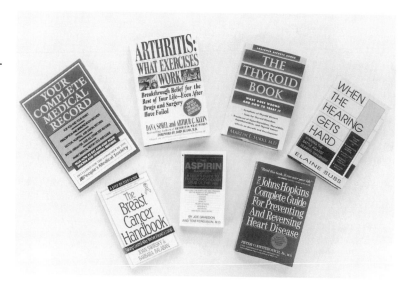

Prostate. *Prostate: Questions You Have . . . Answers You Need* by Sandra Salmans, health writer for *The New York Times* and *Newsweek* magazine, won critical praise as the "best book yet" on the topic. It features basic information on the prostate gland, the disorders that affect it, the treatment of those disorders, and information sources and mutual aid support groups for patients with prostate disorders. (People's Medical Society, 1993. 192 pp. $9.95.)

Stroke. *American Heart Association Family Guide to Stroke: Treatment, Recovery and Prevention* by physicians Louis R. Caplan, Mark L. Dyken, and J. Donald Easton. This clearly written and illustrated sourcebook on stroke includes chapters on warning signs, causes, diagnosis, treatment, rehabilitation, living with disability, and ways to help prevent stroke through diet and lifestyle. (Times Books, 1994. 320 pp. $23.)

Thyroid disease. *The Thyroid Book: What Goes Wrong and How to Treat It* by physician Martin I. Surks. More than 10 million Americans have been diagnosed with thyroid disease. This book discusses diagnosis and treatments for various thyroid disorders. (Consumer Reports Books, 1993. 213 pp. $24.95.) □ Margaret E. Moore

---

Brain and Nervous System

A major advance in research on Alzheimer's disease, a degenerative disorder of the brain that affects many older people, was reported in August 1993 by neuroscientist Elizabeth H. Corder and her associates at the Duke University Medical Center in Durham, N.C. The researchers noted an association between Alzheimer's disease and a gene coding for a protein that transports cholesterol in the blood. The gene is the first to be linked to the form of Alzheimer's disease that occurs mostly after age 65.

Alzheimer's disease is a condition in which *neurons* (nerve cells) in the brain degenerate and die. There are two forms of the disease. One form occurs relatively early in life—before age 65—and has long been recognized as a genetic disorder that runs in families. The other type strikes after age 65 and accounts for more than three-fourths of the Alzheimer's cases in the United States. The scientists' discovery shows that genes are also involved in late-onset Alzheimer's.

Corder and her colleagues found that the risk of developing late-onset Alzheimer's disease increases with the presence of a gene for a protein called Apolipoprotein-E4 (ApoE4). The protein carries cholesterol to body cells, enabling them to construct cell walls.

The researchers found that people with two copies of this gene—one inherited from each parent—are eight times as likely to develop Alzheimer's as individuals with no copies of the gene. Someone with two copies of the gene is almost certain to get Alzheimer's disease by the age of 80.

Only about 2 percent of the population have two copies of the ApoE4 gene. About 1 person in 3, however, carries one copy of the gene. Having a single copy of the gene increases a person's likelihood of developing Alzheimer's by about three times. The scientists could not explain why the gene increases the risk of Alzheimer's disease or how it contributes to the destruction of neurons.

In May 1994, a research team at the University of California at San Francisco reported that perhaps it is not the presence of ApoE4 that is important, but rather the absence of ApoE3, a more common form of the cholesterol-carrying protein. (There are three kinds of apolipoproteins altogether, each produced by a different form of the same gene.)

The scientists grew rabbit neurons in a laboratory dish. They then exposed the cells to a natural substance that induces neurons to send out fibers called neurites that make connections with other neurons. Next, the researchers added either ApoE3 or ApoE4 to the cell cultures. ApoE3 significantly increased the length of neurites, though it decreased the number of neurite branches. ApoE4, however, drastically decreased both the length and branching of neurites. Thus, the researchers said, ApoE3 may be needed by neurons to establish new

261

connections or to maintain existing connections.

When scientists learn how the effects of apolipoproteins relate to the damage seen in the brains of Alzheimer's victims, they may be closer to understanding the cause of this devastating disorder. That knowledge may also bring them closer to a cure. (In the Special Reports section, see COPING WITH ALZHEIMER'S DISEASE.)

Hope for those with diabetes. People with diabetes who maintain their blood sugar at a normal level, rather than just at a level that prevents symptoms, may be able to avoid or delay complications from the disorder—including a serious condition involving the nervous system. That finding was reported in September 1993 by investigators at several medical centers in the United States.

The scientists studied the form of diabetes known as insulin-dependent diabetes mellitus (IDDM). IDDM is an illness that typically develops in childhood and results in the destruction of cells in the pancreas. The pancreas produces the hormone insulin, which controls blood levels of glucose, a sugar used by the body for energy. With IDDM, glucose in the blood can soar to dangerous concentrations.

The disorder is controlled with daily doses of insulin, taken either by injection or from a portable or implanted pump. But the amount of insulin taken

is usually just enough to prevent the acute symptoms of the disease, ranging from excessive thirst to *coma* (prolonged unconsciousness). In most cases, the insulin doses do not reduce glucose to a level equal to that in the blood of nondiabetics.

People with diabetes are prone to a number of health complications from their disorder, including heart disease, kidney disease, and blindness. One of the most disabling complications is a condition called peripheral neuropathy, in which nerve fibers deteriorate and die. Symptoms include arm and leg weakness, numbness, tingling and burning sensations, diarrhea, trouble urinating, and erratic blood pressure. The symptoms usually become progressively worse and can become incapacitating. Some patients suffer excruciating nerve pain.

The researchers studied more than 1,400 people with IDDM. Half the patients were treated with insulin administered either by an external pump or by three or more daily injections of the hormone. The amounts of insulin they received were based on frequent tests of glucose levels and were aimed at keeping blood sugar as close to normal as possible. The other group received insulin in the more conventional way—one or two injections per day, with little variation in the amount.

After following the two groups for about 6½ years, the investigators noted striking differences in the incidence

Does estrogen protect against Alzheimer's?

Taking supplements of the hormone estrogen might help maintain dense connections between brain cells and thus protect against Alzheimer's disease, a degenerative brain disorder that strikes older people. In research reported in early 1994 by scientists at Columbia University in New York City, estrogen produced a marked effect on rat brain tissue grown in the laboratory. Tissue treated with estrogen, *below right,* contains many more connecting fibers than untreated tissue, *below left.*

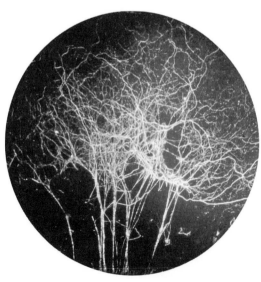
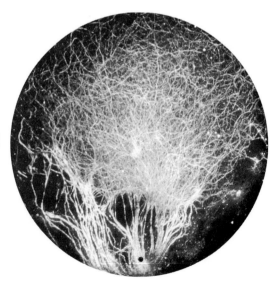

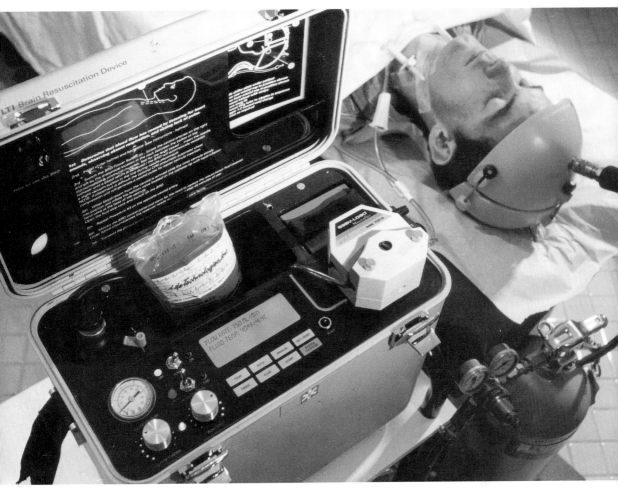

of diabetes complications. The group receiving carefully controlled doses of insulin not only experienced far fewer eye and kidney complications, it also had a 60 percent lower incidence of peripheral neuropathy.

These results offer new hope to people with IDDM who have faced the prospect of developing peripheral neuropathy, as well as other serious complications. Researchers will now attempt to learn if controlling blood sugar by other means would provide the same sorts of benefits for people with adult-onset diabetes, a far more common form of the disorder that usually does not require taking insulin.

The moral center of the brain. How does one make the morally correct decision? Is there a center in the brain devoted to such judgments? Seeking

to answer that question, a team of researchers at several U.S. institutions, led by neurologist Hanna Damasio of the University of Iowa Hospitals and Clinics in Iowa City, analyzed the skull of a man long dead. Their study, reported in May 1994, suggests that there is, indeed, a center in the brain for responsible thinking.

The skull was that of a man named Phineas P. Gage. On Sept.13, 1848, Gage, a 25-year-old railroad construction worker, was involved in a terrible accident. While preparing an explosive charge, he inadvertently tamped down the blasting powder with an iron rod before the powder had been covered with a protective layer of sand. The powder detonated, sending the rod into Gage's left cheek, through his brain, and out the top of his head.

Gage was briefly stunned, but he re-

Cooling the brain
The emerging technology of "brain resuscitation" may soon supplant cardiopulmonary resuscitation for saving the lives of people whose hearts have stopped or who have suffered a stroke or head injury. The technique involves the use of a helmet that lowers the temperature of the head and injected chemicals that limit damage to brain cells while the person is rushed to the hospital.

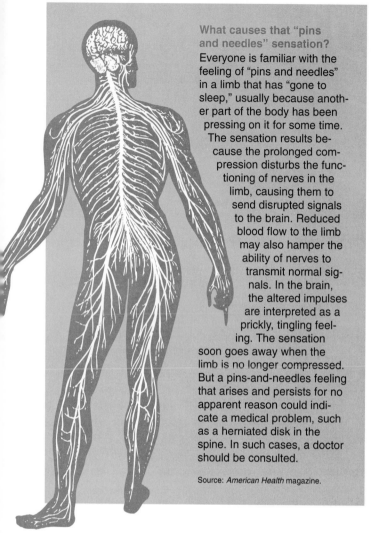

What causes that "pins and needles" sensation?

Everyone is familiar with the feeling of "pins and needles" in a limb that has "gone to sleep," usually because another part of the body has been pressing on it for some time. The sensation results because the prolonged compression disturbs the functioning of nerves in the limb, causing them to send disrupted signals to the brain. Reduced blood flow to the limb may also hamper the ability of nerves to transmit normal signals. In the brain, the altered impulses are interpreted as a prickly, tingling feeling. The sensation soon goes away when the limb is no longer compressed. But a pins-and-needles feeling that arises and persists for no apparent reason could indicate a medical problem, such as a herniated disk in the spine. In such cases, a doctor should be consulted.

Source: *American Health* magazine.

bodily functions. Moral reasoning and social behavior were thought to be functions of the soul.

Several years after Gage's death, his former physician, John Harlow, got permission from the Gage family to exhume the man's skull, as well as the iron bar, which had been buried with the body. Both skull and bar were donated to the Warren Anatomical Medical Museum at Harvard University in Cambridge, Mass. There they lay for over 100 years until Damasio and her associates undertook their study.

The researchers speculated that Gage's antisocial behavior after his accident resulted from damage to a portion of his brain known as the frontal lobes. To demonstrate the site of the man's injury, the investigators carefully photographed the skull and prepared a computer-generated three-dimensional reconstruction of it. They also placed a computer-generated image of a brain into the picture of the skull. Lastly, they passed an image of the rod through the skull and brain at the same angle that the real rod had taken.

The images revealed that the rod had passed through the undersurfaces of both of Gage's frontal lobes, almost certainly destroying that region of the man's brain. This finding supported growing scientific evidence that the frontal lobes are indeed the area of the brain that controls responsible, moral behavior.

Disturbed rhythm. Neuroscientists have long known that there is a "biological clock" in the brain that regulates the body's everyday cycles of activity, known as circadian rhythms. How the clock operates at the molecular level has remained largely a puzzle, though researchers have suspected that genes are involved. In April 1994, neurobiologist Martha H. Vitaterna and her colleagues at Northwestern University in Evanston, Ill., reported finding a gene in mice that controls circadian rhythms.

The scientists injected male mice with a chemical that produced *mutations* (changes) in the DNA of the mice's sperm cells. DNA—deoxyribonucleic acid—is the molecule genes are made of. When the males were mated with normal female mice, the

gained full consciousness and walked away from the accident. From that time on, however, he was a very different person.

Prior to his injury, Gage had been a responsible, hard-working, and considerate young man. After his mishap, though his mental powers were the same and he spoke and moved normally, he became irresponsible and unreliable. He also used profanity continuously and showed no regard for the social conventions that he had once respected.

When Gage died 13 years later, no autopsy was performed to learn what damage to Gage's brain might have caused his striking change in behavior. The medical thinking of the time held that the brain controlled only offspring inherited the mutations in all their body cells.

Of more than 300 mice produced in this way, one had a daily cycle activity of almost 25 hours—about 1 hour longer than that of normal mice. This mouse had inherited a mutation in precisely the gene that the scientists had wanted to locate, one involved with circadian rhythms. The offspring of that mouse were crossbred, resulting in some mice with two copies of the mutated gene. Those mice had a daily cycle of almost 29 hours.

The gene was traced to chromosome number 5 in the mouse cells, which corresponds to human chromosome 4. Presumably the same gene will be found on that human chromosome. Chromosomes are structures in the cell nucleus that carry the genes.

Researchers do not yet know how the newly discovered gene operates to control circadian rhythms. Nonetheless, the finding that an inheritable mutation in a single gene can alter an organism's daily biological cycles is an important advance. The discovery could lead to a better understanding of human disorders, such as severe insomnia, that involve changes in circadian rhythms. □ Gary Birnbaum

In the Special Reports section, see NEW HOPE FOR SPINAL CORD INJURIES. In WORLD BOOK, see BRAIN; NERVOUS SYSTEM.

Cancer

Scientific misconduct by an investigator in a landmark study on the treatment of breast cancer was made public by the *Chicago Tribune* in March 1994. The disclosure triggered widespread criticism of federal government health officials for not reporting the fraud for nearly a year after they discovered it.

The fraud involved the National Surgical Adjuvant Breast and Bowel Project study, conducted by the National Cancer Institute (NCI) from 1976 to 1984. This study had established lumpectomy—removal of the tissue containing a tumor—as a standard treatment for breast cancer. The study had found that lumpectomy followed by radiation therapy is as effective in preventing recurrences of breast cancer as is mastectomy, the removal of the entire breast. In the decade after the study, thousands of breast cancer patients have chosen lumpectomy over mastectomy, based on these results.

Suspicions surrounding data contributed by Roger Poisson, a surgeon at St. Luc's Hospital in Montreal, Canada, first surfaced in routine audits performed by the NCI in June 1990. Poisson had supplied approximately 16 percent of the patients who participated in the study.

At the request of the NCI, the Office of Research Integrity of the Department of Health and Human Services conducted a two-year investigation. A final report in April 1993 concluded that Poisson had enrolled patients who were ineligible for participation in the study for a number of reasons, including the size of their tumors, the date of their diagnosis, and their refusal to grant consent. Moreover, he had altered the data on at least 100 patients he enrolled.

The conclusions of the Office of Research Integrity were not widely known until the newspaper broke the story 11 months later. The newspaper stories alarmed many women who had chosen lumpectomy.

In response, federal health officials scrambled to reassure patients and their doctors that numerous subsequent studies had upheld the effectiveness of lumpectomy. They further asserted that a reanalysis of the data after discounting the fraudulent information led researchers to draw the same conclusions as in the original analysis. As a result of the controversy, the officials pledged to alert the public to suspected fraud in a more timely manner in the future.

The promise of gene therapy for cancer moved a step closer to reality in December 1993. At that time, researchers at the Howard Hughes Medical Institute at the University of Michigan in Ann Arbor reported preliminary findings on a new way of delivering genes that can halt the growth of a severe form of skin cancer.

The therapy involves persuading the body's disease-fighting immune

Defeating Prostate Cancer Through Better Detection

From 1990 to 1993, the number of men diagnosed with prostate cancer in the United States jumped from 106,000 per year to 165,000—an increase of 56 percent. Yearly deaths from the disease increased 17 percent during that time, from around 29,000 to 35,000, according to the American Cancer Society. Cancer of the prostate—a walnut-sized gland between the bladder and the rectum in men—is the second leading cause of cancer death among American men, surpassed only by lung cancer.

Because prostate cancer primarily affects men over age 65, researchers attribute some of the rise in cases to the fact that men are living longer. But the greatest contribution to the rise in cases diagnosed comes from the growing use of a new blood test that can detect prostate cancer in its early stages.

The blood test measures levels of a protein called prostate-specific antigen (PSA), which cells in the prostate produce. Prostate cancer can elevate PSA levels in the blood. A PSA level below 4 *nanograms* (billionths of a gram) per milliliter of blood is considered normal. A level between 4 and 10 is abnormal and may indicate the presence of cancer, and a level above 10 strongly suggests the presence of cancer.

Physicians use the PSA test in addition to a physical examination of the prostate. In this procedure, called a digital rectal examination (DRE), a doctor feels the prostate through the patient's rectum wall for lumps or other irregularities that may signal the presence of cancerous growths.

Any elevation of the PSA level or abnormality in the DRE generally indicates a need for further testing. Physicians may perform a prostate biopsy by removing a small sample of prostate tissue for examination under a microscope. If the tests reveal prostate cancer, physicians take X rays to determine whether the cancer has spread outside the gland. Once the cancer spreads, the chance of curing the disease is low.

Several studies during the 1990's reported on a major advantage of the PSA test: its ability to detect prostate cancer earlier than DRE. In August 1993, researchers at Washington University School of Medicine in St. Louis, Mo., reported the findings of an evaluation of 10,250 men above age 50 who received either a PSA test or a DRE. Detection rates from the PSA test were nearly double those from the DRE. The additional cases of cancer uncov-

ered by the PSA test in general were also less advanced—and thus more treatable—than the cancers detected by DRE.

Results such as these have led physicians to recommend that men over 50 years of age and those who are at greater risk for prostate cancer have a PSA and DRE test every year. African Americans, as well as men with a father or brother who has had the disease, are at higher-than-average risk for prostate cancer.

The PSA test has some drawbacks, however. About 25 percent of men with a noncancerous enlargement of the prostate, a condition common among older men, have an elevated PSA level. This can lead doctors to recommend expensive biopsies for these men. Of much greater concern is the fact that 15 to 20 percent of men with prostate cancer have normal PSA levels.

The standard treatments for prostate cancer are surgery to remove the gland or radiation therapy to kill the cancerous cells. Prostate surgery usually means a hospital stay of less than a week. Radiation therapy is administered on an outpatient basis in daily sessions that continue for six or seven weeks.

Both therapies can have serious side effects, including *impotence* (loss of sexual function) and *incontinence* (involuntary loss of urine). Newer surgical techniques have lowered the risk of both, and radiation therapy, in general, carries less risk of these side effects than surgery.

In some cases, physicians believe that the best initial

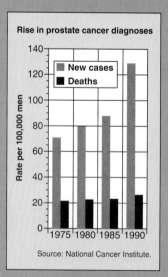

Rise in prostate cancer diagnoses

New cases
Deaths

Rate per 100,000 men

1975 1980 1985 1990

Source: National Cancer Institute.

treatment for early prostate cancer may be no treatment, thus sparing patients the potential side effects. This option is known as watchful waiting.

If the cancer progresses, patients can be treated with drugs that lower levels of the male hormone testosterone. Because testosterone fuels the growth of most prostate cancers, decreasing its level in the bloodstream can slow or halt the cancer's growth. However, hormone treatments cannot cure prostate cancer, and in most cases, the cancer will eventually continue to grow.

A study of 826 men with prostate cancer, reported in January 1994, analyzed the results of this approach. The study, performed by researchers at the University of Chicago Hospitals and other centers, found that, with no treatment, men with small cancers confined to the prostate had as high as an 87 percent chance of survival 10 years after the initial diagnosis.

However, in 40 to 50 percent of the patients, the cancer had spread after 10 years. The findings indicate that men who are unlikely to live another 10 years because of their age or other health problems would make the best candidates for watchful waiting.

The ability to diagnose and treat prostate cancer is improving. Further research will likely increase treatment options and reduce side effects. And improved diagnostic methods may enable physicians to better determine which patients should have surgery, radiation, or a close watch of their cancer.   □ Glenn S. Gerber

system to attack the cancerous tumor as foreign tissue and destroy it. To do so, researchers inserted a new gene into the cancerous cells. The gene produces a protein that sits on the cell surface and marks the cell, much as a uniform marks an enemy soldier, for destruction by white blood cells, the soldiers of the immune system.

Until this experiment, researchers had delivered genetic material to diseased cells by encasing it within deactivated viruses. When the viruses enter cells, they incorporate their own genes—along with any genetic baggage they are carrying—into the genetic material of the cells they infect. But researchers have worried that this technique could backfire and that seemingly harmless viruses could regain some of their power to cause disease. For this reason, they have delivered the viruses into cells that had first been removed from patients. They then injected the cells back into the patients.

In the Michigan study, the researchers placed the genes in a new vehicle, tiny fat globules called liposomes, and delivered them directly to the patient. Liposomes readily slide through a cell's outer membrane and into its nucleus. Doctors injected the gene-loaded liposomes directly into the tumors of five patients with melanoma, a deadly form of skin cancer.

As a result of the new genes, the number of cancer-fighting immune cells attracted to the tumor increased as much as fivefold. In one patient, the gene not only triggered attacks that wiped out the targeted tumor but also initiated assaults on tumors elsewhere in the patient's body. The researchers hope that the new delivery system will expand the possibilities for treating cancer and other diseases.

Guidelines on mammography. In a controversial move, the NCI in December 1993 dropped its recommendation that women under 50 years of age should be screened for breast cancer with a *mammogram* (X-ray examination of the breast) every year or two. The agency stated that scientific data failed to indicate that regular mammograms reduce the number of deaths from breast cancer in women aged 40 to 49.

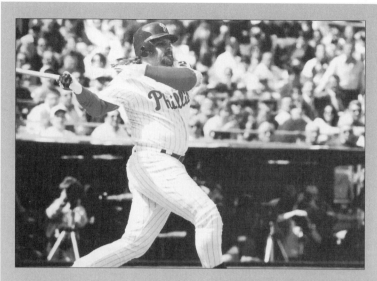

A young man's disease
John Kruk, first baseman of the Philadelphia Phillies, was diagnosed in 1994 with testicular cancer—the most common tumor among men aged 15 to 40. Kruk returned to baseball following surgery and radiation. An estimated 6,800 new cases of this highly curable form of cancer will be diagnosed in 1994. Five years after diagnosis, 93 percent of patients are alive, and recurrence after that is rare. Early detection greatly increases the chances of successful treatment.

- Men aged 20 to 50 should check their testicles monthly for any lumps, enlargement, or changes in consistency.
- Any lump or other change should immediately be checked by a physician.

Source: American Cancer Society.

The NCI continued to recommend that women 50 and older receive annual mammograms, stating that there is clear evidence that mammography lowers death rates from breast cancer by about one-third in this group. The institute replaced its guideline for younger women with a statement advising women under age 50 at high risk for breast cancer to discuss individualized screening plans with their doctors.

The decision by the NCI followed several recent studies that raised questions about the value of mammograms in younger women. A decisive report, published in October 1993, analyzed data from eight large mammography trials conducted since the 1960's. It found no reduction in breast cancer deaths in women in the 40-to-49 age group who were screened every year or two.

Such studies, however, have failed to convince other medical organizations, including the American Cancer Society and the American College of Radiology. These groups continue to recommend regular mammograms for all women, beginning at age 40.

Pain guidelines. New federal guidelines for the management of pain associated with cancer were released in March 1994 by the Agency for Health Care Policy and Research, a branch of the United States Department of Health and Human Services. The guidelines urged physicians to be more aggressive in treating the pain experienced by patients with cancer.

According to a report accompanying the release of the guidelines, at least 60 percent of the 8 million Americans with cancer or a history of cancer have experienced moderate to severe pain. Of the 1,308 cancer patients interviewed at 54 treatment locations, 42 percent reported receiving too little treatment for pain. Women, children, older people, and members of minority groups were particularly vulnerable to undertreatment.

A major barrier to adequate pain relief has been fear of addiction, by both physicians and cancer patients. However, addiction to painkillers among cancer patients, studies have demonstrated, occurs in less than 1 case out of 1,000. Other obstacles to pain relief involve patients' fear that drugs lose their effectiveness when "taken too often," physicians' anxiety over state narcotics regulations, and problems related to insurance company reimbursement of drug costs.

The new guidelines emphasized that the pain of 90 percent of cancer patients can be eliminated by medications ranging from aspirin to morphine. The guidelines encouraged doctors to raise doses based on the patient's own assessment of pain.

Polyps and cancer. The findings of two key studies released in December

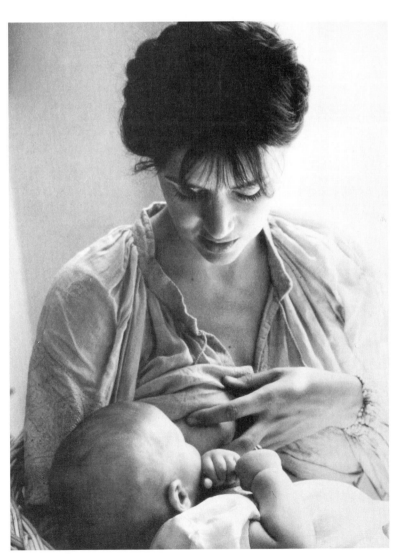

Lowering mother's breast cancer risk
Breast-feeding may provide women with some protection against breast cancer, a group of medical researchers reported in January 1994. The scientists' study of 14,000 mothers found that those who breast-fed their children had a reduced risk of breast cancer before menopause, the time in a woman's life when menstrual periods cease. Women who first breast-fed before age 20 had the lowest incidence of breast cancer. Breast-feeding did not appear to affect the risk of developing breast cancer after menopause, however.

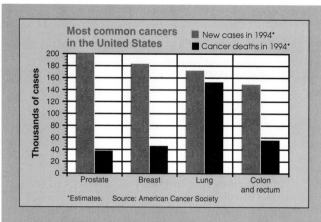

Most common cancers in the United States

- New cases in 1994*
- Cancer deaths in 1994*

Thousands of cases

*Estimates. Source: American Cancer Society

Preventing colon cancer

Cancers of the colon and rectum are the fourth most common types of cancer in the United States but the second leading cancer killers, surpassed only by lung cancer. Some simple steps can lower your risk of developing the disease.

- Maintain a diet high in fiber and low in fat. Dietary fiber, especially that in grain, lowers the risk of colon cancer whereas fat, especially that in red meat, raises the risk.
- Include plenty of fruits, vegetables, vitamin D, and calcium in your diet. All are associated with a reduced risk of colon and rectal cancers.
- Exercise. Studies associate both a sedentary lifestyle and obesity with an elevated risk of colon and rectal cancers.
- After age 40, have an annual rectal examination. After age 50, have a blood stool test annually and an examination of the lower colon every three to five years. Early detection greatly increases the chances of a cure.

Source: American Cancer Society.

1993 armed physicians with new strategies for preventing colon cancer. The National Polyp Study, conducted at Memorial Sloan-Kettering Cancer Center in New York City, found that the removal of growths called polyps from the colon sharply reduces the chances of developing colon cancer. Over time, polyps that sprout from the wall of the large intestine are believed to become cancerous.

In the polyp study, conducted from 1980 to 1990, 1,418 patients had at least one precancerous polyp removed and participated in follow-up examinations for an average period of six years. The follow-up included *colonoscopy* (a visual examination of the colon with a viewing device called a colonoscope).

The study found that the rate of colon cancer was 90 percent lower in patients who had polyps removed than the rate expected in a group that did not undergo the polyp-clearing procedure. The study also supported the view that polyps progress to a cancerous state if not removed.

In a second study of polyps, researchers at Johns Hopkins University School of Medicine in Baltimore worked on perfecting a blood test to detect the gene that places certain individuals at risk for developing polyps. One defective gene leads to familial adenomatous polyposis (FAP)—a rare disorder characterized by the growth of hundreds of colon polyps. Researchers believe that FAP affects 50,000 people in the United States and accounts for about 1 percent of the nation's 150,000 annual new cases of colon cancer.

A new blood test for FAP was developed after researchers discovered that the genetic defect results in a protein that is measurably shorter than the normal gene's protein. The test stimulates production of the protein in quantities large enough to measure. The new test successfully detected the presence of the defective gene in 54 out of 62 patients diagnosed with FAP, an 87 percent success rate. The test will allow physicians to identify people who have the gene and employ such measures as polyp removal or drug therapy to prevent the development of cancer.

News on tamoxifen. Various risks associated with the drug tamoxifen sparked controversy in 1993 and 1994. Tamoxifen is widely prescribed to prevent the recurrence of breast cancer in women who have been treated for the disease.

In September 1993, the developer of tamoxifen reported that the drug was capable of causing liver cancer in rats. Researchers at the company found that rats treated with tamoxifen developed 20 to 35 times more tumors than rats that did not receive the drug. They also found that these tumors spread rapidly.

In March 1994, researchers at Yale University School of Medicine in New Haven, Conn., reported that tamoxifen can foster a deadly form of endometrial cancer, cancer of the lining of the uterus. The Yale researchers studied 53 breast cancer patients who developed endometrial cancer, 15 of whom were taking tamoxifen. They found that two-thirds of the endometrial cancers in women taking tamoxifen were rapidly growing. In contrast, only 25 percent of endometrial cancers in women not taking tamoxifen were of the deadly type. The researchers also found that the interval between the diagnosis of breast cancer and the onset of endometrial cancer averaged 5 years among women who had taken the drug, compared with 12 years among women who had not.

In 1992, the NCI began a cancer prevention trial to determine whether the drug could prevent breast cancer in healthy women at high risk for the disease. The reports of health risks associated with tamoxifen have raised questions over whether the NCI study is jeopardizing participants' health.

In March 1994, NCI reported that 25 of 4,000 women who took tamoxifen after breast cancer surgery had developed uterine cancer. Six of the 25 died. NCI spokespersons insist that the risk of developing uterine cancer from tamoxifen is low and that the drug's benefits in preventing recurrences of breast cancer far outweigh its risks. □ Jill Waalen

In WORLD BOOK, see CANCER.

Child Development

Young children can be made to "remember" events that never happened to them, a study published in the fall of 1993 demonstrated. The study, which was led by developmental psychologist Steven J. Ceci of Cornell University in Ithaca, N.Y., investigated the effect that adult interviewers can have on a child's development of false memories.

The investigators selected 164 preschoolers, ages 3 through 6, and put them into four groups. Each group of children heard stories about a supposedly clumsy adult named Sam Stone.

One group heard twice a week for a month in advance of Sam Stone's visit to the school how Sam had broken someone's Barbie doll, spilled chocolate milk on a white teddy bear, or torn a book. Another group heard for 12 weeks after the man's visit how Sam Stone had broken a doll, spilled milk, and ruined a book during his time at school. A third group heard these stories both during the month before and the 12-week period after the man's appearance at the school. The fourth group received no such misinformation about Sam Stone.

The man called Sam Stone, who was actually one of Ceci's research colleagues, visited the preschool, patted a few children on the head, and left quickly. He spilled nothing and broke nothing.

But the advance publicity had its effect. The children who had been primed in advance to expect bad things from Sam never took their eyes off him. Some of them called out, "Sam, watch out!" or "Sam, don't touch anything!"

When the 12-week period following Sam Stone's visit had ended, a newly introduced investigator asked each of the 164 children, "I wasn't there when Sam Stone came. Can you tell me what happened?" Following a free, undirected narrative from each child, the researcher would ask about specifics, such as broken dolls, dirty bears, or torn books.

The experiment showed that false memories of Sam Stone's clumsiness developed in a large number of the children. This occurred more often among the 3-year-old children than the 5-year-old children. In addition, the children indoctrinated both before and after Sam Stone's visit to the school were most likely to have false memories.

However, when the investigator asked, "Did you see what you've been telling me with your own eyes?" the number of inaccurate memories immediately dropped. When the researcher pressed further, saying "Oh, come on. Really?" the small children tended to abandon their false stories altogether. Only 20 percent of the 3-year-olds and 10 percent of the 5-year-olds clung to their false story after persistent questioning.

This study raises concern that parents' or teachers' comments, or the

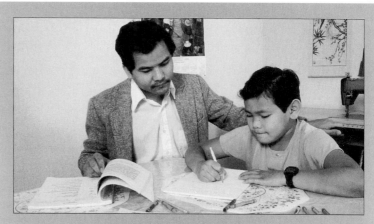

Promoting good study habits

If parents take an active interest in their children's studies, the children learn the importance of achievement, which leads to greater success in school and enhanced emotional growth, according to the American Academy of Pediatrics (AAP). The AAP offers parents the following tips:

- Get to know your child's teachers and what is expected of the child. Attend school events, such as parent/teacher meetings.

- Set up a well-lit, quiet area for doing homework, and designate a regular, nightly homework time.

- Learn how much homework your child is expected to do. The National Education Association recommends no more than 20 minutes of homework each night for children in kindergarten through third grade, and 20 to 40 minutes for children in grades four through six.

- See that your child does his or her own homework. Children learn by thinking for themselves and making their own mistakes. Parents can make suggestions and help a child understand directions, but they should let the child do the learning.

experience of psychotherapy, has the potential to influence children's memories. Repetition of misinformation increases the chances that children will retain faulty memories.

In a number of court cases involving alleged child abuse, the outcome of a case has depended upon the testimony of a child. The question of just how accurate children's memories are often arises.

Professionals and parents dealing with preschoolers should be aware of how open to suggestion these children are. Although experts dealing with abuse cases must be careful not to discourage a child from revealing a true memory, they may succeed in discerning false memories by gently challenging a child.

Sugar and hyperactivity are not related, according to two studies published in February 1994. A popular belief among many parents had maintained that *sucrose* (refined sugar) and the artificial sweetener aspartame caused hyperactivity or other behavioral changes in children.

A group of pediatricians and psychologists from Vanderbilt University, in Nashville, Tenn., and the University of Iowa in Iowa City tested two groups of children. One group consisted of 23 children, aged 6 to 10, who were sensitive to sugar, according to their parents. In the other group were 25 children aged 3 to 5, who were thought to have no such sensitivity. The researchers put the children and their families on three different diets. One diet contained high amounts of su-crose, one contained aspartame, and the third contained saccharin, an arti-ficial sweetener that has not been linked to hyperactive behavior. The subjects were not told which diet they were on.

Each group followed one diet for three weeks, then the second diet for three weeks, and then the third diet. Artificial coloring and additives were excluded from the diets, since some people believe that those substances affect behavior.

Each week, the researchers evaluat-ed the children's behavior and *cogni-tive* (intellectual) skills. Even though all the children ingested large amounts of the three sugary substances, no evi-dence of hyperactive behavior or cog-nitive changes appeared in either of the two groups.

In the second study, conducted by scientists at Yale University in New Haven, Conn., 15 children who had been diagnosed as hyperactive re-ceived very high doses of aspartame. Studies on animals had shown that high doses of aspartame alter the pro-duction of a brain chemical known as catecholamine.

The Yale group theorized that aspar-tame might impair the children's con-centration or self-control—abilities that are associated with catecholamine. However, no such effect surfaced in the study. This was true even though the children were given 10 times the dose of aspartame that a child might ordinarily consume.

Most experts think that these two experiments have all but demolished the hypothesis that associates sugar with hyperactivity. But the question re-mains whether these studies will lay the issue to rest among parents who worry that sugary junk food can cause psychological and behavioral prob-lems in their youngsters. These stud-ies suggest that, so far as sugar goes, parents need concern themselves only with the problems of tooth decay and obesity.

Mozart and the mind. Listening to the music of Austrian composer Wolf-gang Amadeus Mozart may briefly stimulate intelligence. This was the finding of a study published in Octo-ber 1993 by researchers from the Center for the Neurobiology of Learn-ing and Memory at the University of California in Irvine. The researchers suggested that the highly complex and nonrepetitive music of Mozart stimulates the nerve pathways in the brain associated with abstract think-ing—the thought processes used, for example, in solving mathematics problems or playing chess.

The researchers gave 36 college students a standard test of spatial intelligence after they listened to a Mozart composition for piano for 10 minutes. The students also received the same test after listening to a relax-

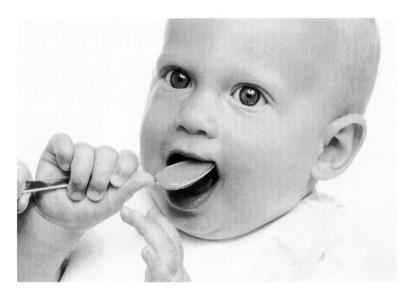

Babies eat greens
Infants aged 4 to 6 months who had never tasted vegetables ate peas and green beans when they were offered the food repeatedly in a study reported in February 1994. The mothers were told to stop offering the food if the infant refused to take it three times. Over 10 days, all 36 babies in the study significantly in-creased their vegetable in-take. Breast-fed babies ate more vegetables than bottle-fed babies.

ation tape for 10 minutes and after 10 minutes of silence.

The students scored an average of 8 or 9 points higher after listening to Mozart than after listening to the relaxation tape or remaining in a silent room. The researchers took the subjects' pulse rates before and after each listening experience and found no indication that physical stimulation had played a role in the higher scores. However, the authors of the study found that the subjects' increased intelligence faded quickly after they had completed the tests.

The researchers expressed an interest in studying other forms of music in the future. They predicted that less complex and more repetitive music would not enhance abstract thinking as Mozart's music did. The researchers also said it would be interesting to test musicians to compare their responses to those of nonmusicians.

Frequent moves cause problems.
Children whose families relocate frequently perform more poorly at school and are affected by more behavioral problems than other children. This was the conclusion of a study published in September 1993 by a group of researchers from the School of Medicine at the University of California at San Francisco.

The researchers examined the results of a 1988 survey of families in the United States. From the survey, they derived data on almost 10,000 children aged 6 to 17 years.

Of the children from families that moved frequently, 23 percent repeated a year in school. In contrast, only 12 percent of children whose families moved infrequently repeated a grade in school. In addition, 18 percent of the children in mobile families exhibited four or more behavioral problems. Only 7 percent of children who rarely moved exhibited that number of behavioral problems.

The researchers concluded that moving is disruptive for children because of the difficult adjustments they face. These include adjustments to new friends, new neighborhoods, and new teachers.

Surveys indicate that American families are twice as likely to move as British or German families. Poor families in America move much more often than affluent families, and families headed by single parents move more frequently than two-parent families. White families move more often than African-American or Hispanic-American families do.

Researchers at the National Institute on Mental Health (NIMH) in Rockville, Md., had previously examined the effects of moving on children. Their 1991 study focused on children with parents in military service who moved frequently among military bases.

The NIMH study found that the severity of emotional and behavioral problems reported among children of military parents did not differ from levels of disturbance reported among children of civilians. In fact, some of the military children reported fewer emotional and behavioral difficulties than did their civilian counterparts.

Although the 1991 and 1993 studies appear to differ in their results, they also differ in the measures they used. The California study looked at failing a grade in school, for example, whereas the NIMH study did not. The California group did not examine signs of emotional distress, whereas the NIMH study did.

Most importantly, the California study took into account the numerous problems that account for repeated moves—evictions, family breakups, substance abuse, lack of money. The NIMH study had included only moves that were based on a job transfer (a military relocation), which is usually not a negative event for a family. The children of military personnel would also have continued to enjoy the advantages of free or low-cost social, recreational, and community services as well as the social support of being among like-minded people.

The California researchers concluded that moving is at least one risk factor among many that can create learning and behavioral problems in children. They recommended that parents and people who work with children be aware of this particular stress in dealing with children.

☐ Lenore Terr

In the Special Reports section, see DR. SPOCK TALKS ABOUT RAISING CHILDREN TODAY. In WORLD BOOK, see CHILD.

Childbirth
See Pregnancy and Childbirth

Contraception
See Birth Control

A new mercury-free material for filling cavities could be ready for use in dental offices within three years, the National Institute of Dental Research (NIDR) announced in October 1993. The silver-tin alloy could replace silver amalgam, a mixture of silver and mercury now used to fill cavities. The NIDR is part of the National Institutes of Health in Bethesda, Md.

NIDR emphasized that dental amalgam containing mercury has been used safely for more than 150 years, and that no scientific evidence links the amalgam with human disease. Although mercury is poisonous, a panel of experts concluded in 1991 that the small amount used in fillings posed no health threat. The NIDR said, however, that public concern about possible harmful effects of amalgam created a need for alternative filling materials.

NIDR funded research on the filling material, which was led by David Lashmore, a metals expert at the National Institute of Standards and Technology. Lashmore noted that it had never before been possible to make a strong, durable, easy-to-use filling material without mercury.

The mercury-free filling was made with new technology for combining, or alloying, metals. It consists of silver and tin powders that a dentist places

Dentistry

Electronic pain control
Dental patients who dislike injections may be happier with a device that uses electric signals to block the sensation of pain. Electrodes are placed on the patient's skin near the site of the dental work, and the patient controls the strength of the signals by means of a small handheld device.

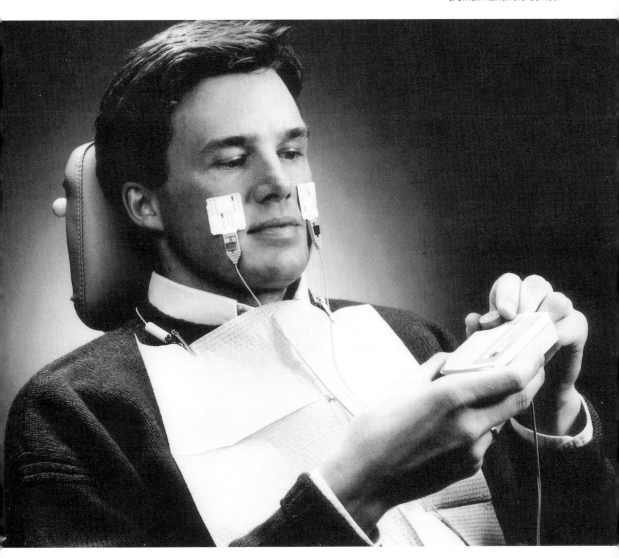

in a prepared cavity, much like a conventional dental amalgam. The powders fuse into a solid plug of metal when subjected to pressure. Lashmore said that the normal pressure a dentist uses to press a filling into a cavity is enough to weld the metals. Patients should notice little difference between the new filling and one containing mercury, except that the new material is shinier.

Gum disease screening. Dentists in October 1993 began adding a new screening test for periodontal, or gum, disease to patients' routine checkups. The periodontal screening and reporting (PSR) test detects early gum disease and gives patients a numerical score for gum health. The PSR test is painless, takes only a few minutes, and will not increase the cost of a routine dental visit, the American Dental Association (ADA) said. The ADA announced the introduction of the test along with the American Academy of Periodontology.

Dentists perform the PSR test with a small probe that measures the depth of spaces between the teeth and gums. They also note other symptoms of gum disease, such as bleeding gums and the presence of *plaque* (sticky deposits made of bacteria, food, and other material). Each patient gets a score ranging from 0 to 4, with 0 meaning no gum disease and 4 meaning advanced gum disease.

Periodontal disease is an inflammation of the gums and other tissues that hold the teeth in the mouth. Affected gums may bleed easily, become swollen and tender, develop infected pockets of pus, and cause bad breath. Although regular flossing, brushing, and professional care can help prevent gum disease, it affects 3 out of 4 Americans and is the leading cause of tooth loss in adults.

Material to heal gum and bone. A powdered glass material that helps heal gum and bone damaged by severe periodontal disease received approval from the Federal Drug Administration (FDA) in November 1993. Called PerioGlas, the material was developed by Larry Hench, a professor of materials science at the University of Florida in Gainesville. It consists of calcium and phosphorus in the proportions found in natural bone, plus silicon and sodium.

Dentists mix PerioGlas powder with sterile water to form a paste. They then surgically pack the paste into deep pockets between the teeth and diseased gums. Body cells recognize PerioGlas as natural bone mineral and grow new bone on it. PerioGlas also encourages new connective tissue to grow in the ligament that holds teeth in the mouth. This ligament is destroyed in severe gum disease.

☐ Michael Woods

In WORLD BOOK, see DENTISTRY.

Diabetes

With the help of a registered dietitian, people with all types of diabetes should create a meal plan tailored just for them, according to new guidelines issued in June 1994 by the American Diabetes Association (ADA). The ADA no longer feels that the standardized "diabetic diet" recommended in 1986 is appropriate for everyone with the disease. Nearly 14 million people in the United States have diabetes.

The new guidelines are based on the results of a landmark study showing that complications of diabetes, including eye and kidney disorders, could be reduced as much as 50 to 75 percent in patients with Type I (insulin-dependent) diabetes through careful control of blood *glucose* (sug-

ar). The guidelines aim at lowering blood glucose to normal or near-normal levels: between 80 and 120 milligrams per deciliter (tenth of a liter) of blood before meals and between 100 and 140 milligrams per deciliter at bedtime.

The new guidelines stress management of the disease by the patient to achieve these levels. In addition to careful meal planning, treatment can include frequent monitoring of blood glucose and regular exercise.

Landmark study results. The Diabetes Control and Complications Trial (DCCT), a 10-year study of the effects of tight glucose control on diabetes, was published in September 1993.

The DCCT researchers from 27 medical centers in the United States and Canada had studied 1,441 people with Type I diabetes, and their findings provided the most solid scientific evidence to date of the benefits of tight control in delaying the onset of diabetes complications.

The patients assigned to tight glucose control measured their blood glucose levels at least four times a day and adjusted their doses of insulin based on the readings. They took insulin either continuously through a tiny pump implanted under the skin or in three or more shots per day. On average, they lowered their blood glucose levels to 155 milligrams per deciliter of blood, compared with 231 milliliters per deciliter for patients in the conventional care group. Those on tight control tended to gain weight, however, and they had two to three times the incidence of severe *hypoglycemia* (low blood sugar) as the conventional care group had.

The researchers found that tight glucose control reduced the incidence of *diabetic retinopathy* (a diabetes-related eye disorder) by 76 percent. For those patients who already had evidence of mild retinopathy when they entered the trial, tight control slowed its progression by 54 percent. The risks of developing two other complications of diabetes, peripheral nerve disease and kidney disease, decreased by 60 percent and 39 percent, respectively, in those who tightly controlled their glucose levels.

Drug therapy. A medication used to treat high blood pressure halts the progression of kidney disease in people with Type I diabetes, according to a study reported in November 1993 by investigators at Rush-Presbyterian-St. Luke's Medical Center in Chicago.

The Chicago researchers gave the drug captopril three times a day to about half of the 409 patients with diabetes, kidney disease, and kidney damage who participated in the study. The rest received *placebos* (inactive substances). People in the captopril group had better kidney function and were less likely to require *dialysis* (a mechanical method of filtering wastes from the blood), receive a kidney transplant, or die of kidney disease. Surprisingly, captopril slowed the rate of loss of kidney function even in participants with advanced kidney disease. The researchers theorized that the drug reduces blood pressure within the kidneys' tiny filters. In people with diabetes, pressure causes scarring of these filters, which leads to kidney failure.

The diabetes price tag. The cost of treating diabetes has risen significantly in recent years, according to an ADA study reported in September 1993. The nationwide cost of diabetes treatment, including the cost to employers

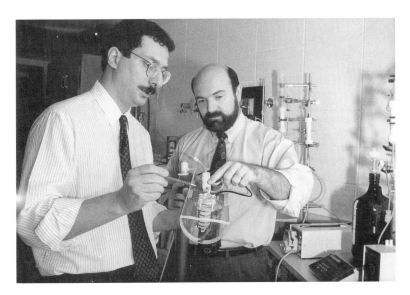

Insulin without shots? Researchers at the Georgia Institute of Technology in Atlanta were testing the insulin-secreting ability of genetically engineered mouse pancreas cells in late 1993. They hope to use the cells in creating an artificial pancreas that would produce insulin in response to the body's changing levels of blood sugar, thus freeing some diabetes patients from daily insulin injections.

when employees with diabetes miss work, was $91.8 billion in 1992, compared with $20.4 billion in 1987. The direct medical cost of treating diabetes was $45.2 billion in 1992, or 5.8 percent of the nation's health care expenditures. The ADA estimated that the annual cost of caring for each person with Type I diabetes was $1,700. The cost would increase to $3,700 with the intensive therapy recommended in the DCCT.

Antibody research. In 1993, researchers in California reported on their discovery that a molecule called glutamate decarboxylase (GAD) stimulates a response in the immune systems of mice that leads to Type I diabetes. This reaction, they said, triggers a cascade of events, called an autoimmune reaction, that results in the destruction of insulin-producing beta cells in the pancreas. Without sufficient insulin, the body is unable to regulate blood sugar levels, and diabetes is the result. But by treating the mice, the scientists were able to block this destructive process, thus preventing diabetes in diabetes-prone mice.

The investigators, at Stanford University and the University of California at Los Angeles, drew blood from mice specially bred to develop Type I diabetes. They mixed various substances with blood samples as the disease progressed in the mice. Tests turned up one substance that the mice react-ed against at all intervals—GAD.

The researchers then injected GAD in mice at three weeks of age, when their immune system was too immature to function well. They hoped to find out if the mouse's immune system could somehow learn not to fight GAD, thus preventing the onset of diabetes. They were able to prevent or minimize the GAD reaction in 75 percent of the mice.

In a second study, reported in January 1994, French researchers found that by treating diabetic mice with a laboratory-produced *antibody* (disease-fighting molecule), they were able to restore the animals' capacity to regulate their blood sugar. The researchers administered the antibody within a week of the first signs of diabetes. Once the antibody was administered, the animals' own immune system cells stopped attacking insulin-producing beta cells, thus halting the progression of the disease. The treated mice stayed disease-free for at least four months after treatment.

When administered to human beings, however, this antibody has caused serious side effects. But investigators are hopeful that just a fragment of the antibody might prove effective in preventing full-blown diabetes without producing adverse effects. □ Richard Trubo

In the Special Reports section, see Understanding Type II Diabetes. In World Book, see Diabetes.

Digestive System

Nicotine delivered through skin patches helps relieve symptoms of ulcerative colitis. That was the conclusion of a study published in March 1994 by gastroenterologist Rupert D. Pullan and his colleagues at the University Hospital of Wales in Cardiff in the United Kingdom.

Ulcerative colitis is an inflammatory disease of the lining of the colon that strikes people primarily between the ages of 15 and 35. The symptoms of the disorder can include rectal bleeding, diarrhea, abdominal cramps, and fever.

The cause of ulcerative colitis is unknown, though gastroenterologists who study the disease suspect that it results when *antibodies* (disease-fight-ing molecules of the immune system) mistake the tissue of the colon for foreign cells and attack it. Medications commonly used in treating the disease include sulfasalazine, hydrocortisone, prednisone, and other agents that help reduce the inflammation by suppressing the activity of the immune system.

Nicotine is a chemical compound found in tobacco plants and is the ingredient in tobacco to which people become addicted. Nicotine patches were designed to help smokers quit their habit by gradually weaning them from nicotine. The patches, which are worn on the skin, deliver a small amount of nicotine directly into the wearer's bloodstream.

Beating the runs

Most cases of diarrhea clear up on their own, but a few simple steps at home can help speed the recovery.

- Drink clear liquids. Water is best, but other options include fruit drinks or juices (not prune juice), caffeine-free soft drinks, gelatin, and broth.
- Drink lots of liquids. Drink at least 8 to 10 glasses of water each day to avoid complications from dehydration and the loss of sodium and potassium.
- Eat low-fiber foods. As symptoms lessen, start to eat low-fiber foods, such as soda crackers, toast, eggs, rice, or chicken. Do not eat greasy or fatty foods, milk, or highly seasoned foods for several days.

See a doctor in the following circumstances:

- The diarrhea lasts more than three days.
- There is severe abdominal or rectal pain.
- A fever rises above 102 °F (38.9 °C).
- There is blood in the stool.
- Little or no urination occurs for 6 hours or more.
- There is repeated vomiting for 12 hours or more.
- There are signs of dehydration, such as little or no urination for six hours or more, severe weakness, excessive thirst, or drowsiness.

Adapted with permission from *The Mayo Clinic Health Letter*, October 1993.

Researchers first noticed a connection between nicotine intake and ulcerative colitis in 1982. At that time, British gastroenterologists noted that rates of cigarette smoking were far lower among people with ulcerative colitis than among the general population. In addition, they observed that colitis symptoms seemed to ease in patients who did smoke. Studies have also found that stopping smoking appears to increase the chances of developing ulcerative colitis.

Pullan's experiment was the first major controlled study of the effect of nicotine treatment on ulcerative colitis, however. For the study, Pullan recruited 72 patients whose colitis was growing worse, despite treatment with anti-inflammatory drugs.

About half the patients received nicotine patches. The remainder received patches containing a *placebo* (inactive substance). All patients continued treatment with anti-inflammatory drugs for the duration of the six-week experiment. The experiment was *double blinded*, meaning that neither the patients nor the physicians knew who had received the nicotine.

Pullan's team reported that colitis symptoms disappeared in nearly twice as many patients in the group that received nicotine as in the group that received the placebo. Symptoms in 16 of the 35 patients in the nicotine group disappeared completely, compared with 9 of 37 in the placebo group.

Physicians are unsure exactly how

nicotine might relieve colitis symptoms, however. And regardless of how nicotine works in such cases, physicians do not recommend that patients with ulcerative colitis resume smoking or take up smoking. Numerous studies have shown that smoking greatly increases the risk of other serious illnesses, including cancer, emphysema, and coronary artery disease.

Treating Crohn's disease. Long-term treatment with the drug cyclosporine may worsen symptoms of Crohn's disease, a chronic inflammatory condition of the small intestine. That was the conclusion of a June 1994 report by a team of gastroenterologists led by Brian G. Feagan of the University of Alberta in Canada.

Medical researchers are unsure what causes Crohn's disease. But many researchers believe that, as with ulcerative colitis, antibodies mistakenly attack the body's own tissue.

The standard treatment for Crohn's disease aims at reducing inflammation in the small intestine. Common medications for reducing inflammation include azathiprine, mercaptopurine, and corticosteroids, which lower the activity of the immune system. Most patients respond well to these drugs, but the drugs can produce serious side effects, including *osteoporosis* (thinning of bone tissue) and inflammation of the pancreas.

Researchers in the early 1990's noted that cyclosporine, which is used to suppress the functioning of the immune system in organ-transplant patients, also relieved symptoms of ulcerative colitis, which closely resembles Crohn's disease. Treatment with cyclosporine has worked well to relieve symptoms in Crohn's patients over a few weeks, but no studies had determined its effectiveness over longer periods.

Feagan's research team treated 151 Crohn's patients with cyclosporine and 154 patients with a placebo for 18 months. Symptoms worsened in 60 percent of the cyclosporine patients, compared with 52 percent of those who received a placebo.

Acid for a deadly cirrhosis. French researchers reported on a potential new treatment in May 1994 for a deadly form of cirrhosis—a disease in which scar tissue forms in the liver. The new treatment slows the progress of the disease and reduces the need for liver transplants.

The form of cirrhosis that the researchers treated—primary biliary cirrhosis (PBC)—progressively destroys narrow tubes called ducts that transport bile from the liver to the small intestine. Bile is a greenish-yellow fluid that helps digest and absorb fat in the small intestine. When PBC destroys bile ducts, acids found in bile and other toxic substances build up in the liver. High concentrations of these toxins can seriously injure liver cells and lead to liver failure. Ninety percent of patients who develop PBC are women in their 40's.

Prior to the French study, the only way of dealing with the progression of PBC was to replace the patient's diseased liver with a transplanted healthy liver. The standard drug treatment for PBC attempts only to alleviate the symptoms of the disease and to prevent certain complications, such as reduced fat absorption in the intestinal tract.

The French researchers reported that ursodeoxycholic (UDC) acid, a bile acid normally present in the liver, slowed the progression of PBC. Gastroenterologist Renée Poupon and her associates in the French Ursodeoxycholic Primary Biliary Cirrhosis Study Group treated 145 patients.

Of those patients, 72 received UDC for two years. The remaining 73 patients received a placebo. The researchers reported that patients in the group that received UDC were three times less likely to need a liver transplant than were patients in the group that received the placebo. The results convinced the researchers to switch the placebo group to UDC treatment two years before the scheduled end of the study.

UDC normally occurs in the liver at smaller concentrations than other, more toxic, bile acids. At increased dosages, UDC helps increase the flow of bile from the liver and neutralizes the effect of the more toxic bile acids on the liver. ☐ James L. Franklin

In the Special Reports section, see BAGGING THE ULCER BUG. In WORLD BOOK, see DIGESTIVE SYSTEM; LIVER.

Drug Abuse
See Alcohol and Drug Abuse

Naproxen sodium, sold as Aleve, reached the market in June 1994. It is the first nonprescription pain reliever containing a new active ingredient to be introduced since the mid-1980's, when the status of ibuprofen was changed from prescription to nonprescription. Naproxen sodium has been available for years as a prescription pain reliever (sold as Anaprox) used to treat arthritis and other conditions associated with mild to moderate pain. The nonprescription product contains a smaller amount of naproxen sodium than the prescription formulation.

Aleve is designed for the temporary relief of minor aches and pains and for fever reduction in adults and children 12 years of age and older. Aleve is administered every 8 to 12 hours, about half as often as other nonprescription pain relievers, because it acts longer in the body. Patients who are allergic to aspirin, ibuprofen, or related drugs should not use Aleve because of the likelihood of a similar reaction.

Treatment for multiple sclerosis.
The first drug approved in the United States to treat multiple sclerosis (MS) became available in October 1993. The drug's manufacturer began providing interferon beta-1b (sold as Betaseron) after the Food and Drug Ad-

---

Comparing nonprescription pain relievers

Over-the-counter pain relievers all reduce pain, but they can cause different side effects and other reactions.

Pain reliever	Aspirin	Acetaminophen	Ibuprofen	Naproxen sodium
Some common brand names	Anacin, Ascriptin, Bayer, Bufferin, Ecotrin, Empirin	Excedrin Aspirin-Free, Panadol, Tylenol	Advil, Ibuprin, Motrin IB, Nuprin	Aleve
Reduces pain and fever	Yes	Yes	Yes	Yes
Reduces inflammation	Yes	No	Not at maximum recommended dosage.	Not at maximum recommended dosage.
Inhibits blood clotting	Yes	No	Yes	Yes
Possible side effects	Gastrointestinal bleeding, stomach upset and ulceration.	Unlikely when taken as directed.	Gastrointestinal bleeding, stomach upset, and ulceration.	Gastrointestinal bleeding, stomach upset.
Special concerns	Do not take if you have an allergy to aspirin or other over-the-counter pain relievers, asthma, bleeding in the digestive tract, or ulcers. Can cause Reye's syndrome in children with chickenpox.	Overdoses can be toxic to the liver. Alcohol may enhance the toxic effect of high doses.	Do not take if you have an allergy to other over-the-counter pain relievers, bleeding in the digestive tract, asthma, kidney problems, or ulcers.	Do not take if you have an allergy to other over-the-counter pain relievers, bleeding in the digestive tract, asthma, kidney problems, or ulcers.

Reprinted with permission from the *Mayo Clinic Health Letter*, April 1994. Reviewed by Daniel A. Hussar.

ministration (FDA) approved the marketing of the drug on July 23, 1993.

MS is a disease of the central nervous system (brain and spinal cord). MS damages the *myelin* (protective covering) that surrounds nerve fibers, disrupting nerve signals that control a variety of body functions. Symptoms of MS include double vision or loss of vision, slurred speech, numbness, muscle weakness, lack of coordination, and tremors. The cause of MS is unknown, but most researchers believe that *antibodies* (disease-fighting molecules of the body's immune system) mistake myelin for foreign tissue and attack it.

Of the estimated 300,000 Americans who have MS, about 100,000 have a relapsing-remitting form of the disease, which is characterized by recurrent attacks followed by periods of partial or complete recovery. Betaseron is intended for use in patients with relapsing-remitting MS who are still able to walk. The new drug is a genetically engineered form of interferon beta, a protein produced naturally by the body that plays an important role in the immune system. Betaseron helps regulate the immune system and reduce the frequency of attacks on the central nervous system, though researchers are unsure exactly how the drug produces this effect.

Although Betaseron is not a cure for MS, the drug's manufacturer—Berlex Laboratories of Richmond, Calif.— claims that the drug can reduce the frequency of MS attacks and decrease the need for hospitalization. Betaseron also reduces the number of *lesions* (damaged areas) that MS produces in the brain.

Betaseron is expensive, however, and supplies are limited. The cost is about $10,000 a year, though very poor or uninsured patients can obtain the drug at a reduced price or without charge from the manufacturer by providing financial information accompanied by a physician's referral. The initial supply of Betaseron did not meet the demand for the drug, and Berlex asked physicians to register patients for whom they wished to prescribe the drug. Berlex then conducted a lottery to determine who would receive the drug. The company said it hoped to produce enough Betaseron by the end of 1995 to treat all patients who might benefit from it.

New cystic fibrosis treatment.
The FDA approved dornase alfa (also known as DNase) on Dec. 30, 1993, for the treatment of cystic fibrosis. The approval marked the first new approach to treating cystic fibrosis in 30 years. The drug is manufactured by Genentech Inc. of South San Francisco and is sold as Pulmozyme.

Cystic fibrosis is an inherited disorder that affects about 30,000 Americans. It is the most common fatal genetic disease among Caucasians. Because of a faulty gene, certain cells of the body produce thick, sticky secretions of mucus that clog the lungs and make breathing difficult. The secretions also become a breeding ground for bacteria, resulting in prolonged infections that damage lung tissue and ultimately lead to death from respiratory failure. People with cystic fibrosis live to an average age of 29 years.

DNase is a copy of an enzyme that occurs naturally in the body. Patients inhale the drug by means of a device that converts a liquid form of the drug into a mist. In the lungs, DNase thins the mucous secretions so that they can be coughed up. According to Genentech, DNase improves lung function and reduces by 27 percent the frequency of respiratory infections requiring treatment with antibiotics. Preliminary investigations indicate that DNase may also be effective against some complications of chronic bronchitis, a lung disorder resulting primarily from smoking.

Alzheimer's drug approved. The FDA approved tacrine hydrochloride (sold as Cognex) on Sept. 9, 1993, for the treatment of Alzheimer's disease. Tacrine is the first drug to be approved for treating Alzheimer's. Alzheimer's disease afflicts about 4 million older Americans and is characterized by a progressive decline in memory, judgment, and reasoning ability.

The new drug is designed to treat mild to moderate symptoms of Alzheimer's. For some patients, it appears to provide a small but significant improvement in memory and reason-

Over-the-counter medications and children

In giving cold medications and other over-the-counter drugs to children, it is important to remember that a child is not simply a small adult. Reduced dosages can have unintended side effects in children, the United States Food and Drug Administration (FDA) warns. In addition to reading the labels carefully, the FDA advises parents and other caregivers to:

- Use child-resistant caps to prevent accidents, and do not leave caps off containers.
- Store medicines as instructed in a safe place and out of reach of children.
- Do not cut an adult dose in half or increase the dose without consulting a physician.
- Do not use medications for purposes that are not listed on the label.
- Do not try to remember the dose used during a previous illness. Read the label each time.
- Do not guess when converting measurements—for instance, teaspoons (tsp.) or tablespoons (tbs.) to ounces (oz.).
- Examine dose cups carefully. Cups may be marked with various units of measurements, such as tsp., tbs., oz., or drams. Others may not use standard abbreviations.
- Check with a physician before giving a child more than one medicine at a time.
- Check with a physician before giving a child aspirin products. Aspirin should not be given to a child who has chickenpox or the flu, because aspirin use can lead to Reye's syndrome, a rare disorder of the nervous system.

ing ability. Tacrine is not a cure for Alzheimer's disease, and its benefits are effective for only about six months, after which mental functioning continues to decline. But tacrine represents an important advance in the management of a disorder for which no effective treatment was previously available.

Tacrine produces side effects in more than one-third of patients, however. Many people taking it experience nausea, vomiting, diarrhea, and abdominal pain, and it may cause damage to the liver. Physicians can usually detect liver problems by checking patients' liver function every week for the first 18 weeks of treatment and periodically thereafter. Tacrine may also increase the activity of certain other drugs, such as the asthma drug theo-

phylline, and the dosage of these drugs may have to be reduced. Food may significantly reduce the effectiveness of tacrine, and so it is generally recommended that the patient take the drug at least an hour before a meal.

New epilepsy drugs. The first new antiepileptic drug since 1978 went on sale in August 1993. The FDA approved the new drug—felbamate (sold as Felbatol)—on July 29, 1993. About 2.5 million Americans have epilepsy, a form of brain dysfunction characterized by recurrent seizures. Seizures occur in various forms, ranging from a brief loss of consciousness to severe *convulsions* (violent muscle contractions) and are caused by an uncontrolled discharge of electrical energy by brain cells.

Although existing medication adequately relieves symptoms in many epilepsy patients, between 20 and 30 percent continue to experience seizures despite the use of medication. In studies of epilepsy patients, felbamate significantly reduces the frequency of seizures when taken by itself or in combination with other antiepileptic drugs. In combination with other antiepileptic drugs, felbamate has also effectively treated seizures associated with Lennox-Gastaut syndrome, which occurs mostly in children. Lennox-Gastaut syndrome involves many types of seizures and may cause mental retardation.

Felbamate produces fewer side effects than most other antiepileptic drugs. If it is used with other antiepileptic agents, however, felbamate may increase the risk of adverse effects from those agents.

On Dec. 30, 1993, the FDA approved a second new antiepileptic drug— gabapentin (sold as Neurontin). Gabapentin is intended for use with other antiepileptic drugs to treat partial seizures—seizures that affect limited areas of the body—in patients over 12 years of age.

Gabapentin is more likely than felbamate to cause side effects such as sleepiness and dizziness, however. But gabapentin has an advantage over felbamate and many other anti-epileptic drugs, because it is not likely to interact with and change the activity of other drugs with which it is used.

New drug for enlarged prostates. On Sept. 29, 1993, the FDA approved terazosin hydrochloride (sold as Hytrin) to treat symptoms of benign prostatic hyperplasia (BPH), a noncancerous enlargement of the prostate gland. The prostate is a walnut-sized gland in males that surrounds the *urethra* (urinary tube) just below the bladder. The prostate produces fluid that helps nourish sperm.

More than 10 million men over 50 years of age in the United States suffer from urinary problems due to BPH. Symptoms of BPH include frequent urination, urinary hesitancy, dribbling, impairment in size and force of urinary stream, and the sensation of incomplete bladder emptying.

Hytrin has been marketed in the United States since 1987 for the treatment of high blood pressure. Researchers found that the drug also increased urinary flow in approximately 70 percent of the patients who took the drug to lower high blood pressure. Terazosin is only the second drug to be approved for the treatment of BPH, joining finasteride (Proscar), which came on the market in 1992.

☐ Daniel A. Hussar

In the Special Reports section, see MEDICINES FOR THE MIND. In WORLD BOOK, see DRUG.

Ear and Hearing

Some people who suffer from tinnitus—a persistent ringing, buzzing, or hissing in one or both ears—are at high risk for committing suicide. That finding was reported in January 1994 by researchers at several institutions in the United Kingdom.

The investigators studied 28 tinnitus sufferers who had committed suicide. They wanted to discover what other factors besides tinnitus might have been involved in the patients' suicides. Such information would aid physicians in identifying patients with tinnitus who could be at high risk for taking their lives.

The researchers found that 20 (71 percent) of the suicide victims were male, and most were elderly and socially isolated. Nearly all of them had experienced psychiatric problems, including 20 who had been depressed. Five of the victims had made a suicide attempt within the previous year. More than half the individuals had had tinnitus for at least a year.

The researchers concluded that tinnitus—both chronic, long-term tinnitus and tinnitus of shorter duration—was a significant factor in the suicides. They said that a tinnitus patient, especially an older man who is alone and is suffering from psychiatric problems, should be considered a suicide risk.

Drug for relief of tinnitus. A drug called alprazolam provides relief for some patients with tinnitus, investiga-

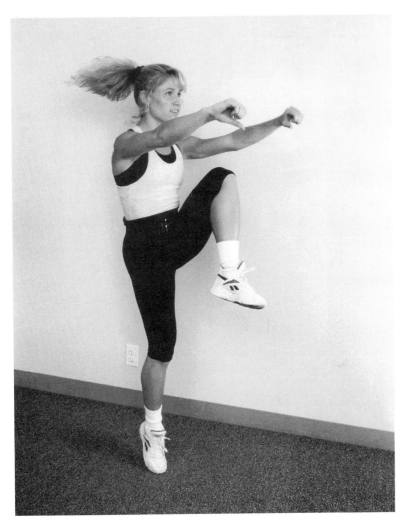

Ear-damaging aerobics
High-impact aerobics can lead to damage of inner-ear structures governing balance, according to a study reported in early 1994 by neurologist Michael I. Weintraub of New York Medical College in Valhalla. Weintraub said anyone doing high-impact aerobics who starts experiencing dizziness or sensations of disorientation should cease the exercises. He added that if the symptoms do not go away, the individual should see a doctor.

tors at the Oregon Health Sciences University in Portland reported in August 1993.

Physicians have had little success in relieving tinnitus. One drug, lidocaine, has been somewhat effective against the condition, but it is not a practical remedy because it must be given intravenously and does not provide lasting relief.

The Oregon doctors tested alprazolam with 36 adult patients who had been bothered by constant tinnitus for at least one year. The participants were divided into two groups. One group of 17 patients received alprazolam, and the other 19 patients were given a *placebo* (inactive substance).

Thirteen of the patients receiving alprazolam (76 percent) had a reduction in the loudness of their tinnitus. Only one of the patients who received the placebo showed any improvement.

Screening infants' hearing. All infants should be screened for hearing impairment in the first three months of life and preferably before being discharged from the hospital, a panel of ear specialists at the National Institutes of Health (NIH) in Bethesda, Md., recommended in September 1993. The panel said routine screening would help ensure that babies born with hearing problems would be helped before the impairments began to hinder the children's development.

One out of every 1,000 infants is born deaf or with a severe hearing disorder. Fewer than half of the infants with these impairments are identified until the condition has already affected speech and language development.

Currently, only infants with certain risk factors, such as low birth weight, a family history of hearing problems, or abnormalities of the face or head, are screened for hearing impairment. The NIH panel said this approach misses 50 to 70 percent of children with hearing impairment. The average age when a hearing problem is identified is close to 3 years.

Other screening guidelines. The NIH panelists also recommended that children who are recovering from bacterial meningitis have their hearing tested because there is a 5 to 30 percent incidence of profound hearing loss associated with the disease. Other conditions that can cause hearing loss in children, the experts said, include head injuries, viral encephalitis, excessive exposure to loud noise, and repeated episodes of middle-ear infection in which there is a discharge from the ears.

The panel said that any child who has had one or more of those problems should be tested. It also recommended that all children be tested when they start school, as that will provide another opportunity for identifying hearing loss.   □ Julie Foreman
In WORLD BOOK, see DEAFNESS; EAR.

Environmental Health

News that low levels of lead may not be as dangerous to children as previously thought, and new evidence that even legal limits of some forms of air pollution may be deadly, highlighted environmental health topics in late 1993 and early 1994. Research on the effects of estrogenlike compounds in the environment also made news.

Lead poisoning risk overstated?
Unsound research methods flawed two key studies demonstrating adverse effects of very low levels of lead in children. That was the March 1994 conclusion of researchers at the Office of Research Integrity, an arm of the United States Department of Health and Human Services. The original studies were performed by Herbert Needleman, a professor of pediatrics and psychology at the University of Pittsburgh. Needleman published his studies in 1979 and 1990.

Scientists have known for many years that high concentrations of lead can delay mental development and stunt physical growth in children. The government forbids lead in gasoline, paint, and food, but many homes still contain lead in older painted surfaces and have water pipes with lead solder. Until Needleman's study, scientists had performed few studies on the

Lethal air pollution
Emissions from factories and power plants may be lethal though legal, according to a study released by Harvard University researchers in December 1993. The study said that legal levels of *particulates* (small airborne particles) above some cities cause respiratory and other health problems that lead to the premature death of 50,000 to 60,000 people in the United States each year.

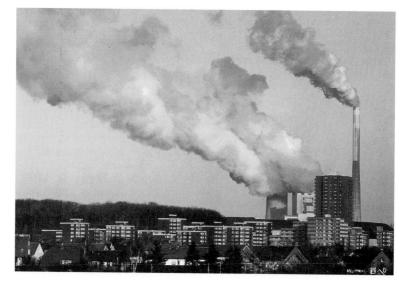

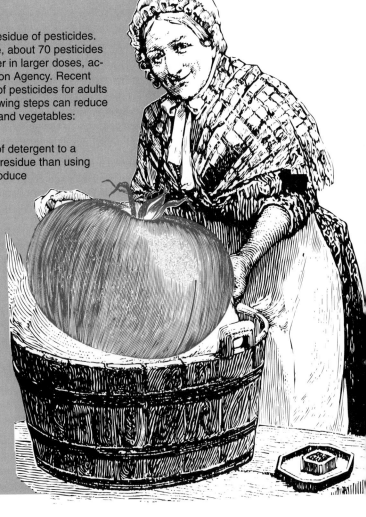

long-term effects of low levels of lead on children, however.

Needleman's studies reportedly showed that very low levels of lead in children's blood—on the order of 10 micrograms per *deciliter* (tenth of a liter)—can cause a three- or four-point reduction in children's intelligence quotient (IQ). Largely on the basis of these studies, the Centers for Disease Control and Prevention in Atlanta, Ga., issued new guidelines in October 1991, lowering the permissible level of lead in children's blood from 25 micrograms per deciliter to 10 micrograms.

Many public health authorities have also issued frequent calls for mandatory screening of all children for lead, arguing that as many as 4 million children under the age of 6 are at risk under the new guidelines. This figure compares with 250,000 children under the old guidelines.

The Office of Research Integrity said that it was unclear from Needleman's studies how his sampling of lead levels in the blood of 270 Boston children reflected lead levels in larger populations. The research office also said that Needleman failed to accurately describe his methods for choosing subjects and for classifying lead levels. In 1993, an ethics panel at the University of Pittsburgh also said that Needleman "was deliberately misleading in the published account of the procedures used in the 1979 study."

Needleman has denied the charges. Because his research has not been duplicated by other researchers, how-

Estrogen Mimics in the Environment

Modern farms are able to feed millions of people in part because of the heavy use of chemicals to kill pests that threaten crops. Some scientists now suspect that these pesticides, which infiltrate the food chain, may threaten the very people they helped feed.

In April 1994, an apparent, though weak, link between the presence of the chemical DDE in a woman's blood and her risk of developing breast cancer was reported by researchers at Mount Sinai School of Medicine in New York City and the Kaiser Foundation Research Institute in Oakland, Calif. DDE results from the breakdown of DDT, an insecticide that was once widely used on crops.

Although the U.S. Environmental Protection Agency (EPA) banned most uses of DDT in 1972, the insecticide is still used in many other countries. Moreover, DDT decays slowly and still turns up in plants, in animals that eat the plants, and in tissues of people who eat the contaminated plants and animals.

The researchers looked at levels of DDE in blood samples from 150 women, of whom a third were African American, a third were white, and a third Asian American. (The samples were taken during the 1960's as part of another study.) Each of the 150 women subsequently developed breast cancer. DDE levels in their blood were compared with those in an equal number of women from the same racial or ethnic group who did not develop cancer.

The link between DDE levels and breast cancer was strongest among African-American women and weaker among white women. In Asian-American women, surprisingly, higher levels of DDE were linked to a lower risk of breast cancer. The researchers found the trend worrisome and deserving of further study.

Other studies have reported a stronger link between DDE and breast cancer. Another study from Mount Sinai, which appeared in April 1993, monitored 229 women in the New York City area. That study found that women with high blood levels of DDE faced four times the risk of breast cancer that women with low levels did. A smaller study of Canadian women, published almost 10 months later, reached much the same conclusion.

Why should DDT residues be tied to breast cancer? No one knows for certain. But during 1993 and 1994, one theory emerged as the front-runner in scientific discussions and papers. The theory proposes that DDT and certain other environmental pollutants may promote cancer and other problems by masquerading as the female hormone estrogen.

Estrogen is the animal kingdom's primary feminizing hormone. Although both males and females need estrogen to function normally, too much estrogen can prove a problem for members of either sex.

Studies have shown, for example, that a high lifetime exposure to estrogen is a primary risk factor for breast cancer in women. In male animals, too much estrogen can disrupt sexual development, especially among those exposed to the hormone as fetuses.

Inside the body, estrogen enters cells by binding with molecules called estrogen receptors located on the surface of cells. Some pesticides and other chemicals that resemble estrogen in chemical structure can also fit onto estrogen receptors in the breast tissue and tissues elsewhere in the body.

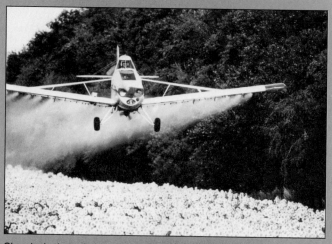

Chemicals that mimic estrogen include some pesticides.

These so-called estrogen mimics may cause abnormal cell growth, scientists speculate.

Since the 1950's and 1960's, wildlife researchers have observed the results of estrogen-mimicking pollutants in nature. For example, researchers have found DDT to be responsible for thin, fragile eggshells that led to the deaths of many incubating birds, especially bald eagles. In sea gulls, DDT has led to gender mix-ups. Some male sea gulls have carried reproductive organs usually seen only in females. Female sea gulls, which should have had reproductive organs only on their left side, were found to carry a small set on their right side as well. With both sexes overly feminized, sea gull reproduction rates plummeted.

Similar changes have been witnessed in other animals exposed to pesticides. And the list of estrogenlike pollutants is expanding.

Some changes observed in animals exposed to environmental estrogens have also been seen in people. In the 1990's, medical scientists have reported growing numbers of reproductive abnormalities in men, including undescended testicles in newborns, malformation of the penis at birth, and low sperm production. A 1992 study by Danish investigators found a 50 percent drop worldwide in men's sperm counts from 1938 to 1991.

Evidence of the pesticide-hormone relationship is still circumstantial. However, it does raise concerns about the reproductive health of future generations.   □ Janet Raloff

ever, many experts now believe that the dangers of low levels of lead have been overstated. The hazards of higher levels remain unquestioned.

Pollutants affect males. Pollutants that mimic the female sex hormone estrogen within the body may interfere with male reproductive systems. That was the conclusion of a study reported in early 1994. Industrialized societies produce a variety of chemicals that resemble estrogen in their chemical structure, which enables them to latch onto estrogen receptors in the body. Such chemicals include many pesticides, herbicides, industrial wastes, and commercial chemicals.

These chemicals can exist even in public water supplies that have been treated to remove bacteria and other contaminants. In February, researchers at the Royal Free Hospital School of Medicine in London reported that men who drank treated water from the Thames River were significantly more likely to produce abnormal sperm than men who drank water from cleaner sources. The researchers reported a high concentration of estrogenlike pollutants in the Thames.

A false suspect? A report published in March 1994 disputed the findings of an earlier study that had linked radiation from the United Kingdom's largest nuclear power complex with leukemia in children who lived near the plant. The 1994 report was prepared by Sir Richard Doll, a cancer epidemiologist at Oxford University in England.

The suspect plant is named Sellafield, and it is located 2 miles (3.2 kilometers) from the town of Seascale in northeastern England. A nationwide survey discovered that, from 1951 through 1991, 10 times more children than expected for a town of Seascale's population developed leukemia, a cancer of the blood-forming tissues.

A 1990 study by English epidemiologist Martin J. Gardner reported that childhood cases of leukemia in Seascale appeared to be associated with fathers who worked at Sellafield. The study speculated that fathers who worked at the plant would have been exposed to elevated levels of radiation and that the radiation could have damaged the men's sperm. This damage, in turn, could have led to genetic defects in the men's children, defects that later developed into leukemia. Gardner's report stated that all the children who developed leukemia had been born in Seascale and had been conceived after their fathers began working at Sellafield.

Doll argued that this analysis was wrong. When his team looked at data covering the children of all 9,000 men who worked at Sellafield, they found no higher-than-expected incidence of leukemia. Moreover, several cases of leukemia had developed in the nearby town of Egremont in children whose fathers did not work at the plant, according to Doll.

The Oxford researchers also noted that men who survived the bombing of the Japanese cities of Hiroshima and Nagasaki at the end of World War II (1939-1945) did not pass along a susceptibility to leukemia to their children, even though the men were exposed to much higher doses of radiation than the Sellafield employees.

Deadly (but legal) air pollution?
Some 50,000 to 60,000 people in the United States may die prematurely each year as a result of breathing fine particulates—very small airborne particles and tiny droplets containing sulfuric acid. This was the conclusion of a study reported in December 1993.

Particulates enter the air in emissions from factories and power plants.

The U.S. Environmental Protection Agency (EPA) set a limit for particulate pollution in 1987, and states have passed laws regulating particulate levels based on the EPA limit. Yet even legal levels of particulates may be lethal, according to researchers at the Harvard School of Public Health in Boston.

The Harvard team, led by epidemiologist Douglas W. Dockery, studied daily levels of fine particulates in six cities for 11 to 26 years. The cities were Harriman, Tenn.; Portage, Wis.; Topeka, Kans.; Watertown, Mass.; St. Louis, Mo.; and Steubenville, Ohio. Researchers picked the cities to represent a range of pollution levels. The researchers recorded how many people died from lung cancer, lung disease, and heart disease among 8,111 study participants in those cities.

After taking into account other health risks, such as cigarette smoking, the researchers reported that higher levels of fine particulates were associated with higher death rates due to lung disease, lung cancer, and heart disease. Death rates were 26 percent higher in the most polluted city—Steubenville—than in Portage, the least polluted city, even though both cities met federal air quality standards.   □ Thomas H. Maugh II

In WORLD BOOK, see ENVIRONMENTAL POLLUTION.

Exercise and Fitness

Strenuous physical activity may trigger a heart attack, particularly in people who exercise infrequently, according to studies reported in December 1993 by researchers at the Harvard Medical School in Boston and at the University of Berlin in Germany.

The American Heart Association has recommended regular exercise to reduce the overall risk of heart attack. But when ordinarily inactive people engage in strenuous physical activity—such as jogging, playing tennis, or shoveling snow—their risk of heart attack increases significantly, the study results showed.

Exercise and heart attacks. In each study, researchers interviewed more

than 1,000 patients who had recently suffered a heart attack. The patients described their usual patterns of physical activity and their activities in the hours prior to their heart attack. The responses showed that patients were as much as six times more likely to have suffered a heart attack during or just after strenuous activity than they were during light activity or rest. Patients who were regularly active, however, were from 10 to 50 times less likely to have a heart attack during strenuous activity than were patients who were not generally active.

These studies suggest that although strenuous physical exertion may occasionally trigger a heart attack, regular exercise greatly reduces that risk during such exertion. The reports also pointed out that the overall risk of a heart attack during vigorous activity is fairly low. For a person who is generally inactive, the risk is about 1 in every 10,000 hours of exertion.

Changes in physical activity over time affect the factors that put people at risk for *cardiovascular* (heart and blood vessel) damage, according to an August 1993 report from Stanford University in California.

Researchers studied 380 men and 427 women whose risk factors and patterns of physical activity had been recorded in 1979 and again in 1985. The study showed that people whose activity decreased during that period had lower levels of high-density lipoprotein (HDL) cholesterol in their bloodstreams. Doctors believe that HDL, sometimes called "good cholesterol," clears the blood of artery-clogging cholesterol, which contributes to cardiovascular disease.

Reduced activity was also associated with increased obesity, another risk factor for heart disease. On the other hand, women who had become more physically active showed a lower resting heart rate, which reflects a healthy cardiovascular system.

The connection between changes in activity and cardiovascular risk factors was most distinct among men under 50 years of age and women who had not reached *menopause,* the time of life when menstruation stops.

Preventing osteoporosis. Regular exercise during the years immediately following menopause may help women prevent *osteoporosis* (a thinning of bone tissue), according to a study reported in September 1993 by researchers at the University of Florida in Gainesville. Most cases of osteoporosis develop among women during the first years after menopause, when they produce far less estrogen, a hormone that helps maintain bone mass.

The University of Florida researchers studied 55 women who had reached menopause and were similar in age, weight, and physical ability. The women were divided at random into a group that either exercised by walking three times a week or that participated in no aerobic exercise.

The researchers measured the bone density of the women in each group regularly for one year. At the end of that time, they found that the women who exercised had about 50 percent less bone loss than did the women who did not exercise.

The onset of menstruation. Exercise, nutrition, and other factors may influence when girls begin menstruating, researchers in Germany reported in August 1993. The researchers sought to identify factors that influence the onset of menstruation because previous studies have suggested that girls who begin menstruating at an earlier age have a greater risk of

Get in shape first
Shoveling snow has long been considered risky for the out-of-shape. A December 1993 report by German researchers established a scientific basis for that notion, finding that engaging in strenuous physical activity temporarily increases the odds of a heart attack—especially among people who exercise infrequently. Regular exercise largely protects against the elevated risk.

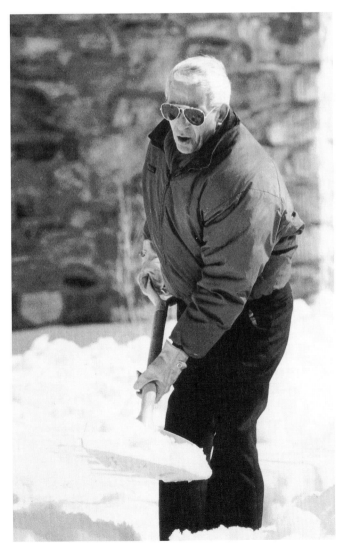

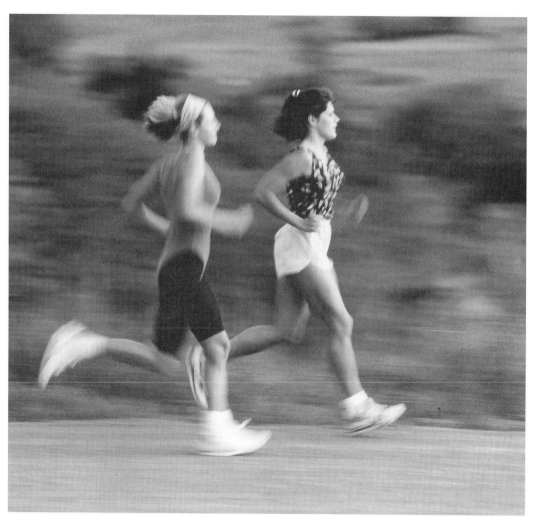

Heading toward trouble?
Female athletes—espe-
cially adolescents—are at
risk for a group of disorders called "the female
athlete triad," according to
a 1993 report by a panel
of sports physicians. The
problem begins when the
athlete develops an eating
disorder while trying to
maintain an unrealistically
low weight. The eating
disorder may lead to the
cessation of menstrual periods and to *osteoporosis*
(bone thinning).

breast cancer later in their lifetime.

The study concentrated on 261
girls, from 8 to 15 years of age, who
had participated in a German survey
of nutrition and activity from 1985 to
1988. The researchers asked the girls
to complete a questionnaire recording
information on their physical development, activity, and nutritional habits
from 1988 to 1989. For the following
two years, girls who had not begun
menstruating continued to record their
habits until menstruation began.

The researchers found that the more
active girls generally began menstruating later. Girls whose diet was higher
in fat generally began menstruating
earlier. The researchers pointed out
that other factors, such as total body
weight and the percentage of body

weight that is fat, may influence the
onset of menstruation. Moreover, the
influence of such factors as physical
activity and fat intake varies according
to other factors, such as changes in
body weight and percentage of fat.

Previous studies have shown that a
late onset of menstruation is common
among young female athletes and ballet dancers. However, the German
study is the first to show that less intense physical activity also influences
when girls begin to menstruate.

Flexibility of arteries. Regular exercise may help maintain the flexibility of
arteries, scientists at the Gerontology
Research Center in Baltimore reported
in October 1993. A study conducted
by the scientists revealed that physi-

cally fit people have less stiffness in their arteries than do people who are generally inactive. Artery walls tend to harden and thicken as people age, and this process contributes to heart disease.

The researchers assessed the physical fitness of 146 men and women, aged 21 to 96 years, who did not exercise regularly. They also measured the stiffness of each person's arteries. The researchers performed similar tests on a group of 14 men, aged 54 to 75 years, who jogged an average of 30 miles a week.

The study suggested that physically fit people have more flexible arteries than do people of the same age who are out of shape. The men who regularly jogged had a 30 percent lower average level of arterial stiffness than their peers in the other group. But the study also supported the view that people show increased stiffness in their arteries as they grow older.

The researchers noted that this study does not prove that exercise reduces the hardening of arteries. Another explanation of the results says that flexibility of arteries and a tendency toward physical fitness could be inherited qualities that complement each other. □ David S. Siscovick

In the Special Reports section, see EXERCISE: THE GAIN MADE PLAIN. In WORLD BOOK, see PHYSICAL FITNESS.

Eye and Vision

People who wear contact lenses overnight significantly increase their risk of developing a disorder called ulcerative keratitis, researchers at Johns Hopkins University in Baltimore reported in February 1994. Ulcerative keratitis is an inflammation of the cornea, the transparent membrane that forms the front of the eye. The inflammation is usually caused by an infection in the tissues that cover the cornea.

A previous study at Johns Hopkins revealed that wearers of disposable soft contact lenses have a much higher risk of developing ulcerative keratitis than do wearers of nondisposable soft lenses. The new report suggests that the habits of the wearers, rather than the material of the lenses, increases that risk.

The researchers at Johns Hopkins studied 40 patients who had ulcerative keratitis associated with contact lens wear, and compared their records with 180 patients who had received contact lens prescriptions from the same physicians on the same dates. They found that the risk of developing ulcerative keratitis was eight times greater among patients who wore their contact lenses overnight.

The study showed that such high levels of risk could develop in as few as one to three nights of wear. Special

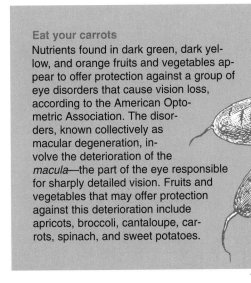

Eat your carrots
Nutrients found in dark green, dark yellow, and orange fruits and vegetables appear to offer protection against a group of eye disorders that cause vision loss, according to the American Optometric Association. The disorders, known collectively as macular degeneration, involve the deterioration of the *macula*—the part of the eye responsible for sharply detailed vision. Fruits and vegetables that may offer protection against this deterioration include apricots, broccoli, cantaloupe, carrots, spinach, and sweet potatoes.

lens materials or meticulous lens care did not reduce the risk. The researchers concluded that from 49 percent to 74 percent of ulcerative keratitis cases associated with contact lenses could be prevented by eliminating overnight wear.

Improved cataract surgery. A new surgical technique to remove *cataracts* (clouding of the lens of the eye) improves treatment success and speeds recovery, the American Academy of Ophthalmology reported in February 1994. Cataracts afflict many people over age 65.

When a cataract causes significant loss of vision, surgeons remove the clouded lens and replace it with an artificial one. Cataract removal is the most commonly performed surgical procedure in the United States.

With the new technique, surgeons break up the clouded area of the lens with ultrasound, a focused beam of high-pitched sound waves, and remove the lens fragments by suction through a narrow tube. An artificial lens, specially designed for flexibility, is then inserted into the eye.

This type of cataract surgery requires an incision of about 0.12 inch (3 millimeters), eliminating the need for stitches. Traditional cataract surgery, in which the entire lens is removed, creates a 0.4-inch (10-millimeter) incision and requires stitches.

Eye implants in children. Children have successfully tolerated artificial eye implants with few complications, according to a February 1994 report from researchers at Thomas Jefferson University in Philadelphia. The placement of artificial eye implants in children is uncommon because physicians are customarily hesitant to experiment with new surgical materials or techniques on children.

Artificial eye implants are used to replace an eyeball that has been removed. In most cases involving children, the eyeball is removed to treat malignant tumors in the eye. If untreated, the tumors can spread into the brain, where they become fatal.

The researchers at Thomas Jefferson University studied 60 children under age 10 who had received artificial eye implants. They found that the chil-

dren were able to adapt physically to the implants with few complications. The implants also showed good movement and had a satisfactory cosmetic appearance.

Myopia may be hereditary. Myopia, commonly called nearsightedness, may be an inherited condition, a study by researchers from the University of California at Berkeley suggested in May 1994. The researchers found that children with nearsighted parents show physical characteristics of nearsightedness before they actually develop the condition.

To a nearsighted person, distant objects appear fuzzy. In most cases, however, nearsighted people are able to see objects clearly up close. The reason for this is the elongation of the eyes in nearsighted people, which makes the distance from the lens to the *retina* (the light-sensitive area at the back of the eye) too long for normal vision. Instead, light rays from distant objects focus before they reach the retina and result in fuzzy images.

The researchers at Berkeley studied the size and shape of the eyes in 716 children aged 6 to 14 years. They found that children with a family history of nearsightedness had elongated eyes, even before they became nearsighted. The eyes of children with two nearsighted parents were more elongated than the eyes of children with only one nearsighted parent.

About 25 percent of adults in the United States are nearsighted. Nearsightedness in children, known as juvenile onset myopia, is less common and usually develops between the ages of 8 and 14. Scientists have disagreed about whether the condition is entirely inherited or whether it might be brought on by certain visual activities, such as reading heavily or watching television.

Eye surgery risk for diabetics. Cataract surgery may aggravate an eye condition called diabetic retinopathy, researchers from St. Mary's Hospital and Medical Center in San Francisco reported in March 1994.

Diabetic retinopathy occurs among people who have long-standing diabetes mellitus—a disease in which the body fails to produce or properly use

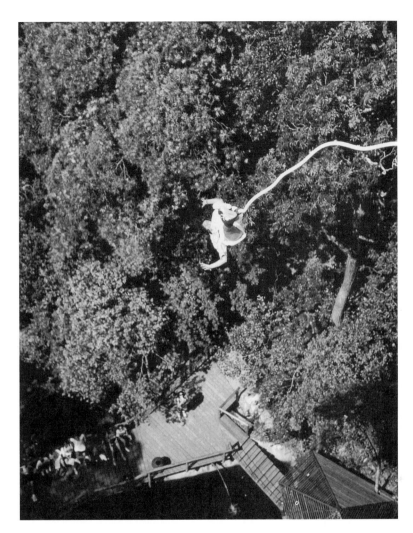

Vision hazard
Thrill seekers should add potential vision loss to the risks of bungee jumping, in which a person leaps off a bridge or high platform and bobs above the ground at the end of an elastic cord. In February 1994, British researchers reported treating a young woman who suffered bleeding within the eyeballs and vision loss after bungee jumping. The scientists suspected that other leapers could suffer temporary or permanent visual impairment as well.

the hormone insulin. Diabetic retinopathy is characterized by a growth of abnormal blood vessels and fibrous tissue in the retina. As the condition progresses, these vessels may burst and cause clouded vision. In more severe cases, the retina can become detached from the back of the eye, eventually leading to blindness.

The medical records of 32 diabetic patients who had cataract surgery in one eye were compared with the records of 32 diabetic patients who had not had cataract surgery. Patients in both groups had diabetic retinopathy. The records covered a 14-year period, during which conditions of the eye and symptoms and treatment of diabetes were detailed.

According to the study results, pa-tients who had undergone cataract surgery had poorer vision and more severe diabetic retinopathy in their surgically affected eye than in their other eye. The affected eyes were also in worse condition than those of the patients who had no surgery.

The researchers recommended that ophthalmologists warn patients with diabetes about the potential risks of cataract surgery. They also suggested that diabetics—particularly those with retinopathy—consider postponing or entirely avoiding cataract surgery.

Eye treatment reduces rate of MS.
Injections of drugs used to treat an eye condition called optic neuritis may also slow the development of multiple sclerosis (MS), according to a Decem-

ber 1993 report by researchers from 15 medical centers associated with the Optic Neuritis Study Group.

Optic neuritis is an inflammation of the optic nerve, which connects the eye to the brain. It impairs vision and makes eye movement painful. Optic neuritis is often one of the first symptoms of multiple sclerosis, a disease of the nervous system. From 45 to 80 percent of people diagnosed with optic neuritis eventually develop MS.

The researchers originally conducted the study to determine whether steroid treatment with corticosteroids—hormones secreted by the adrenal glands—could help patients recover from attacks of optic neuritis more rapidly. The study included 389 patients who had optic neuritis but had not been diagnosed with MS. Researchers divided them into three groups. One group received corticosteroids through injections and pills, a second group took only corticosteroid pills, and the third was given *placebos* (pills with no active ingredients).

The study showed that steroids had an insignificant effect on patients' recovery from optic neuritis. But the researchers discovered that after two years, only 7.5 percent of patients who took intravenous steroids had developed MS. In contrast, 14.7 percent of those who took steroid pills and 16.7 percent of those who took

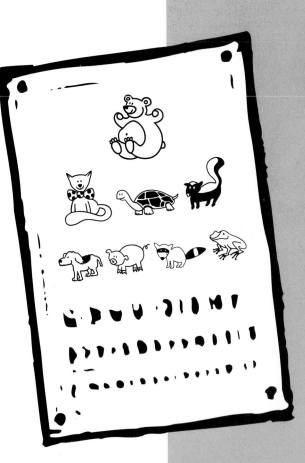

Spotting eye problems in the young

Vision problems in young children often go undetected—at least until a child is old enough to read an eye chart. But parents can watch for some signs of eye trouble that suggest an eye examination is in order. A pediatrician can conduct a preliminary exam, but the child should see an ophthalmologist if a problem is found, according to the American Academy of Pediatrics. Signs of eye trouble include the following:

- A failure to stare at things, respond to visual stimulation, or follow a moving light at 3 months of age or more.
- A tendency to examine objects very close to the eyes.
- An inability to see distant objects that others can see.
- A tendency to rub the eyes, squint, or blink when looking at distant objects.
- Unusual clumsiness, difficulty going up or down stairs, trouble throwing or catching a ball or tying shoelaces, though these difficulties can also signal problems of muscular coordination.
- A tendency to tilt or turn the head when looking at something, as if to bring it into focus.
- A dislike or avoidance of work done close-up.
- Complaints of headaches when doing work close-up.

Source: American Academy of Pediatrics.

placebos developed MS within two years. Patients from all three groups developed MS at the same rate after the next two years.

Scientists know of no cure for MS. Treatment is usually aimed at its symptoms.

A new glaucoma treatment that uses a special enzyme was developed by researchers at the Weizmann Institute in Rehovot, Israel, as reported in March 1994. Glaucoma is a disease in which fluid that fills the eye does not drain properly. Pressure from the fluid can eventually destroy the optic nerve and result in blindness.

The Israeli researchers tested their new treatment on laboratory animals afflicted with glaucoma. They placed on the animals' eyes a plastic disk the size of a contact lens that contained an enzyme called collagenase. The enzyme thins the eye's surface tissue, allowing the fluid to drain, thus relieving pressure. Researchers found that in some cases the enzyme treatment drained the eye in just a few hours.

The enzyme treatment has not yet been approved for testing on people, however, and is not likely to become available in medical practices for several years. □ Julie Foreman

In the Health Matters section, see WHAT YOU SHOULD KNOW ABOUT CATARACTS. In WORLD BOOK, see EYE.

Food
See Nutrition and Food

Genetic Medicine

Three genes involved in the development of human cancers were discovered in late 1993 and early 1994 by researchers in the United States and Europe. These discoveries lent further support to the long-standing belief among biologists that cancer is essentially a genetic disorder. They also provided some clues to the prevention and treatment of cancer, one of the leading causes of death in the United States.

The newly found cancer genes control critical mechanisms in cell division, the process by which cells reproduce. Cancer is characterized by uncontrolled cell division, with cancerous cells ultimately invading and damaging other tissues. This rampant proliferation of cells results from the loss of the normal mechanisms that regulate cell growth—mechanisms that are under genetic control.

Genes and DNA reproduction. Two of the recently identified cancer genes are involved in the *replication* (reproduction) of DNA. DNA (deoxyribonucleic acid) is the molecule genes are made of. The research was reported in December 1993 and March 1994 by geneticists in Boston; Baltimore; Helsinki, Finland; and elsewhere.

Just before a cell divides, its DNA replicates by making a complete and precise new copy of itself from raw materials in the cell. DNA replication ensures that each of the newly formed cells ends up with exactly the same genetic material as the cell from which it arose. But sometimes mistakes in DNA replication occur. Such errors can result in *mutations* (changes) in genes that produce malfunctioning proteins. The end result can be disease, including cancer.

Fortunately, cells have evolved a number of mechanisms, under the control of specific genes, that enable replication mistakes to be identified and repaired. That is the function of the normal form of the two genes reported on in December and March.

Colon cancer research. The identification of those genes stemmed from earlier work on one form of hereditary colon cancer, which pointed to problems with DNA replication. That study, reported in May 1993 by investigators at Johns Hopkins University in Baltimore and the University of Helsinki, identified a colon cancer gene on chromosome 2. Chromosomes are structures in the cell nucleus that carry the genes. The scientists knew that the gene was involved in altered DNA replication, but they were unable to pinpoint the gene.

In December 1993, the Johns Hopkins researchers, working with a team at Harvard University's Dana-Farber Cancer Institute in Boston, succeeded in isolating the gene. The investigators determined that the gene is responsible for checking the accuracy of DNA replication and fixing errors. When the gene is mutated, DNA errors multiply.

French genetic map
Molecular biologist Daniel Cohen of the Center for the Study of Human Polymorphism, in Paris, explains the most complete map so far of all human *chromosomes* (structures in the cell that carry the genes). Although it needed to be refined, the map, announced in December 1993, was a milestone in the Human Genome Project, an international effort to map all the 50,000 to 100,000 human genes.

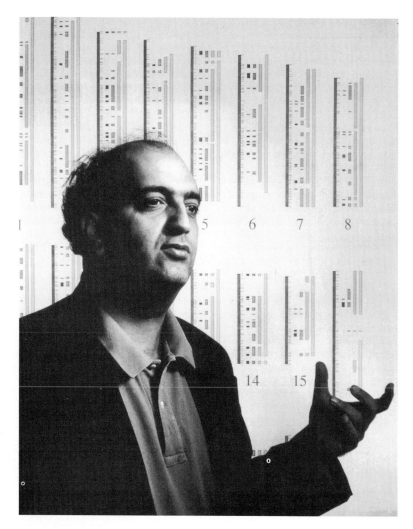

The errors eventually affect genes involved in cell division, leading to colon cancer. The gene is implicated in about 60 percent of all hereditary colon cancers and can also lead to several other types of cancer.

In March 1994, the Boston and Helsinki researchers, joined by scientists at Karolinska Hospital in Stockholm, Sweden, and at several U.S. institutions, reported the discovery of a second colon cancer gene. This gene, located on chromosome 3, also proved to be involved in repairing errors in DNA replication, showing that defects in such genes may be a fundamental cause of cancer.

Together, the two DNA repair genes account for a large number of cancers, including about 90 percent of hereditary colon cancers. More work is needed to identify the causes of the remaining 10 percent of colon cancers that run in families.

Cancer gene test. Isolation of the two colon cancer genes opened the way for the development of a genetic test to identify people who carry those genes. At least one commercial firm had begun such testing by the summer of 1994.

Some geneticists and cancer specialists said, however, that large-scale screening for the genes should wait until the complex tests have been perfected. When such testing is begun, they said, it should be accompanied by education and counseling for people who are found to have the mutated genes. Researchers say many of those people could be saved from developing fatal cancers by undergoing regular checkups to catch cancers in their earliest stages.

The identification of the primary mechanism in colon cancer also provides some promise for a treatment. Geneticists say that it might be possible, for example, to identify abnormal cells and destroy them before they become cancerous.

Tumor suppressor gene. In April 1994, researchers at the University of Utah in Salt Lake City reported the discovery of a third gene that may be implicated in a large number of malignancies, ranging from breast cancer to melanoma, a severe cancer of the skin. This gene, called p16, is a tumor suppressor gene, a gene that in its normal role keeps cell division under control. Mutations in the p16 gene may result in a loss of that control and the subsequent development of cancer.

After identifying the mutated gene in melanoma cells, the researchers looked for p16 mutations in other kinds of cancer cells grown in laboratory cultures. They found evidence of p16 mutations in more than 50 percent of the cancer cells. That finding indicated that p16 is one of the most common cancer genes in the body.

But in June, at least two other groups of researchers in the United States questioned the p16 findings. Those investigators reported that their own research failed to find much evidence of a mutated p16 gene in tumor cells taken from cancer patients, an indication that the gene may not play a major role in the development of cancer. The researchers added that the presence of p16 mutations in laboratory cells might result from the techniques used to grow the cells. Geneticists predicted that the uncertainty would be cleared up by late 1994 or early 1995.

If p16 is confirmed as an important cancer gene, it may be possible to use gene therapy to counteract the mutated form of the gene. For example, if copies of the properly functioning gene could be delivered to cancer cells, the cells might stop proliferating. Another possibility would be to give patients a drug that substitutes for the abnormal protein produced by the mutated gene.

Gene-mapping milestone. The first comprehensive map of all the chromosomes in a human cell was announced in December 1993 by researchers at the Center for the Study of Human Polymorphism in Paris. The French map, though somewhat rough and incomplete, was a milestone in the Human Genome Project, an international effort to map the estimated 50,000 to 100,000 human genes and decipher their functions.

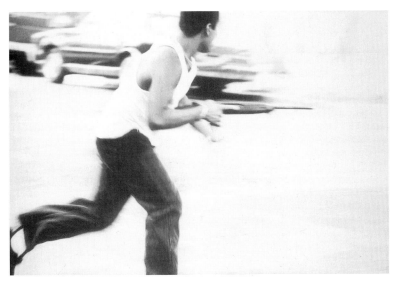

Violence in the genes? Scientists in the Netherlands reported in October 1993 that they had found an abnormal gene that may predispose some people to violent behavior. The gene, the investigators said, allows a build-up in the brain of several chemicals that help the body respond to stressful situations. In people with a normally functioning gene, those chemicals are broken down when they are no longer needed.

The so-called physical map made by the French scientists consists of thousands of chromosome segments. The map gives the sequence in which the segments are arranged in an intact cell. Although it provided an incomplete picture of the human *genome* (all the genetic material in a human cell), the map was hailed by many geneticists as an important tool. Researchers around the world will now refine the map, constructing an ever more detailed picture of humanity's shared genetic makeup.

Genetic clue to violent behavior?

The discovery of an abnormal gene that may be related to aggressive behavior was reported in October 1993 by geneticist Hans Brunner and his colleagues at University Hospital in Nijmegen, the Netherlands. The finding seemed sure to renew the controversy about the relative contributions of heredity and environment in molding human behavior.

The researchers studied a Dutch family in which several men had a history of aggressive and impulsive behavior, including violent outbursts, attempted rape, and exhibitionism. The men also had borderline mental retardation, with IQ's of about 85.

Urine samples from the affected men contained higher-than-normal amounts of several brain chemicals that help the body respond to stressful situations—the so-called fight-or-flight response. Those chemicals have several effects, including increasing the heart rate and sending more blood to the muscles. Ordinarily, the chemicals are later broken down by an *enzyme* (substance that initiates or speeds up chemical reactions) called monoamine oxidase type A (MAOA).

The investigators theorized that MAOA in the men's brains was not working properly, and was thus allowing the stress chemicals to persist. If so, the men could be in a continuous state of tension, perhaps predisposing them to aggressive behavior. The most likely cause of faulty MAOA in several related individuals, they reasoned, is an abnormal gene.

Brunner and his colleagues identified a region of the X chromosome—one of the two chromosomes that determine a person's sex—that includes the gene for MAOA. They discovered that the gene contained a mutation that drastically altered the structure of the MAOA molecule. Researchers will now try to find the same mutation in other families in which aggressive behavior is common. But even if the mutation is found to be relatively common, some experts said, it would be unwise to discount the contribution of environmental factors to the development of a violent personality.

☐ Joseph D. McInerney

In the Health Studies section, see GENETIC MEDICINE: WHAT IT'S ALL ABOUT. In WORLD BOOK, see CELL; GENETICS.

Glands and Hormones

A study published in November 1993 brought good news to people with Type I diabetes, a disease in which the body cannot produce insulin. Insulin is a hormone that regulates the level of *glucose* (sugar) in the blood. Even though people with Type I diabetes inject insulin daily, many of them develop serious complications, including damage to the eyes, kidneys, and nerves in the arms and legs.

A medication commonly used to reduce high blood pressure can slow the progression of kidney disease in patients with Type I diabetes, according to the study by doctors at Rush-Presbyterian-St. Luke's Medical Center in Chicago. Cases of kidney failure and deaths from kidney disease were 50 percent lower among a group of patients who received the drug captopril over three years than among a group that received a *placebo* (substance with no active ingredients). In February 1994, the United States Food and Drug Administration approved the use of captopril for the prevention of kidney damage in people with diabetes. (See also DIABETES.)

Scanning for tumors. Several research groups in late 1993 and early 1994 announced progress in the detection of very small cancerous tumors by tracing a radioactive artificial hormone called octreotide. Octreotide attaches to cells at the same sites as does the natural hormone somatostatin, which is responsible for slowing the secretion of growth hormones.

Doctors can inject a patient with the radioactive octreotide, which seeks to bind to specific *receptors* (binding sites) on the surface of cells. Some tumors that form on glands or in the brain have such receptors, and the radioactive octreotide finds them. A scanning device detects the radiation emitted by the radioactive substance, enabling doctors to locate the tumor.

In the spring of 1994, researchers from the Netherlands and France reported using this approach for the first time to detect tumors that produce a hormone called ACTH. Such tumors are extremely small and difficult to locate. A team of investigators from the universities of Cologne and Stuttgart, both in Germany, reported in early 1994 success in finding certain brain tumors with this method. The procedure offers a major advantage in allowing doctors to diagnose these tumors, as well as their spread in the body, without surgical procedures.

Detecting thyroid cancer. A group of researchers based in various U.S. institutions reported in early 1994 a new method for detecting recurrences of thyroid cancer. The thyroid is a small gland in the throat that secretes hormones which regulate the rate of *metabolism* (the conversion of nutrients into energy). Thyroid cancer strikes 12,500 Americans each year.

In a standard procedure for recovering thyroid cancer patients, physicians inject the patients with radioactive iodine. The iodine travels through the blood and is taken up by any cancerous thyroid cells that have spread to other parts of the body. The radiation from the iodine can then be detected by a special scanning device.

This procedure has a major disadvantage, however. After the removal of cancerous thyroid tissue, most patients produce too little thyroid hormone and take thyroid hormone supplements to restore normal hormone levels. Several weeks before the procedure, patients must stop taking their supplements. Discontinuing the hormone supplements allows levels of thyroid-stimulating hormone (TSH), secreted by the pituitary gland, to rise, which helps concentrate the iodine

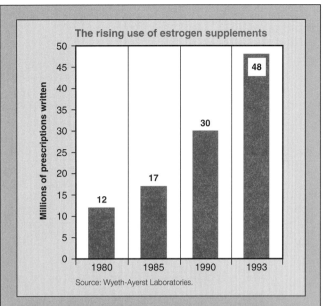

The rising use of estrogen supplements

Source: Wyeth-Ayerst Laboratories.

Weighing the evidence
Many women take supplements containing the hormone estrogen, either alone or in combination with the hormone progesterone, after they reach menopause, the time when their estrogen production drops. From 1980 to 1993, the number of prescriptions written for estrogen supplements in the United States quadrupled. Hormone supplements can relieve hot flashes and other symptoms of menopause. Moreover, studies show that they also can prevent *osteoporosis* (a loss of bone tissue) and that they may reduce the risk of heart disease. However, the supplements also may raise a woman's risk of developing cancer of the breast or uterus. Studies of the long-term effects of hormone supplements are now underway.

in any remaining cancerous tissue.

Discontinuing the supplements, however, also leads to hypothyroidism, a lowering of the rate of metabolism resulting from insufficient thyroid hormone. Patients also risk accelerated growth of cancerous tissue.

The researchers sought to sidestep the hormone withdrawal. They injected patients with a synthetic version of TSH prior to performing the total body scan. This artificially and briefly increased TSH levels while allowing the patients to continue taking their hormone supplements. The results of the study showed that cancerous tissue could effectively be detected in this way.   □ Andre J. Van Herle

In WORLD BOOK, see DIABETES; GLAND; HORMONE; THYROID GLAND.

Health Care Issues

Health care reform remained a prominent political issue in the United States during 1993 and 1994, as President Bill Clinton and other proponents of reform faced a legislative road that proved rocky. After months of promises, debate, and surprises, Congress approached its August 1994 recess with the fate of the nation's health care system unresolved.

Meanwhile, national health care statistics continued to paint a bleak picture. In December 1993, the Employee Benefit Research Institute in Washington, D.C., reported that 38.5 million Americans were not covered by health insurance during 1992. A U.S. Bureau of the Census report issued in March 1994 said that 25 percent of all Americans—about 60 million people—were uninsured for at least one month from 1990 to 1992.

As part of its annual industry forecast, the Department of Commerce predicted in January 1994 that total health costs in the United States would rise to more than $1 trillion during 1994. This rate would mark about a 12 percent increase from 1993.

The President's proposal. President Clinton unveiled a widely anticipated plan to restructure the nation's health care system in an address to Congress on Sept. 22, 1993. The primary goal of the plan was to provide universal health insurance coverage for all Americans by 1998. In his speech, Clinton described his proposal in terms of six principles: security, simplicity, savings, choice, quality, and responsibility.

The Task Force on National Health Care Reform, headed by Clinton's wife, attorney Hillary Rodham Clinton, developed the plan with the help of more than 500 advisers. The task force presented its reform proposal in a document of more than 1,300 pages, which the President delivered to Congress on October 27.

Clinton's plan guaranteed a standard medical benefits package to every American, regardless of health or job status. The package included most services that are medically necessary, such as doctor's office visits, tests and screenings, hospitalization, prescription drugs, and immunizations. It also covered eye and ear examinations, mental health care, and certain types of home treatment.

The plan required employers to pay 80 percent of their employees' health insurance, with the employees to pay the rest. Businesses with fewer than 50 employees were to receive federal subsidies to help pay for insurance. The federal government was also to pay for covering unemployed workers and the poor. Funds to pay for the expanded coverage were to come from reductions in spending on Medicaid (the government-run health program

Reno decries media violence
At an October 1993 Senate hearing, U.S. Attorney General Janet Reno displays a letter from a first grader who wrote that violence on television "makes me feel rotten." Reno criticized the television industry for not taking immediate steps to reduce the amount of violent programming. Days earlier, a motion picture and a TV program had been blamed in the deaths of several youngsters who attempted to imitate dangerous or violent scenes.

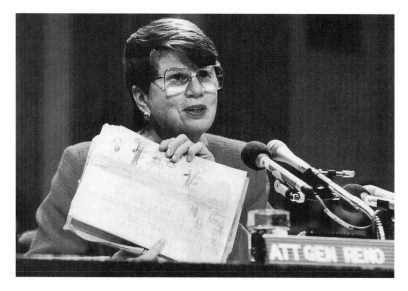

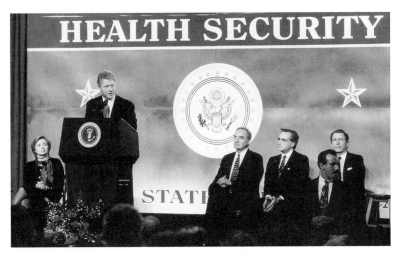

**Introducing
health care reform**
Standing in front of a giant
"health security card,"
U.S. President Bill Clinton
explains his version of
health care reform to a
Pennsylvania audience in
November 1993. The
Administration's plan, designed to guarantee a
standard medical benefits
package for every citizen,
soon came under fire from
critics in Congress and
special-interest groups.

for the poor and disabled) and on
Medicare (the government-run insurance program for older people).
Funds would also have come from
taxes on corporate and personal income and a higher tax on cigarettes.

Under the Clinton plan, most people
would be required to join large insur-
ance-purchasing groups called health
alliances, which were to negotiate with
insurance companies and other health
plans, such as health maintenance organizations (HMO's). The plans, in
turn, would negotiate for services from
health care provider organizations.

The Clinton plan also called for the
creation of a National Health Board,
which was to have broad powers, including managing the nation's total
health care budget. In addition, the
plan required caps on annual increases in insurance premiums. The goal
was to cut health care cost increases
in half—to less than 4 percent per
year—by 1999.

Opposition and debate. Almost immediately after its introduction, Clinton's plan was buffeted by criticism
from conservative and liberal sources
and from a variety of interest groups.

Senate Minority Leader Robert Dole
(R., Kans.) quickly became the key
spokesman for Republican opponents
of the plan. Dole argued that requiring
employers to pay for insurance would
put an unnecessary financial burden
on business and harm the nation's
economy. He also described the
health alliances as government bu-

reaucracies with too much potential
power. Dole and many others raised
doubts about the methods of funding
outlined in the plan, and predicted
that actual costs would run much
higher if Clinton's plan were adopted.
Many opponents criticized proposed
regulations, such as caps on insurance premiums, while others claimed
that reduced funding would harm
Medicare and Medicaid beneficiaries.

Interest groups that actively op-
posed Clinton's plan included the
Health Insurance Association of America, which represents many commercial insurers. The association ran a series of television ads intended to fuel
public concern about the merits of the
plan. The Chamber of Commerce and
a group of influential firms called the
Business Roundtable also refused to
support the plan.

The President's plan also faced
competition from other health care reform proposals. A bill sponsored by
Representative James H. Cooper (D.,
Tenn.) proposed a system that would
rely on market competition to control
medical costs. Representative Jim
McDermott (D., Wash.) and Senator
Paul D. Wellstone (D., Minn.) led a
group of legislators who supported a
"single-payer" plan—similar to the Canadian health care system—in which
a single government agency would
pay for all insurance coverage. The
single-payer system would be funded
primarily by corporate and personal
income taxes. Variations of this plan
were supported mainly by Democrats.

Republican-sponsored health care bills included a plan backed by Senator Phil Gramm (R., Tex.), which would offer tax credits to employees and other individuals who purchase coverage. Senator John H. Chafee (R., R.I.) and a group of moderate Republicans introduced a plan based on an "individual mandate," which would require every American to purchase health insurance personally.

In his State of the Union address on Jan. 25, 1994, President Clinton responded to such alternative proposals by vowing to veto any legislation that did not include universal coverage. But he reemphasized his willingness to compromise on other issues, to ensure that a bill would be passed.

The health subcommittee of the House Ways and Means Committee voted against the President's plan on March 28, 1994, but approved a compromise bill that included some elements of his proposal. It was widely reported that the committee's influential chairman, Representative Dan Rostenkowski (D., Ill.), could help bring about passage of the subcommittee's bill or a similar one. But Rostenkowski was forced to resign his chairmanship on May 31, when he was charged in federal court with 17 counts of corruption.

The Senate Labor and Human Resources Committee, chaired by Senator Edward M. Kennedy (D., Mass.), approved a Clinton-style bill on June 9,

but it received almost no support from Republicans. On June 11, Dole threatened to block any bill that required employers to pay for insurance. By mid-June, Clinton and his top aides had begun to discuss alternatives to the employer mandate and to universal coverage. Senate Majority Leader George J. Mitchell (D., Maine) unveiled a compromise bill on August 2, which aimed at covering 95 percent of the population and required employers to pay 50 percent of the cost of insurance for their workers.

State reform efforts, in many cases, suffered from the same debate and deadlock as did national reform. In Vermont, legislative disagreement over how to fund universal coverage halted progress on a preliminary health care reform plan that had been approved in 1992. Ambitious reform proposals put forward by Florida Governor Lawton M. Chiles, Jr., and Missouri Governor Mel Carnahan also stalled as their state legislatures adjourned without action on health care.

Other states, however, saw progress in health care reform. Among the most notable was Tennessee, where in November 1993 Governor Ned Ray McWherter won approval from the U.S. Department of Health and Human Services to replace the state's Medicaid program with a program called TennCare. The new program was designed to reduce health care

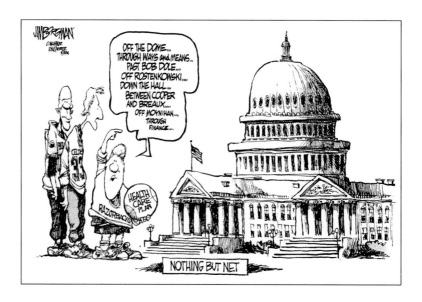

costs while insuring more people. The state projects that by 1996, 500,000 previously uninsured people will be added to the 1 million already covered by Medicaid. Despite severe criticism from physicians and hospital administrators, more than 900,000 people were enrolled in TennCare by April 1994.

In another development in health funding, the states of Florida and Mississippi filed lawsuits in 1994 against several major tobacco companies, seeking to reclaim millions of dollars in expended state Medicaid funds. The states claimed that tobacco-related health problems dramatically raised expenses for Medicaid patients.

Gulf War syndrome. A mysterious set of symptoms known as Gulf War syndrome, which has afflicted thousands of veterans of the Persian Gulf War (1991), raised the issue of government sensitivity to veterans' health in 1994. Jesse Brown, secretary of the Department of Veterans Affairs, proposed in June that federal disability benefits be extended to veterans suffering from symptoms attributed to Gulf War syndrome. Representative G. V. (Sonny) Montgomery (D., Miss.), chairman of the House Veterans Affairs Committee, introduced a bill providing such assistance, and the Clinton Administration quickly endorsed it.

Physicians have been unable to identify the cause of Gulf War syndrome, making it difficult to prove that the symptoms are related to service in the war. Symptoms include skin rashes, illness resembling influenza, joint pain, headache, and depression. Some tumors in veterans and birth defects in the children of veterans have also been attributed to the syndrome. Reports have cited pollution from oil well fires and exposure to various chemicals or to uranium in shells as possible causes of the illness.

The Lakeberg twins. A case that raised questions about the limits of Medicaid coverage came to a close in June 1994 with the death of Angela Lakeberg, who had been surgically separated from her twin, Amy, in August 1993. The Lakeberg twins had been joined at the abdomen and shared an abnormal heart and fused

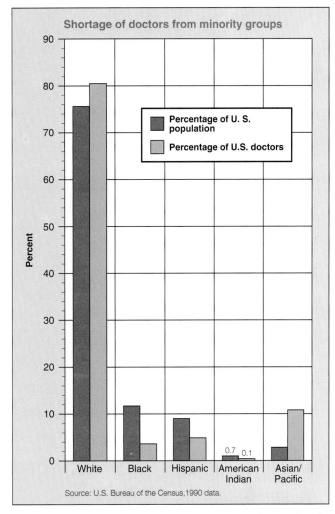

Shortage of doctors from minority groups

Legend:
■ Percentage of U. S. population
□ Percentage of U.S. doctors

Source: U.S. Bureau of the Census, 1990 data.

liver. Their parents were beneficiaries of Medicaid. Physicians at the hospital in Maywood, Ill., where the twins were born estimated that neither girl had more than a 1 percent chance of survival. However, surgeons at Children's Hospital of Philadelphia believed they could save one of the twins.

During the surgery, which took place on Aug. 20, 1993, the shared heart was removed from Amy, who died immediately. Angela survived and was placed on a respirator, which she required until her death, on June 9, 1994. The medical costs for the Lakeberg twins, paid for in part by Medicaid, eventually exceeded $1 million.

☐ Emily Friedman

In the Health Matters section, see THE MANAGED CARE PRESCRIPTION.

Increasing the number of doctors from minority groups, health care experts agree, is crucial to improving health care for the poor. The high cost of medical school, which leaves many students in debt, has been cited as a major deterrent to entering the profession for members of minority groups.

Hearing
See Ear and Hearing

Heart and Blood Vessels

A surprising link between heart disease and cancer was suggested in 1994 by studies on the effectiveness of balloon angioplasty, a procedure for opening blocked coronary arteries. Three studies in late 1993 found that in as many as 40 percent of angioplasty patients, the procedure had to be repeated. A study reported in July 1994 offered a possible explanation for the angioplasty failure rate, involving a mechanism also implicated in the development of cancer.

Angioplasty or bypass surgery. Three studies reported in November 1993 found angioplasty as successful as bypass surgery in treating multiple coronary artery disease. Unlike surgery, however, angioplasty often has to be repeated. The coronary arteries, which carry blood to the heart, can become blocked by fatty deposits that restrict blood flow, causing chest pain and, in some cases, heart attacks.

In performing angioplasty, a heart specialist inserts a thin, flexible tube called a catheter into an artery in the patient's arm or leg and threads it into the clogged artery. A balloon at the end of the catheter is then inflated, crushing the fatty deposits. Angioplasty usually is performed on patients with blockages in only one of the three coronary arteries.

Patients with more than one blockage usually undergo bypass surgery, in which veins or arteries taken from another part of the body are grafted to the coronary arteries above and below the blockage. As a result, blood to the heart bypasses the blockages. While a bypass requires open-chest surgery, angioplasty involves only puncturing the skin to insert the catheter.

The first study, conducted in London, followed 1,055 patients with multiple diseased coronary arteries. Half were treated with angioplasty, half with bypass surgery. After a year, the same number of people in both groups had died or had a heart attack. Those who needed repeat treatment, however, made up 40 percent of the angioplasty group but only 9 percent of the surgery group.

Similar findings were reported in another study of patients in England. Of 1,011 patients with multiple coronary artery disease, half received angioplasty and half bypass surgery. The groups showed the same rate of death and heart attack after an average of 2½ years. Repeat treatment was needed by 38 percent of the angioplasty group but only 11 percent of the surgery group.

The third study, the Emory Angioplasty Versus Surgery Trial (EAST) involved 392 people with multiple coronary artery disease in Atlanta, Ga. As in the other studies, half the patients underwent angioplasty and half bypass surgery. After three years, these groups also had the same rate of death and heart attack. Repeat treatment was needed by 22 percent of the angioplasty group and 1 percent of the surgery group.

Angioplasty is initially less expensive than surgery, but hospitalization for repeat treatment raises its cost to that of surgery. Despite the frequent need for repeat procedures, angioplasty involves less discomfort and inconvenience than surgery, and a shorter recuperation period. Because both treatments can produce the same medical results, many patients may opt for angioplasty in the future.

Cancer link? A study reported in July 1994 offered a possible explanation of why as many as 40 percent of the clogged arteries that are unblocked by angioplasty become blocked again within six months. The study, which also suggested a surprising link between heart disease and cancer, was led by Stephen E. Epstein, chief of the cardiology branch at the National Institutes of Health (NIH) in Bethesda, Md., and Edith Speir, also in the cardiology branch.

The process that leads to clogged arteries begins with the proliferation of cells that line artery walls. The researchers found that a protein called p53, which normally controls cell growth, failed to function properly in about a third of the angioplasty patients whose arteries had reclogged. This is the same protein that fails to function in halting many cancers.

Atherosclerosis treatment. Drugs can slow the development of atherosclerosis, a condition in which fatty deposits called plaques form on the insides of arteries and hamper blood flow. This was the conclusion of two studies reported in November 1993.

The study by the NIH treated 919 people who had high levels of the fatty substance cholesterol in their blood and a carotid artery thickened by cell growth and plaques. The carotid arteries, which run along both sides of the neck, carry blood and oxygen to the brain.

Some of the patients in the study were treated with the cholesterol-lowering drug lovastatin; some with warfarin, a drug that prevents blood clotting; and others received no therapy. The anticlotting drug is given to ath-

erosclerosis patients to prevent clots from forming at the site of plaques and closing off the artery.

After six months, those taking lovastatin had reduced their blood cholesterol and carotid artery wall thickness by 28 percent. The group treated with warfarin showed no change in the thickness of the artery wall. The artery wall had grown thicker in people receiving no treatment. Also, the group receiving no treatment had a higher rate of heart attacks and death than those treated with the drugs.

The Montreal Heart Institute in Canada reported in February 1994 on a study in which 331 patients with high blood cholesterol received either

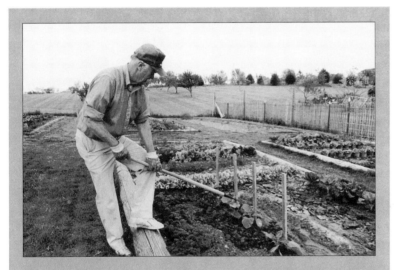

Why people get heart disease
Each year, some 1.5 million people in the United States are newly diagnosed with coronary heart disease, and more than 500,000 die of it. Although heart disease can arise from a combination of factors, doctors may pinpoint one or more particular factors, such as obesity or smoking, as the main reasons a patient developed a heart condition. A report on people who died of heart disease in 1986, issued in September 1993 by the Centers for Disease Control and Prevention in Atlanta, Ga., broke the deaths down by primary causes:

- High cholesterol—253,194 deaths
- Lack of adequate exercise—205,254
- Obesity—190,456
- High blood pressure—171,121
- Smoking—148,879

Source: *FDA Consumer.*

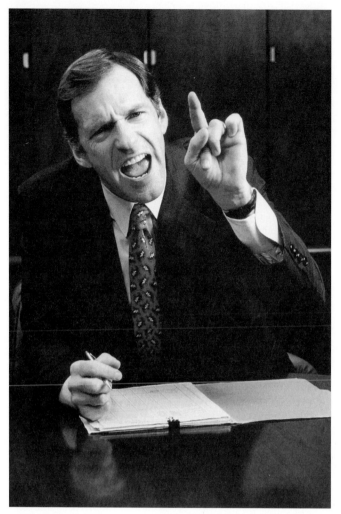

ter 35 days, 7.3 percent of the patients had died. However, for patients who received a dilating drug known as an ACE (angiotensin converting enzyme) inhibitor, the death rate dipped to 6.9 percent. This difference, though small, was statistically significant.

A separate project in Italy tracked almost 19,000 patients at 200 hospitals. Half of the patients received ACE inhibitors. After 42 days, 6.3 percent of those who received the ACE inhibitor had died, compared with 7.1 percent of the other group. This constituted a 12 percent reduction.

Gender and bypass results. The death rate of women after coronary artery bypass surgery is more than twice that of men, researchers reported in November 1993. The researchers, from Dartmouth-Hitchcock Medical Center in Lebanon, N.H., tracked 3,404 women who underwent bypass surgery between 1987 and 1989. The death rate for women was 7.1 percent, compared with 3.3 percent for men.

Previous explanations for this disparity included the fact that women are often older than men at the time of bypass surgery. Coronary artery disease generally does not develop in women until after their reproductive years. Another theory was that women are more likely than men to have other diseases, such as diabetes, that raise their risk of dying during surgery.

Although the women studied by Dartmouth-Hitchcock tended to be older and to have a higher rate of diabetes, a statistical analysis showed that these two factors did not explain their higher risk of dying. What the researchers found was that larger people—both men and women—had a higher survival rate than did smaller people. Men and women of the same size had the same death rate.

Among the patients who died, bypass grafts had failed in 12 percent of the men and 40 percent of the women. The graft, which bypasses a diseased artery, consists of a vein or artery taken from elsewhere in the body. The higher rate of failure in women could be because women's arteries are smaller than men's, and therefore less able to handle sufficient blood flow from the graft.

Watch that temper
Outbursts of anger double the chances of having a heart attack, according to a study reported in March 1994 by researchers at Harvard Medical School in Boston. In the study, the researchers asked 1,623 heart attack patients to rate their anger at various times, including two hours before their heart attack. To understand how anger might bring on a heart attack, the researchers said, requires further study.

lovastatin or no therapy. After two years, the patients taking lovastatin had a 21 percent decrease in blood cholesterol. Fatty deposits in the coronary arteries grew in both groups but less so in the group receiving the drug. New fatty deposits formed in 32 percent of untreated patients but only 16 percent of the treated patients.

Dilating drug increases survival. A drug that *dilates* (widens) blood vessels slightly increases the survival rate of heart attack patients if administered immediately after the attack. This finding, from two European studies, was reported in November 1993.

A study by researchers in Oxford, England, followed 58,000 heart attack patients in more than 30 countries. Af-

The researchers recommended that heart specialists take this factor into account when deciding whether to perform bypass surgery or another procedure, such as angioplasty, on a patient. Moreover, certain alterations in the procedure might lessen the grafts' failure rate. For example, in women and small men, surgeons could use grafts made from arteries, which tend to stay open better than do the more commonly used, and more expendable, veins.

Antihistamines and sudden death. The U.S. Food and Drug Administration warned physicians in late 1993 against using terfenadine, a nonsedating antihistamine sold as Seldane, in combination with certain antibiotics, such as ketoconazole (sold as Nizoral). The antibiotics interfere with the breakdown of the antihistamine, which can lead to toxic reactions in some individuals. In the most serious cases, *arrythmia* (irregular heartbeat) led to sudden death.

Antihistamines are drugs used to treat a variety of ailments, including asthma and hay fever. Many of them cause sleepiness. Terfenadine and other newer antihistamines lack this effect and so are popular with people who need to work or pursue other activities that require alertness.

Vitamin E and beta carotene. Small studies have suggested that vitamin E and beta carotene, a nutrient from which the body produces vitamin A, may protect against heart disease and cancer. However, a large study comparing people who took these nutrients with those who did not cast doubt on their value—at least in supplement form—in April 1994.

The study, conducted by researchers in Finland, followed almost 30,000 middle-aged Finnish male smokers. The men were divided into four groups: One received vitamin E alone, one beta carotene alone, one a combination of both, and one no treatment. The investigators concluded that treating male smokers for five to eight years with vitamin E and beta carotene does not protect against heart disease or cancer.

Because the study focused on smokers, the findings do not mean that the nutrients would not help other people at less risk of cancer or heart disease. In addition, the researchers used a smaller dose of vitamin E than has been used in studies that have found a beneficial effect in reducing heart disease. More studies are needed using larger doses of vitamin E. In the meantime, doctors recommend that people at risk for heart disease should concentrate on reducing more powerful contributing factors, such as smoking, high blood pressure, and high levels of blood cholesterol.

☐ Michael H. Crawford

In WORLD BOOK, see HEART.

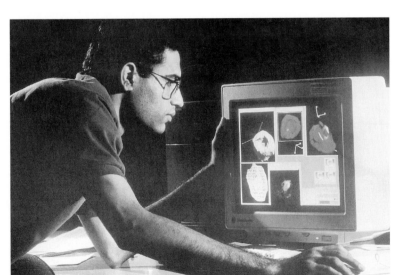

A matter of the heart
A computer program may someday assist cardiologists in diagnosing heart disease and making treatment recommendations. The experimental program, developed at the Georgia Institute of Technology in Atlanta, interprets three-dimensional images that show how well blood is flowing through the heart muscle.

Infectious Diseases

Major declines occurred during 1993 in reported cases of several childhood diseases, the United States Centers for Disease Control and Prevention (CDC) in Atlanta, Ga., announced on Feb. 4, 1994. The CDC said that the number of cases of six diseases in 1993 was at or near the lowest levels ever reported. The diseases were measles, polio, rubella (German measles), tetanus, diphtheria, and congenital rubella syndrome (CRS). CRS produces birth defects in infants born to women infected with the rubella virus during the first three months of pregnancy.

The biggest drop occurred in the cases of measles reported in 1993, down from 2,231 cases in 1992 to 281 in 1993. No cases of diphtheria were reported in 1993, compared with 3 in 1992. And, as in 1992, no cases of polio were reported.

The CDC attributed the decline to wider use of vaccines, noting that diseases such as measles tend to decline when vaccination rates go up. But the CDC warned that the immunization of children must continue at the same or higher levels, or the number of cases will surge again. Experts noted that the incidence of measles had fallen to very low levels in the 1980's. But a measles epidemic began in 1988 when the number of childhood vaccinations dropped.

The CDC announced on Oct. 28, 1993, that measles had virtually disappeared. Only 167 cases of measles occurred during the first half of 1993. That figure was a 99 percent decrease from the first half of 1990.

Progress against polio. The World Health Organization (WHO), an agency of the United Nations, on April 8, 1994, reported progress toward its goal of eliminating polio globally by the year 2000. Polio results from a viral infection and causes inflammation of the brain and spinal cord, which can lead to paralysis. The disease primarily strikes children. Polio was widespread before scientists developed a vaccine for it in the 1950's.

WHO said that the number of polio cases worldwide dropped by 50 percent from 1992 to 1993, falling from 15,911 cases to 7,898. The number of countries reporting no cases of the disease rose to 141—the highest ever. WHO said that the entire Western Hemisphere has been polio-free since September 1991.

The decline has occurred because of widespread polio vaccination programs. WHO said that intensified vaccination efforts are needed to control polio in Pakistan, Sudan, and other Asian and African countries where the disease still strikes.

The last smallpox virus? Infectious disease experts in December 1993

Flesh-eating bacteria
A physician examines a man infected with a particularly nasty strain of streptococcus bacteria in New York state in June 1994. The bacteria release a *toxin* (poison) that destroys flesh and muscle and can cause death if not treated. The deadly bacteria killed 11 people in England in May 1994. U.S. health officials reported one death and scattered cases of infection but noted that infection with this strain was uncommon.

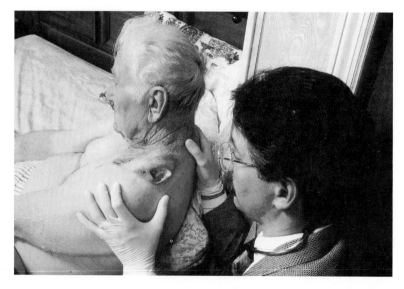

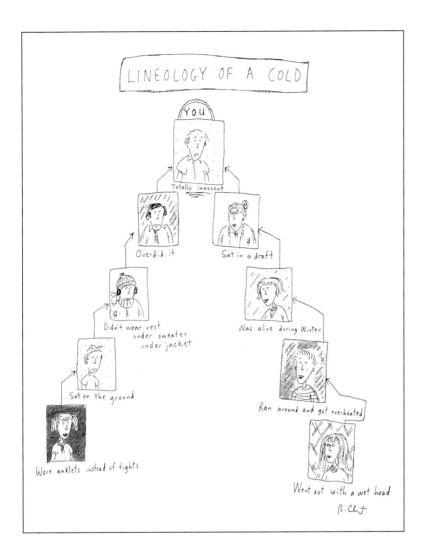

decided to delay destruction of the world's last stocks of smallpox virus, the cause of one of the most feared diseases of all time. Destruction of the virus would have been the first deliberate elimination of a biological species from the planet.

Samples of the smallpox virus are stored at the CDC and in the Research Institute for Viral Preparations in Moscow. Countries transferred their stocks of the virus to these high-security central storage facilities after medical science totally eliminated smallpox as an infectious disease in 1980.

In 1990, a special WHO panel recommended that all smallpox viruses be destroyed by Dec. 31, 1993. But WHO also advised destroying the virus only after researchers sequenced the virus's genes and only if scientists raised no serious objections. Sequencing involves determining the order of the chemical subunits in the virus's genetic material. This information could be used in research on smallpox and perhaps to re-create the virus for future research.

American and Russian scientists completed sequencing the two major strains of the virus by late 1993. But work on a third strain, which caused a mild form of smallpox, continued past the deadline.

WHO said that destroying the virus would prevent infections among laboratory personnel and prevent the virus's use by terrorists or in biological warfare. Some scientists objected to the destruction, arguing that further research on the virus could provide information about other viral diseases.

New vaccine technology. Researchers at the University of California at Los Angeles (UCLA) said on March 18, 1994, that they had developed a new technology for making vaccines against viral diseases. UCLA pathologist Nir Kossovsky said the process involves tricking the body's disease-fighting immune system into mounting a response to harmless "decoy" viruses and thereby developing an immunity to infection from them in the future.

A virus contains a core of genes wrapped in a coating of sugar and protein that is unique to that viral *strain* (subtype). When the immune system recognizes this coating as an *antigen* (foreign material), it responds by producing disease-fighting molecules called antibodies that attack the antigen. The body develops an immunity to a specific viral strain because some antibodies remain that can destroy future invaders before they cause infection.

The researchers created harmless "decoy" viruses by wrapping tiny particles of ceramic material in an outer coating identical to that of an actual virus. Animal experiments show that the immune system recognizes the decoy as an actual virus and develops antibodies against it. Kossovsky said the technology could be the basis for

a vaccine against 7,000 to 8,000 viruses.

Four Corners virus isolated. Scientists in November 1993 isolated the virus responsible for a mysterious outbreak of a fatal, flulike disease that began in the U.S. Southwest in April 1993. The scientists also confirmed that the virus is a member of the hantavirus family, as health officials had believed. Researchers from the CDC and the U.S. Army Medical Research Institute of Infectious Diseases at Fort Detrick, Md., also reported successfully growing the virus in the laboratory. They said the step could lead to better ways of detecting the virus in human beings and in the deer mice that transmit the disease to humans.

Now known as hantavirus pulmonary syndrome, the respiratory disease was first reported among Navajo Indians in New Mexico. The disease begins with symptoms similar to influenza, but serious breathing problems soon develop as fluid accumulates in the lungs. Most cases of the disease occurred in the "Four Corners" area where New Mexico, Arizona, Colorado, and Utah converge. As of July 1994, 80 cases had occurred in 18 states, claiming 45 lives, according to the CDC.

☐ Michael Woods

In the Special Reports section, see THE ORIGIN OF NEW DISEASES. In WORLD BOOK, see VIRUS.

Kidney

Restricting the amount of protein in the diet appears to offer a slight benefit to people with chronic kidney disease, according to the March 1994 report of the Modification of Diet in Renal Disease Study, a research project conducted at several medical centers in the United States. The study also found that reducing blood pressure below the level typically recommended slowed the loss of kidney function in most kidney-disease patients. Tests in laboratory animals had indicated that both strategies could delay the progression of kidney disease.

The new study involved 585 patients with various types of kidney disease. All had only 25 to 50 percent of

normal kidney function. One group of patients consumed an average amount of dietary protein, and another group of kidney patients consumed about one-third less protein. In addition, most subjects were prescribed blood-pressure medication. About half of the patients maintained their blood pressure below the levels usually recommended.

During the first four months of the study, the patients on the low-protein diet and those who had stringent blood pressure control lost more kidney function than people receiving the usual therapy. Thereafter, however, kidney function was lost at a slower rate in the low-protein-diet and low-blood-pressure groups. When the study ended three years later, the low-protein, low-blood-pressure groups had a slight advantage in kidney function compared with the other patients.

Researchers noted that the study included patients with many types of kidney disease, and that future studies may find that low-protein diets and strict blood-pressure control provide a clearer benefit to patients with certain types of kidney disease. Meanwhile, because following a low-protein diet requires extensive nutrition counseling and significant changes in eating habits, some experts said they would not recommend the therapy for every patient.

Transplant benefit confirmed.

Kidney-transplant recipients have a lower risk of death than kidney patients on dialysis. (Dialysis is a mechanical means of filtering wastes from the bloodstream, normally a function of the kidneys.) Researchers at the Michigan Kidney Registry and the University of Michigan, both in Ann Arbor, reported this finding in the Sept. 15, 1993, issue of the *Journal of the American Medical Association*.

The researchers compared survival odds for people who received kidney transplants and for patients on dialysis who were considered healthy enough for a kidney transplant. The comparison showed that those who received a transplant were much more likely to die during the first four months after

transplantation, because of the risks of surgery and the side effects of medications intended to prevent rejection of the new kidney. By the end of one year, however, the group of transplant patients had a lower overall risk of dying than the group of dialysis patients.

The long-term survival benefit of transplantation was especially pronounced for people with kidney failure due to the complications of diabetes mellitus, the most common form of diabetes. Among people with kidney failure from certain other causes, however, the study could find no benefit from transplantation.

Taxol for cystic kidney disease.

The anticancer drug taxol can prevent the formation of kidney *cysts* (fluid-filled sacs) in laboratory mice. That was the April 1994 finding of researchers at the University of California at Los Angeles and the Institute of Child Health in London. The report was significant because kidney cysts are the primary feature of the most common form of inherited kidney disease in the United States, autosomal dominant polycystic kidney disease (ADPKD).

Although the kidneys of people with ADPKD usually appear normal at birth, the organs begin to grow cysts that distort and destroy the surrounding normal kidney tissue. ADPKD patients account for 3 to 4 percent of

**Sea squirts
show kidney stones**
California biologist Mary Beth Saffo holds an underwater structure covered with tiny sea squirts, *below left,* the only known animals that develop *renal* (kidney) stones naturally and regularly. A stone is visible in the renal sac of a transparent sea squirt, *below right.* In 1994, Saffo was devising ways to use the sea squirt as an aid to studying the development of kidney stones in human beings.

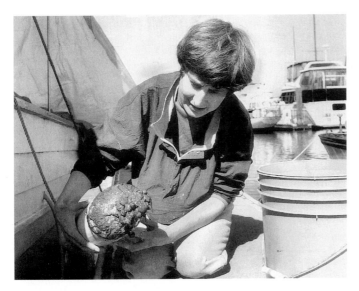

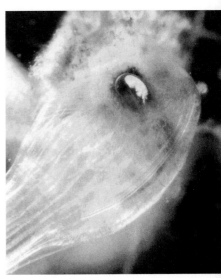

those who develop kidney failure and start dialysis.

The British and American scientists tested taxol in a strain of mouse that develops polycystic kidneys. The drug was able to prevent new cysts from forming in young mice that had not yet developed multiple kidney cysts. The mice, which normally die of kidney failure within one month, did not die for more than six months.

Much research is needed to determine whether taxol therapy is safe or useful for ADPKD patients. Such treatment would not benefit patients who already have kidney failure, but it might prevent kidney damage in those who are not already severely affected.

Preventing kidney damage from diabetes mellitus is possible through tighter control of patients' blood sugar levels, according to the September 1993 findings of the Diabetes Control and Complications Trial. The study involved 1,441 patients treated in 29 centers throughout the United States from 1983 through 1989. And in November 1993, researchers reported that a study of 409 diabetes patients treated in the United States and Canada showed that a drug called captopril could reduce a patient's risk of substantial loss of kidney function. For more information, see DIABETES.

□ Jeffrey R. Thompson

In WORLD BOOK, see KIDNEY.

Medical Ethics

The ability to manipulate the beginnings of life raises fundamental ethical questions about the limits of science and the wisdom of interfering with natural reproductive processes. Two events in late 1993 fueled debate over the ethics of using technology to manipulate human reproduction.

Cloning. Researchers at the George Washington University Medical Center in Washington, D.C., reported in October 1993 that they had *cloned* (produced an identical copy of) a human embryo. This procedure may eventually help infertile women become pregnant. Cloned embryos could be used for *in vitro fertilization*, a process in which an egg is fertilized in a laboratory and then placed in a woman's uterus, where normal pregnancy continues. By cloning a fertilized egg, a physician could implant several embryos, improving a woman's chances of becoming pregnant.

Although cloning is common in veterinary medicine, similar experiments with human embryos have caused controversy. Critics of the technique warn of potential abuses, such as the sale of embryos or the use of selective cloning to produce certain genetic traits. Supporters of the research argue that parents should have the sole right to make reproductive choices.

Postmenopausal mothers. The French Parliament proposed legislation in January 1994 to restrict artificial

fertilization of postmenopausal women, following reports that two women had become pregnant through artificial means after menopause—the time when menstrual periods cease. A 59-year-old British woman gave birth to twins in December 1993, after fertilized eggs had been implanted in her uterus at a clinic in Rome. A 62-year-old Italian woman became the world's oldest new mother in July 1994, after treatment at the same clinic.

The French legislators argued that pregnancy at an advanced age is immoral as well as dangerous to the health of the mothers and children. Critics of the legislation have pointed out that older fathers are ordinarily considered acceptable, even though the risk of birth defects is higher among the children of older fathers.

Radiation experiments. A series of reports published in November 1993 in *The Albuquerque Tribune* described radiation studies conducted by the United States government on human patients from the 1940's to the 1970's. Many of the projects arose at a time when the United States knew little about the long-term effects of the radiation released in a nuclear explosion. The revelations set off public outcry and inspired further investigation into similar government activities.

One of the most dramatic revelations concerned a series of experiments conducted between 1945 and 1947, in which 18 patients were injected with large doses of the toxic radioactive element plutonium. The study was designed to determine the effects of radiation exposure on government workers in nuclear research. Study records claim that only terminally ill patients were selected so that they would not be subject to long-term effects and so that autopsies could be performed to compile results. However, several patients suffered the effects of radiation for more than 20 years, and autopsies were performed on only a few patients.

Other experiments conducted or approved by the U.S. Atomic Energy Commission (now part of the Department of Energy), involved injecting hospital patients with uranium, exposing the testicles of prison inmates to X rays, and giving radioactive iron to pregnant women and radioactive calcium to mentally retarded teen-agers.

Critics of the studies have argued that many patients were not properly informed of experimental risks or were not informed of their participation at all. Furthermore, researchers rarely tracked the health of the subjects after the experiments ended, leaving many people mystified by the ailments they developed. In response to the public outcry, the Administration of President Bill Clinton established a special agency and a nongovernmental advisory committee to investigate harm caused by the studies.

Hepatitis B drug tests. After 5 of 15 participants died in a test of an experimental drug for hepatitis B, the Food and Drug Administration (FDA) announced new rules in November 1993 requiring medical researchers to report all patient deaths or serious side effects. The test of the experimental drug Fialuridine, or FIAU, was conducted by the National Institutes of Health (NIH) in Bethesda, Md. Other patients in the study suffered severe side effects. Hepatitis is a disease of the liver caused by a virus.

During an investigation, the FDA found that some participants in an earlier NIH study of the drug had also died. The researchers had not reported these deaths to the FDA because they did not believe they were related to the test drug. The FDA criticized the way the study was conducted, but

an NIH review found no evidence of wrongdoing.

Unfair tests on the mentally ill. The U.S. Congress held hearings in May 1994 on the treatment of mentally ill patients in clinical trials, after a federal investigation found that a study of schizophrenic patients at the University of California at Los Angeles was conducted unethically. In the study, people with schizophrenia were not told that their medication would be withdrawn and that without medication they were likely to suffer a relapse of mental illness. In some cases, patients were given drugs to worsen their symptoms before a test drug

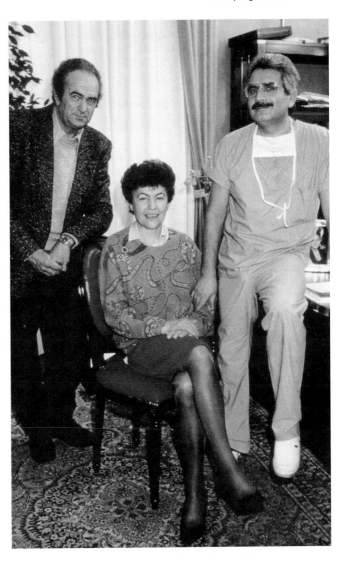

World's oldest new mother
Rossana Dalla Corte poses with her husband, *far left,* and with a physician who helped perform a medical procedure in which she became pregnant despite having passed *menopause* (the time when menstruation ceases). She gave birth in July 1994, at age 62. Her case, and that of a 59-year-old woman who gave birth to twins in December 1993, sparked debate over the ethics of "retirement pregnancies."

was administered. One patient killed himself. Some patients may have suffered mental damage and others became severely ill. As a result of these and other studies, some medical ethics experts have recommended that a national board be established to set ethics guidelines and to review potentially unethical procedures.

Physician-assisted suicide. On May 2, 1994, a Michigan jury cleared retired physician Jack Kevorkian of charges that he had violated a state law against assisted suicide by helping Thomas W. Hyde, Jr., kill himself in 1993. Hyde had suffered from a fatal disease of the nervous system. Michi-

gan passed a law in 1992 that made it a felony to assist in a suicide. The jury cleared Kevorkian on the grounds that he was relieving a patient's pain, which is allowed under the law. Kevorkian has fought for the right to help terminally ill people commit suicide since 1990. As of mid-1994, 20 people had done so with his assistance.

In a related case, a federal judge in May struck down a Washington state law banning assisted suicide. In her ruling, the judge held that the right of terminally ill people to end their suffering is guaranteed by the constitutional right of privacy. □ Carol Levine

In WORLD BOOK, see MEDICINE. See also HEALTH CARE ISSUES.

Mental Health

New drugs to treat mental disorders continued to appear on the market in 1994. Among the most promising were a drug for the treatment of schizophrenia, the most devastating of psychiatric conditions, and a drug to treat depression.

Schizophrenia drug. In January 1994, the United States Food and Drug Administration (FDA) approved the drug risperidone, which is marketed as Risperdal, for the treatment of schizophrenia.

Many people with schizophrenia suffer from *delusions* (irrational beliefs) and hear disturbing or threatening voices, a phenomenon known as hallucination. In addition, they often have problems forming coherent thoughts and maintaining close relationships. Over time, schizophrenia leaves its victims less and less able to function.

About 2 million Americans suffer from schizophrenia, and people with the disorder occupy about one-fourth of the nation's total hospital beds. Unfortunately, many people suffering from schizophrenia do not receive adequate care, and they make up a sizable percentage of the homeless population in the United States.

Because schizophrenia exacts a tremendous toll on its victims, new and effective medication is welcomed. Clozapine, which came on the market as Clozaril in 1990, was hailed as a breakthrough because it could stop hallucinations, paranoia, and unrealis-

tic thinking. But clozapine also has disadvantages, the main one being its price tag of about $4,200 a year per patient. Patients on clozapine also need a weekly blood test to ensure that they do not develop a potentially fatal depletion of certain white blood cells. Because of these problems and some other serious, though rare, side effects, doctors recommend clozapine for a patient only after other drugs have failed.

Risperidone, though, can be used during an initial attack of schizophrenia. Its cost ranges from $1,900 to $2,400 per year. No blood tests are necessary, which constitutes an important advantage for schizophrenic people who often are suspicious and forgetful and fail to comply with their doctors' requests.

New depression drug. In December 1993, the FDA approved venlafaxine hydrochloride, sold as Effexor, for the treatment of major depression. Major depression is characterized by a continuous depressed mood, a loss of interest or pleasure in most activities, an increase or decrease in appetite, a tendency to sleep too much or too little, loss of energy, feelings of worthlessness or inappropriate guilt, indecisiveness or an inability to concentrate, and thoughts of death or suicide.

Venlafaxine hydrochloride is chemically unrelated to other antidepressants. However, it is similar in its action to the widely prescribed antidepressant fluoxetine, commonly known by its trade name Prozac, in that it increases the effectiveness of an important brain chemical called serotonin. It also acts on another chemical, norepinephrine. Disruption in the activity of these chemicals is believed to play a role in depression.

Although Effexor has not been proven superior to other antidepressant medications in treating depression, it carries one significant advantage. It does not appear to curb sexual desire, as do Prozac and certain other antidepressants in some patients. Effexor does, however, cause *impotence* (loss of sexual ability) or other sexual problems in about 6 percent to 12 percent of men who take it. The most frequent side effects noted in the clinical trials of Effexor were nausea, constipation, loss of appetite, sleepiness, dry mouth, dizziness, insomnia, and nervousness. Effexor has not been tested for use in children.

Stress and hypertension. A study published in November 1993 offered clues to a possible link between psychological stress and *hypertension* (high blood pressure disease). The researchers used data from the Framingham Heart Study, a large-scale project that has tracked the health of a group of subjects since the 1950's. The team was headed by Jerome Markovitz at the University of Alabama School of Medicine, in Birmingham.

The researchers looked at data on 1,123 men and women who had had normal blood pressure levels 18 to 20 years ago to see if people with high levels of anxiety and anger were more prone to hypertension than others. They found that middle-aged men who developed hypertension had higher anxiety levels than those who did not develop hypertension.

However, the researchers also found that the increased risk occurred only among middle-aged men with very high levels of anxiety. No correlation was found between hypertension and anxiety levels in women or in older men.

Stress and cancer. Seeking to determine a link between cancer of the colon or rectum and stress, Joseph

G. Courtney of the School of Public Health at the University of California at Los Angeles teamed up with researchers in Sweden. The researchers had access to a large database of patients from the Stockholm area who suffered from colorectal cancer.

The researchers, who reported their results in September 1993, compared 569 Swedish patients who had colorectal cancer with 510 randomly selected cancer-free adults. Each person answered a series of questions about stressful events. The team found that severe job pressure increased the risk of developing colorectal cancer. The finding held even after the researchers took into con-

Depression in children

Children who suffer from depression are likely to do so again as adults, according to a study reported in 1994. Moreover, depression often goes unrecognized in children, though it can be treated. The American Psychiatric Association offers some guidelines for recognizing a chronic form of depression known as dysthymia and a more severe major depression.

Dysthymia is a depressed mood that affects a child most of the time for at least two years. Additional symptoms of dysthymia in children include:

- Feelings of hopelessness
- Low self-esteem
- Pessimistic attitude
- Fatigue
- Irritability
- Insomnia or oversleeping
- Poor appetite or overeating
- Difficulty concentrating or making decisions
- Poor social skills
- Poor school performance

Signs of major depression in children are a depressed mood accompanied by four or more of the following symptoms during a two-week period:

- Feelings of sadness most of the time; tearfulness; irritability
- Feelings of worthlessness or excessive, inappropriate guilt
- Loss of interest or pleasure in most activities
- Fatigue or low energy nearly every day
- Agitation or sluggishness most of the time
- Insomnia or oversleeping nearly every day
- Weight loss or gain, or not making expected weight gains
- Poor concentration or indecisiveness nearly every day
- Recurrent thoughts of death or suicide; suicide attempts

Source: *Diagnostic and Statistical Manual of Mental Disorders*, Fourth Edition.

After the Quake: Post-Traumatic Stress Disorder

At 4:31 a.m. on Jan. 17, 1994, a powerful earthquake rumbled across northern Los Angeles, tearing down freeways and damaging hundreds of buildings. Even when the aftershocks subsided, many of those who had felt the quake remained shaken by the event and had problems sleeping at night and focusing their attention during the day. Months later, nightmares and vivid recollections of the terror felt during the initial tremor continued to plague some quake survivors.

Such responses are common among survivors of natural disasters or such traumatic events as airplane crashes, military combat, and violent personal assault. Researchers estimate that about 30 percent of trauma survivors experience some emotional problems. Most gradually regain their emotional equilibrium and return to normal functioning. However, some develop post-traumatic stress disorder (PTSD), an anxiety disorder that develops in response to a life-threatening event.

PTSD usually develops in three stages. In the first stage, right after the trauma, individuals may feel greater anxiety than others, or they may become preoccupied with the experience. In the second stage, about four to six weeks after the traumatic event, they start to feel helpless and out of control and begin to relive the trauma through flashbacks. In the final stage, individuals with PTSD suffer from depression, chronic anxiety, and emotional numbness.

To be diagnosed with PTSD, an individual must exhibit re-current flashbacks and certain other symptoms of psychological distress for more than one month. In addition to flashbacks, symptoms include avoidance of people, places, or situations that might trigger painful memories; feelings of isolation or intense fear; and extreme irritability. Some individuals cannot recall an important aspect of the traumatic event. Others may have difficulty concentrating or completing tasks.

Depending on the type of trauma, PTSD sufferers may feel rage at those responsible for the trauma, resentment toward those who were not harmed in the event, or shame over their own helplessness. Some feel remorse over what they did during the event or guilt because they survived and others did not. Many turn to alcohol or drugs to escape their painful memories and block out their negative feelings and emotions.

Typically, individuals with PTSD also experience physical symptoms, including constant agitation and jumpiness. Some of them have difficulty sleeping. Children often experience stomachaches and headaches.

PTSD can occur at any age. Individuals who have experienced previous emotional or behavioral problems or such traumas as childhood abuse tend to be especially vulnerable to the disorder. Those who suffer severe physical injury or witness shocking scenes, such as the deaths of others, are also far more likely to develop PTSD than those spared such traumas. PTSD also tends to be more intense and longer lasting when the stress results from a deliberate act of human malice, such as torture or rape, rather than from chance.

Prompt intervention immediately following the trauma is the best way of preventing PTSD. Survivors benefit most from comforting, help with decision making, and protection from further harm. Talking about what happened with someone who has shared the

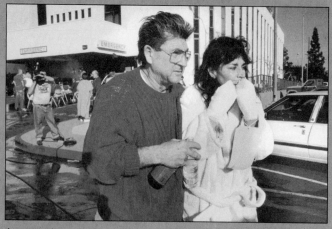

A woman is comforted after the 1994 Los Angeles earthquake.

experience can help survivors begin to deal with the trauma.

The recommended treatment for most cases of PTSD is psychotherapy. Therapy sessions begin with patients recounting the events before, during, and after the trauma and then working to interpret the events and to express their emotions about them. This insight into their feelings helps people overcome the trauma.

Hypnosis can be an especially effective treatment for PTSD. During a hypnotic trance, PTSD sufferers can recall memories and thoughts they may have blocked out. The process helps survivors face traumatic memories and put them into perspective.

Support groups made up of others who have experienced a similar trauma offer another avenue of treatment. Such groups can provide understanding and encouragement.

In some cases, medication can help treat PTSD. Psychiatrists have reported that antidepressants reduce nightmares, flashbacks, and anxiety.

The odds of recovering from PTSD are best for those who receive strong emotional support from family and friends and for those who exhibited good physical and mental health before the trauma. Without treatment, PTSD can last for years, with symptoms intensifying during periods of stress. With treatment, individuals with PTSD can feel increased control over their frightening memories and feelings. In time, they come to accept what happened as a tragedy of the past that does not have to affect the future. □ Dianne Hales

sideration differences in diet and other factors that are linked to these malignancies.

Japanese researchers reported in September 1993 their findings that chemical changes that can lead to cancer occur in the *DNA* (genetic material) of liver cells in rats who are subjected to psychological stress. The chemical changes are known as DNA lesions.

The researchers at Saitama Medical School in Japan placed young laboratory rats in boxes where they shared close quarters with rats that received periodic electrical shocks. They wanted to test the physical responses of the nonshocked rats after witnessing the trauma of their neighbors. After two to four days of continuous stress, the nonshocked rats had developed DNA lesions.

The researchers found that the rats' livers healed rapidly. However, other studies have shown that such lesions accumulate in aging animals and that these defects may not be repaired as quickly as they are in younger animals.

Diagnostic manual revised. In May 1994, the American Psychiatric Association published the fourth edition of the *Diagnostic and Statistical Manual of Mental Disorders,* commonly abbreviated as *DSM-IV.* First published in 1952, the *DSM* provides guidelines for psychiatrists, psychologists, and other mental health and medical professionals to use in diagnosing mental disorders.

Other people use the *DSM* as well. Lawyers and judges, for example, rely on the *DSM* in reaching decisions in legal cases that involve the mental state of a defendant or victim. Insurance companies rely on the *DSM* in deciding whether to cover a particular condition or whether and how to insure individuals. Researchers rely on the guide for uniform psychiatric terms.

The researching, testing, and writing of *DSM-IV* took five years. Committees of doctors reviewed and revised each large category of disorders. Although the fourth edition of the *DSM* contains some important changes, it presents no entirely new categories of disease.

Nervous System

See Brain and
Nervous System

Changes in psychiatric terms.

Some changes in the *DSM-IV* are intended to clarify the nature of specific psychiatric conditions. For instance, the term *multiple personality disorder* (MPD) has been confusing to the general public. Does it mean "split personality" and therefore signify schizophrenia? Does *multiple* mean possibly hundreds of separate personalities? The *DSM-IV* now terms MPD *dissociative identity disorder* (DID) to emphasize the patient's problem with his or her own identity. Dissociation refers to the divided nature of a normally integrated identity.

The heading *Delirium, Dementia, Amnestic, and Other Cognitive Disorders* replaced *Organic Mental Disorders* because the old wording implied that other mental conditions had no biological or chemical basis. Most psychiatrists now believe that depression, mania, obsessive-compulsive disorder, panic, schizophrenia, and other mental disorders have a strong biochemical component.

Acute stress disorder. The *DSM-IV*

describes a new condition called acute stress disorder in which a person who has been exposed to a traumatic event experiences such psychiatric symptoms as lack of emotion, loss of awareness, and amnesia within a month of the event. Psychological reactions that last longer than a month may indicate the presence of post-traumatic stress disorder (PTSD).

DSM-IV also narrowed the criteria for PTSD. Mental health experts had found that the condition was being overdiagnosed. The criterion that a person must have responded to a traumatic event with "intense fear, helplessness, or horror" replaces the requirement that the traumatic event be "outside the range of normal human experience." See Mental Health (Close-Up).

A once popular diagnosis, passive-aggressive personality disorder, lost its place in the *DSM* after mental health experts decided that *passive-aggressive* describes a single character trait rather than an entire personality. The term applies to a way of handling anger and assertiveness in which a person expresses aggressive or angry feelings through concealed actions rather than direct confrontation.

The *DSM* has also added for the first time a number of conditions formerly not considered suitable as the focus of psychiatric treatment. These conditions include neglect or maltreatment as a child; problems in relationships; religious or spiritual problems; difficulty with *acculturation* (adapting to a new culture); noncompliance with therapies; and a decline in memory, reasoning, and other mental abilities that is associated with aging.

☐ Lenore C. Terr

In the Special Reports section, see MEDICINES FOR THE MIND. In WORLD BOOK, see MENTAL ILLNESS.

Seeking support

Studies have shown that people who are coping with a serious problem can benefit from a support group in which they can address their concerns openly, share their feelings, and receive insight and information from others who have had similar experiences. There are support groups for a large variety of health problems. To find a group that can help you, try these sources.

- Hospitals and other health care organizations.

- Newspaper columns or advertisements listing meeting times for self-help groups.

- Churches, libraries, and other public meeting places may have bulletin boards that list meeting times.

- Organizations formed to address a particular health concern or disease, such as the American Cancer Society or American Heart Association. Many of these organizations have local chapters. Check your local telephone book.

- The list of toll-free telephone numbers to call for information and referrals that appears on pages 40 and 41.

- Self-help clearinghouses that publish directories and can help you start a group yourself. They include:

  American Self-Help Clearinghouse
  St. Clares-Riverside Medical Center
  25 Pocono Road
  Denville, NJ 07834
  (201) 625-7101

  National Self-Help Clearinghouse
  Room 620
  25 West 43rd Street
  New York, NY 10036
  (Send a letter with a self-addressed stamped envelope.)

Sources: *Mayo Clinic Health Letter* and *Prevention* magazine.

Men who eat large amounts of animal fat, particularly fat from red meat, may have an increased risk of developing advanced prostate cancer. That finding was reported in October 1993 by investigators at several research institutions, including Brigham and Women's Hospital and Harvard Medical School, both in Boston. The prostate is a walnut-sized gland in males at the juncture of the bladder and the urethra. Prostate cancer is second only to lung cancer as a leading cause of cancer deaths among men.

The study examined prostate cancer rates and dietary habits among 47,885 men aged 40 to 75 who participated in a large-scale research project called the Health Professionals Follow-Up Study. All of the participants were healthy at the start of the study in 1986. By 1990, 300 had been diagnosed with prostate cancer, and 126 of them had developed advanced forms of the disease.

The investigators found that the men's total fat intake was related to their likelihood of developing advanced prostate cancer. The men who reported the highest fat intake had a 79 percent greater risk than the men with the lowest fat intake.

Eating large amounts of red meat was associated with an even higher level of risk. The men who ate the most red meat were 164 percent more likely to develop advanced prostate cancer than the men who ate the least red meat.

Medical researchers are not sure exactly how dietary fat might be linked to prostate cancer, but there are many theories. One possibility is that dietary fat may affect a man's levels of sex hormones, which may be responsible for the increased prostate cancer risk.

Broccoli's anticancer chemicals.
A compound that is found in broccoli and other cruciferous vegetables—such as cabbage, kale, and Brussels sprouts—can inhibit the growth of cancerous tumors in animals, according to an April 1994 report by a group of researchers at the Johns Hopkins School of Medicine in Baltimore. In laboratory research two years earlier, the same research group had discovered that the chemical, called sulforaphane, could increase the activity of cancer-fighting compounds from the human immune system.

In the new study, the scientists fed sulforaphane or one of three artificial compounds in its same chemical class to one of two groups of laboratory rats. Then all the rats were force-fed a substance that causes *mammary* (breast) cancer.

The researchers found that the development of mammary cancer was delayed or prevented in the rats fed sulforaphane or the related compounds. In the animals that were giv-

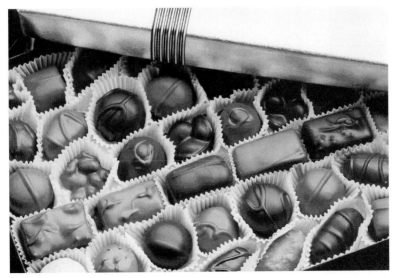

Eat chocolate and spare the heart
Saturated fats raise cholesterol levels, potentially clogging arteries and elevating the risk of heart disease. And chocolate's luscious taste comes from cocoa butter, a highly saturated fat. But according to a 1994 study, cocoa butter consists chiefly of a fatty acid that the body quickly converts into a monounsaturated fat with no effect on cholesterol. Even so, chocolate remains high in calories.

A Genetically Engineered Cow Hormone Sparks Consumer Ire

A controversy over genetically engineered foods gathered force in the United States in February 1994 when the Monsanto Company of St. Louis, Mo., began selling a synthetic hormone that boosts milk production in dairy cows. The substance, called bovine growth hormone (BGH), was being used to produce an estimated 15 percent of the U.S. milk supply by late winter 1994.

But some consumer groups were not happy about it. They charged that BGH, which is sold under the name Prosilac, causes health problems for cows and could also pose a threat to human health.

BGH is a synthetic form of a natural growth hormone, bovine somatotropin (BST), that stimulates milk production in cows. The synthetic hormone is called either BST or BGH.

Monsanto makes BGH by inserting copies of the natural somatotropin gene into bacteria, which then produce the hormone. When cows get extra doses of somatotropin in the form of BGH injections, their milk production increases by 10 to 20 percent.

The synthetic hormone underwent almost 10 years of scientific testing before receiving the approval of the U.S. Food and Drug Administration (FDA) in November 1993. The FDA concluded that milk from BGH-treated cows is chemically indistinguishable from the milk of untreated cows and has the same nutritional value.

By then, BGH had received other endorsements. The National Institutes of Health, the Congressional Office of Technology, the American Academy of Pediatrics, and the American Dietetic Association all gave BGH their blessing.

But tests and reassurances from government agencies and health groups left many people unconvinced. Consumer groups claimed the use of BGH carried hazards that were not being adequately addressed.

They questioned whether the hormone would remain in milk. The FDA said that although studies had shown that traces of BGH do show up in milk, so do small amounts of the natural hormone. But, the FDA added, 90 percent of either hormone is broken down during the pasteurization process, and whatever remains is destroyed by chemicals in the human digestive tract.

Another concern involved the possibility of antibiotic residues in milk. Consumers Union, the publisher of Consumer Reports magazine, claimed in February 1994 that cows treated with BGH are more likely to develop an in-flammation of the udder that requires treatment with antibiotics. The organization said milk from BGH-treated cows is more likely to contain unsafe antibiotic residues.

People who drink the milk, the argument went, might harbor bacteria in their bodies that could develop a resistance to the antibiotics. The people would then be more vulnerable to hard-to-treat infections.

The FDA denied that consumers faced any such risk. It said studies showed that the hormone produced no significant adverse health effects on cows or their calves. Furthermore, it said, federal inspectors and dairy producers routinely test milk for antibiotics, and milk found to contain unsafe drug residues is discarded.

Perhaps the biggest controversy surrounding BGH was whether milk and other dairy products produced with the hormone should carry special labels for the benefit of consumers who want to avoid

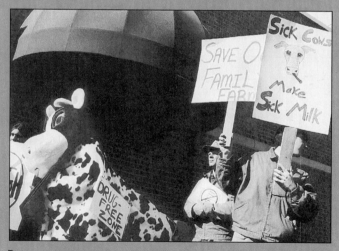

Demonstrators protest synthetic bovine growth hormone.

those products. In March, the governors of Vermont and Maine signed laws requiring such labels, and other states were considering similar laws.

The FDA had convened scientific panels in May 1993 to consider the labeling issue. Based on the panels' recommendations in favor of BGH and its own long-term studies of the synthetic hormone, the agency decided that there was no reason for mandatory labels. The FDA said, however, that dairies and food companies could voluntarily label such products. The agency's only stipulation was that labels must be written so as not to mislead consumers.

FDA guidelines stated that it would be untruthful to label milk products as "BST-free" because all milk contains BST. The agency also advised caution in using the term "rBST-free," in which the r stands for the recombinant DNA (gene-splicing) methods used to make the hormone. Calling milk rBST-free, the FDA said, wrongly implies that it is safer or of higher quality than milk from hormone-treated cows.

In 1994, Monsanto warned dairy companies against using labels that tout milk products as being BGH-free unless the labels also state that studies have found no difference between milk produced with BGH and ordinary milk. To show that it meant to play hardball, Monsanto filed suit against two dairy producers for labeling that it found unacceptable. At the same time, the company agreed to monitor dairy products from BGH-treated cows to ensure that the products contain no antibiotic residues and are causing no adverse health effects. ☐ Michael Woods

en the highest dose of the anticancer compounds, only 35 percent developed tumors, compared with 68 percent of the rats that were not fed any of the protective compounds. One of the synthetic chemicals proved to be even more effective than sulforaphane. Only 25 percent of the rats given that compound grew tumors.

Scientists are not sure exactly why sulforaphane and its chemical cousins have a protective effect, though the researchers' previous work showed that sulforaphane may encourage the body to produce natural cancer-fighting compounds. Researchers also do not know how much sulforaphane is in cruciferous vegetables other than broccoli and whether eating any of the vegetables can provide a protective effect.

Caffeine and miscarriage risk.
Pregnant women who consume caffeine may have an increased risk of miscarriage, according to a December 1993 report by researchers at McGill University in Montreal, Canada. The McGill researchers interviewed 331 women who had been hospitalized because of miscarriage. The health habits of the women were then compared with those of women whose pregnancies were normal.

While making the comparison, the investigators took into account a variety of factors that can affect pregnancy, including the age of the women; whether they had medical conditions such as high blood pressure; and their histories of smoking, alcohol use, and exposure to chemicals at work. The scientists also compared the two groups' consumption of beverages containing caffeine, such as cola, tea, and coffee.

The researchers found that pregnant women who consumed the amount of caffeine in 1½ to 3 cups of coffee per day before and during their pregnancy were twice as likely to have suffered a miscarriage as the women who consumed no caffeine. Drinking more than 3 cups was associated with a tripled risk of miscarriage. The study thus supported health officials' previous recommendations that pregnant women—and those who may become pregnant—reduce their consumption of caffeine.

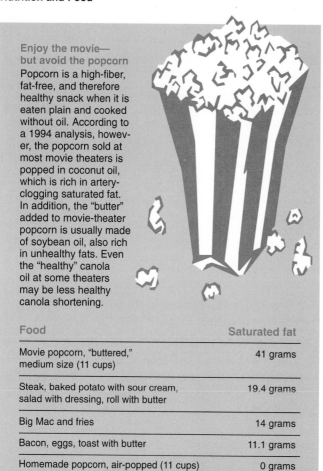

Popcorn is a high-fiber, fat-free, and therefore healthy snack when it is eaten plain and cooked without oil. According to a 1994 analysis, however, the popcorn sold at most movie theaters is popped in coconut oil, which is rich in artery-clogging saturated fat. In addition, the "butter" added to movie-theater popcorn is usually made of soybean oil, also rich in unhealthy fats. Even the "healthy" canola oil at some theaters may be less healthy canola shortening.

Food	Saturated fat
Movie popcorn, "buttered," medium size (11 cups)	41 grams
Steak, baked potato with sour cream, salad with dressing, roll with butter	19.4 grams
Big Mac and fries	14 grams
Bacon, eggs, toast with butter	11.1 grams
Homemade popcorn, air-popped (11 cups)	0 grams

Sources: Center for Science in the Public Interest; U.S. Department of Agriculture; McDonald's.

Questions about beta carotene.

Nutritionists and physicians were forced to reevaluate the general wisdom about beta carotene supplements after a study released in April 1994 appeared to link the nutrient to an increased risk of lung cancer. The study was undertaken by a group of scientists led by researchers with the National Public Health Institute in Helsinki, Finland, and the National Cancer Institute in Bethesda, Md.

Beta carotene is an antioxidant, a type of compound capable of blocking the destructive effects of molecules called free radicals. In the body, free radicals can cause damage to cells, including the genetic damage that may lead to cancer.

The new study was designed to ex-amine the potential protective effects of beta carotene and another antioxidant nutrient, vitamin E, in a group of Finnish men at high risk for developing lung cancer. The researchers divided 29,133 male smokers aged 50 to 69 into four groups. One group took 50 milligrams of vitamin E per day. Another was given 20 milligrams of beta carotene per day. A third group took both supplements, and the last received a *placebo* (substance with no active ingredients).

The health of the men was then monitored for five to eight years. The researchers found that the men who took vitamin E supplements did not have a lower risk of lung cancer than the men who received placebos. A more startling finding was that the group of men taking beta carotene supplements had an 18 percent higher incidence of lung cancer and an 8 percent higher death rate than the group of men who did not take that supplement.

Nutritionists and other health experts said that the Finnish study was by no means the final word on beta carotene and cancer. Indeed, no other study, whether using human beings or laboratory animals, has shown that beta carotene is linked to higher rates of cancer. In fact, dozens of studies suggest that beta carotene may protect against various types of cancer and heart disease.

The authors of the Finnish study pointed out that their results could be due simply to chance. In addition, medical experts said that the duration of the new study might have been too short. Because it takes decades for lung cancer to develop, few scientists believe that an antioxidant could have a rapid protective effect against cancer in long-term smokers.

Many experts were nonetheless taking a cautious approach, recommending that people obtain beta carotene not by taking supplements but through foods rich in beta carotene, such as carrots, sweet potatoes, and apricots

Cranberry juice remedy. Drinking cranberry juice has long been a home remedy to treat or prevent urinary tract infections. In March 1994, a study conducted by researchers in

Boston scientifically established the beverage's healthful effects.

The researchers, from Brigham and Women's Hospital and Harvard Medical School, gave 153 older women either a cranberry juice drink or a drink that looked like cranberry juice, every day for six months. Each month, nurses checked urine samples from the women for bacteria and white blood cells, both of which indicate the presence of an infection.

Over the six months of the study, the women who drank cranberry juice had a 42 percent lower risk of contracting a urinary tract infection than the women who drank the look-alike beverage. And among women who did develop an infection, those who received cranberry juice were one-fourth as likely as those in the noncranberry group to still have the infection the next month.

The researchers speculated that cranberry juice probably contains substances that restrict or prevent the growth of bacteria in the urinary tract. Previous experiments have shown that cranberry and blueberry juices reduce the ability of bacteria to stick to the lining of the urinary tract.

☐ Jeanine Barone

In the Special Reports section, see CAN VITAMINS HELP PREVENT CANCER? In the Health Matters section, see WHICH FATS ARE WORSE THAN OTHERS?

Occupational Health
See Environmental Health

Pregnancy and Childbirth

A pregnant woman infected with the human immunodeficiency virus (HIV), the virus that causes AIDS, can reduce the chances of passing the virus to her baby by taking the drug zidovudine (AZT). That risk can be lowered from about 26 percent to 8 percent, according to a study reported in February 1994. The study was conducted by the United States National Institutes of Health (NIH), in Bethesda, Md., in collaboration with French public health officials.

The researchers, who began the study in 1991, tested the effects of AZT therapy on 477 women. Some women received a *placebo* (inactive substance) whereas others received AZT during pregnancy and labor. Because of the therapy's success, the researchers ended the study earlier than scheduled, and public health officials recommended that doctors consider prescribing AZT for pregnant HIV-infected patients.

The short-term side effects of AZT among the mothers and babies in the study were minor and included mild anemia—an easily treated condition—in the babies. The long-term side effects of AZT are unknown, however, and patients receiving the drug continue to be monitored.

An estimated 7,000 HIV-infected women give birth annually in the United States. About 25 percent of these babies are infected with HIV. Health experts have estimated that by the year 2000, 10 million children globally will have been infected by the AIDS-causing virus.

Routine ultrasound not needed.
The routine use of ultrasound, a scanning technique that enables physicians to observe a fetus in the womb, does not improve a healthy woman's chances of having a healthy baby, according to a study published in September 1993 by the National Institute of Child Health and Human Development, part of the NIH. The results of testing more than 15,000 pregnant women at low risk for problems during pregnancy showed that although ultrasound helped detect problems early, it did not change the outcome of a pregnancy.

Ultrasound relies on high-frequency sound waves that are sent into the uterus and turned into an image of the fetus by a computer as they bounce back. Doctors use this technique to check for birth defects or multiple fetuses or to assess the growth and age of the fetus.

The NIH and the American College of Obstetricians and Gynecologists (ACOG) have argued against routine use of ultrasound for several reasons: the high cost, the risk of overtreating women because of false indications of problems, and the lack of evidence that ultrasound affects the pregnancy's outcome. Most pregnant women in the United States are at low risk for problems during pregnancy.

The researchers divided the study

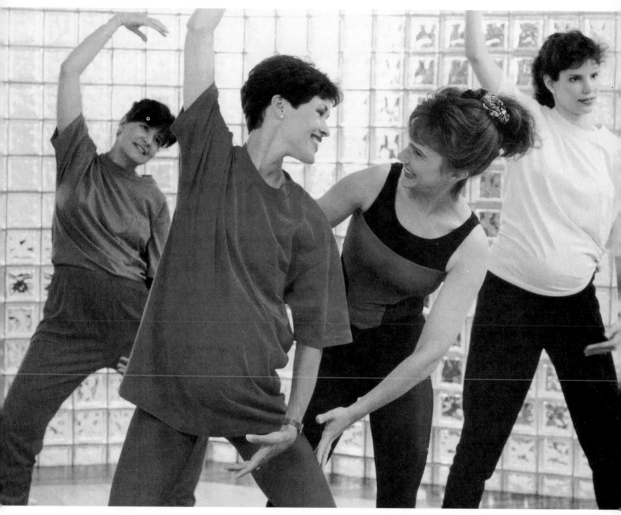

Exercise benefits pregnant women

There are no medical reasons why most women should not continue to exercise during pregnancy, according to new guidelines issued by the American College of Obstetricians and Gynecologists in February 1994. The benefits of moderate exercise during pregnancy include regulation of blood sugar levels and weight gain, and improved emotional well-being.

participants into two groups. One group received ultrasound examination twice during pregnancy, and the other group received ultrasound only if the doctor suspected a problem. Both groups displayed the same rates of premature births, low birth-weight babies, and babies with birth defects. Although doctors could detect more birth defects with ultrasound than without, the health at birth of the baby remained the same in either group. The researchers concluded that the use of ultrasound as a routine procedure adds considerably to the overall cost of health care without an improvement in childbirth results.

Down syndrome testing guideline.

Blood tests to detect a woman's risk of having a baby with Down syndrome

should be offered to pregnant women under age 35, according to an August 1994 recommendation by the ACOG. The tests, known as maternal serum screening, measure certain substances in a pregnant woman's blood that may indicate the presence of Down syndrome or various other birth defects in her fetus.

Down syndrome is a genetic disorder characterized by mental retardation and certain physical features. Because the risk of having a baby with Down syndrome increases with the age of the mother, doctors routinely test pregnant women over age 35. However, 80 percent of children with Down syndrome are born to mothers under age 35, because women in that age group give birth to the majority of babies. Most of these women do not have risk factors for delivering a child with the condition and therefore are not usually tested for it.

The maternal serum tests are performed at 15 to 18 weeks of pregnancy and can give a preliminary indication if a woman has an above average risk of having a baby with a defect. If the tests find substances in the blood that indicate a possible abnormality, an additional procedure called amniocentesis can confirm the presence of the defect. In this procedure, a sample of the amniotic fluid that surrounds the fetus in the mother's uterus is withdrawn and the cells are examined for abnormalities.

The advantages of the maternal serum tests are that they are easy to perform, they carry no risk, and the results are available within a week. The ACOG predicts that maternal serum testing can help detect up to 60 percent of Down syndrome cases in fetuses of women under age 35.

Breast-feeding and breast cancer.
Breast-feeding slightly lowers a woman's risk of developing breast cancer before menopause, the time when a woman's menstrual periods cease. This was the finding of a January 1994 report by researchers based at the University of Wisconsin in Madison. The researchers studied nearly 6,000 breast cancer patients and about 8,000 women without the disease to determine if breast-feeding provided any protection against breast cancer.

The researchers found that the risk of breast cancer before menopause was lowest for women who were 20 years of age or younger when they first breast-fed their infants. In addition, the risk kept decreasing the longer a woman breast-fed her infant. Breast-feeding did not appear to lower a woman's risk of developing breast cancer after menopause, the time when the majority of cases occur.

The researchers speculated that the protective effect of breast-feeding may result from the hormonal changes or interruption of ovulation that occurs during breast-feeding. They estimated that if all mothers breast-fed for 24 months or longer, breast cancer among premenopausal women could be reduced nearly 25 percent. This re-

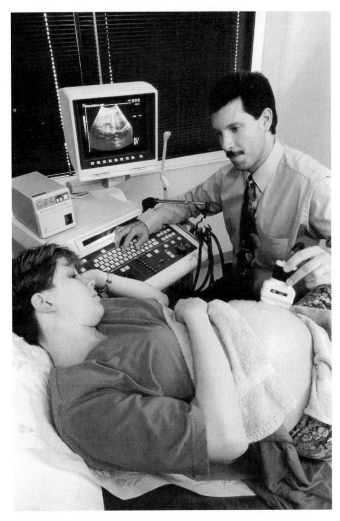

duction in risk would be even greater among women who breast-fed for the first time at an early age.

Exercise and pregnancy. Women who have exercised prior to pregnancy should safely be able to continue that level of exercise through pregnancy and the postpartum period, according to new guidelines issued in February 1994 by the ACOG. The new recommendations reflect several studies that indicate there is no real risk in exercising during pregnancy. The report states that, in the absence of complications, women can continue to exercise during pregnancy and derive benefits that exercise brings.

□ Rebecca D. Rinehart
See also NUTRITION. In WORLD BOOK, see PREGNANCY.

Overused procedure?
A woman not known to be at risk for problems during pregnancy does not need routine screening by ultrasound, according to a study published in September 1993. Ultrasound is a technique that uses sound waves to produce an image of the fetus. The study found that low-risk women were just as likely to give birth to healthy babies whether they received ultrasound screenings or not.

Respiratory System

Health care workers can reduce the number of drug-resistant tuberculosis (TB) cases by supervising patients to make sure they take their medication. That was the conclusion of a study reported in April 1994 by endocrinologist Stephen E. Weis and colleagues at the University of North Texas Health Science Center in Fort Worth.

Tuberculosis is an infectious disease caused by bacteria. TB most often strikes the lungs and respiratory system, but it can affect any organ of the body. Since 1985, TB has been making a comeback in the United States. In 1993, 25,313 new cases of TB were reported, down from the 26,673 new cases in 1992 but well above the 1985 low of 22,201 cases, according to the Centers for Disease Control and Prevention (CDC) in Atlanta, Ga.

Even more alarming than the number of new cases is the appearance of strains of TB that resist treatment with the antibiotic drugs typically used against the disease. Scientists attribute the increase in drug resistance in part to patients' failure to complete the standard course of treatment, which lasts from six to nine months. When a patient stops taking the antibiotics too soon, some bacteria better able to resist the drug survive and multiply. In time, the drug-resistant bacteria take over.

Weis compared the effectiveness of the standard, unsupervised treatment

in 379 TB patients with the treatment of 578 TB patients who received daily visits from health care workers to make sure they took their antibiotics. Weis reported that no patient who underwent supervised therapy from the beginning to the end of treatment developed drug resistance. That compared with 39 patients who developed resistance during the unsupervised treatment. Moreover, the proportion of people who were already infected with a drug-resistant strain at the time of diagnosis dropped from 13 percent to 6.7 percent.

Hantavirus isolated. Researchers in November 1993 isolated the virus responsible for an outbreak of severe respiratory illness that began in the Southwestern United States in April 1993. Infection with the virus had caused 45 deaths in 18 states by July 1994, according to the CDC. The virus—a previously unknown form of hantavirus—struck first in the Four Corners area, where New Mexico, Arizona, Colorado, and Utah converge.

The new hantavirus causes a flulike illness that scientists have termed the hantavirus pulmonary syndrome. The illness can quickly progress to respiratory failure and death.

Deer mice carry the hantavirus and spread it through their droppings and urine. When the excrement and urine dry, they break into fine particles and

Colds affect sinuses, too
On the basis of computerized tomographic (CT) scans, researchers at the University of Virginia at Charlottesville reported in January 1994 that mucus clogs the sinuses *(arrow, left)* as well as the nasal passages *(asterisk)* in people with colds. An uncongested sinus and nasal passage appear on the right. The finding overturned a theory that bacterial infection causes sinus congestion after a cold.

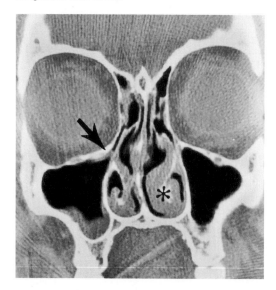
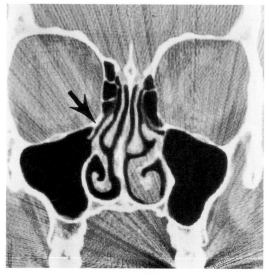

disperse in the air. People contract the virus when they breathe in the airborne particles.

Researchers from the CDC and several health care institutions in New Mexico published a detailed description of hantavirus pulmonary syndrome in April 1994. The researchers based their description on studies of the first 17 people with confirmed infections with the virus.

The researchers noted that the disease struck patients ranging in age from 13 to 64, with an average age of 32. The initial symptoms of the illness included fever, muscle aches, cough, headache, nausea, and vomiting that continued for about five days before the patients were hospitalized. In most cases, fluid built up rapidly in the patients' lungs, and they suffered from severe reductions in blood pressure and the failure of major organs as a result of insufficient oxygen. Of the initial 17 patients, 13 died.

Antioxidants and lung cancer. Vitamin E and beta carotene supplements may not offer smokers any protection against lung cancer, according to a study reported by Finnish researchers in April 1994. Past studies have suggested that diets rich in these compounds may reduce a person's risk of developing the disease. In the Finnish study, by contrast, taking beta carotene appeared to actually increase the chances of developing lung cancer.

Researchers from the Finnish Public Health Institute in Helsinki studied 29,133 male smokers from 50 to 69 years of age, for five to eight years. The participants were divided into groups. Some took daily supplements of beta carotene or vitamin E. Others took both beta carotene and vitamin E or a *placebo* (inactive substance).

Vitamin E and beta carotene are *antioxidants*—compounds that are thought to help slow or halt certain chemical reactions involving oxygen in the body. Scientists believe these reactions may contribute to the development of some cancers.

The Finnish study, however, found no significant protection against lung cancer from taking vitamin E supplements. At the same time, it showed a surprising rise in risk among those who received beta carotene. Only 2 percent fewer cases of lung cancer developed in the group that took vitamin E than in the group taking the placebo. But the participants who took beta carotene had an 18 percent higher incidence of lung cancer than did the group that received the placebo. In addition, the death rate for the beta carotene group was 8 percent higher than that for the placebo group.

Some researchers criticized the study, because the participants took the antioxidants for a relatively short time and at low dosages. Participants also continued to smoke during the study, a behavior that may have reduced the beneficial effect of the antioxidants, according to some critics.

New clue to near-fatal asthma.
People who have had life-threatening attacks of asthma may have trouble perceiving the severity of their symptoms. A group of Japanese internists at the Tohoku University School of Medicine in Japan reported this finding in May 1994.

Asthma, which afflicts between 9 million and 12 million people in the United States, is characterized by attacks of wheezing and difficulty breathing brought on by the narrowing and inflammation of the bronchial tubes. In many cases, asthma results from an allergic reaction.

The study measured participants' perceived difficulty in breathing on a scale of 1 to 10 as researchers gradually increased the effort required to breathe by narrowing the diameter of a breathing tube that the participants used. The study involved 11 patients who had a history of near-fatal asthma attacks, 11 patients with asthma who had not had near-fatal attacks, and 16 people without asthma.

The researchers said that people who have had life-threatening asthma attacks demonstrated a significantly decreased sensation of breathlessness, compared with other study participants. This deficiency could cause a dangerous delay before asthmatics feel that they need medical help, the researchers said.

□ Robert A. Balk

See also INFECTIOUS DISEASES; ALLERGIES AND ASTHMA. In WORLD BOOK, see ASTHMA; LUNG; RESPIRATION.

Safety

The number of Americans who died in injuries at work declined by 23 percent during the 1980's, according to a National Institute for Occupational Safety and Health (NIOSH) study issued in November 1993. Researchers said it was the most comprehensive study ever conducted on deaths from job-related injuries.

NIOSH, an agency of the United States Centers for Disease Control and Prevention (CDC), based in Atlanta, Ga., found that 63,589 workers died from on-the-job injuries during the 10-year period from 1980 through 1989. The number of deaths decreased from a high of 7,405 in 1980 to 5,714 in 1989. The death rate per 100,000 workers declined by 37 percent, from 8.9 per 100,000 in 1980 to 5.6 per 100,000 in 1989.

Motor vehicle accidents were the leading cause of occupational fatalities, responsible for 23 percent of all on-the-job deaths. Accidents involving machinery were next (causing 13 percent of all deaths), followed by homicides (12 percent), falls (10 percent), electrocutions (7 percent), and being struck by falling objects (7 percent).

The study showed that males, who tend to work in more dangerous occupations, accounted for about 94 percent of workplace deaths. Their fatality rate was 12 times higher than the women's rate. Most men died in accidents. But homicide was the leading cause of workplace death for women. Murders accounted for 41 percent of workplace deaths for women, compared to 10 percent for men.

Miners had the highest fatality rate, followed by construction workers; employees in the transportation/communication/public utilities sector; and workers in agriculture/forestry/fishing. States with the highest occupational fatality rates were, respectively, Alaska, Wyoming, Montana, Idaho, West Virginia, Mississippi, and South Dakota. States with the lowest fatal workplace injury rates were Connecticut, Massachusetts, and New York.

Researchers said that although injury deaths at work are declining, an average of 17 workers still die each day. The new study data, they said, will help reduce the toll by identifying occupations most in need of injury-prevention programs.

Crayons. The U.S. Consumer Product Safety Commission (CPSC) on April 5, 1994, warned that certain crayons imported from China can cause lead poisoning if eaten by children. CPSC identified the crayons in a nationwide study, begun after an infant in Phoenix developed lead poisoning from eating a crayon.

The CPSC issued a recall order for 750,000 boxes of contaminated crayons, most of which already had been sold. It advised parents to discard the crayons or return them to the store for a refund. CPSC tests

Press, don't pump
Motorists driving vehicles with antilock brakes should apply steady pressure to the brakes during emergency stops, rather than pumping the brakes, the Highway Loss Data Institute warned in January 1994. Pumping reduces the brakes' effectiveness.

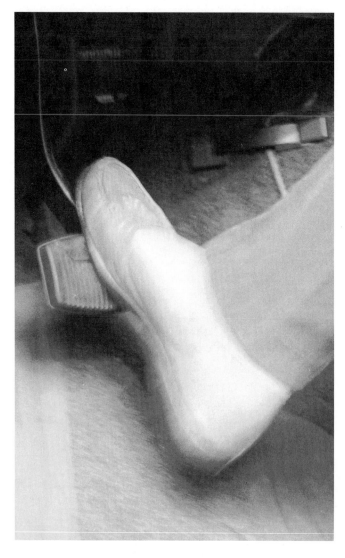

found that Crayola crayons, the most popular brand in America, were safe. But other brands sold in the last four years, the CPSC said, contained enough lead to cause poisoning. The brands were "12 Jumbo Crayons," "Safe 48 Nontoxic I'm a Toys 'R' Us Kid! Crayons," "12 Crayons Glory," and "18 Crayons That Paint."

Eight other brands of imported crayons also contained lead, though not enough to cause poisoning. Experts at CPSC, however, said those brands still posed a hazard, especially for children who swallow lead from other sources. These sources include water from pipes sealed with lead solder and dust or chips of lead-based paint in old, run-down housing. CPSC advised parents and schools to buy only crayons with a label stating that they conform to "ASTM D-4236." The phrase means that the crayons have been tested and do not pose a lead-poisoning hazard.

Sudden infant death. Researchers reported in January that rebreathing exhaled air may have contributed to the deaths of some infants diagnosed as having died from sudden infant death syndrome (SIDS)—also known as crib death. SIDS, which kills 6,000 to 7,000 infants in the United States each year, is a mysterious condition in which infants stop breathing while asleep. Previous studies showed that infants put to sleep facedown have a higher risk of SIDS. The American Academy of Pediatrics in 1992 began advising parents to put healthy infants to sleep on their back or side.

In the new studies, researchers from Washington University in St. Louis, Mo., placed sedated experimental animals facedown on a beanbag cushion. The animals inhaled their own exhaled air while they slept. Carbon dioxide in the stale air accumulated to fatal levels in the animals' blood, and they suffocated. Researchers said parents should be aware that soft bedding can trap exhaled air, so that infants placed facedown inhale it. Researchers cited the importance of using proper infant bedding, such as a firm crib mattress covered with a sheet.

The findings led the CPSC on January 5 to issue a safety alert advising

Calcium supplements carry lead risk
People who take calcium supplements may be ingesting hazardous amounts of lead, according to research published in August 1993. Many women take the supplements to ward off the loss of bone tissue known as osteoporosis, and the products are also a popular source of calcium for children who are allergic to milk and other calcium-rich foods. But lead is a poison that is especially dangerous to children and developing fetuses, for whom even small quantities can lead to learning disabilities and behavioral problems. In the 1993 research, scientists analyzed 70 brands of calcium supplements sold in the United States and Canada. They found that 17 brands, or 24 percent, contained lead in concentrations greater than 6 micrograms per day—the maximum daily intake that the U.S. Food and Drug Administration considers safe for children under age 7. Supplements made from bone meal had the highest lead levels, followed by those made from the fossilized shells of mollusks such as oysters. The brands with the lowest lead content were made from purified calcium carbonate and carried the USP (United States Pharmacopeia) seal of approval.

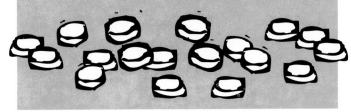

that parents not place infants to sleep on soft bedding products, such as soft mattresses, sheepskins, plush comforters, or infant beanbag cushions. The CPSC had previously banned the sale of infant beanbags as an infant suffocation hazard.

Infants and automobile safety.
Parents should not place an infant safety seat in the front seat of an automobile equipped with a passenger-side airbag, the National Highway Traffic Safety Administration (NHTSA) warned on February 18. Many parents put infants in the front seat, where it is easier to tend a baby who fusses or cries. But in an accident, the passenger-side airbag may slam into the back of an infant safety seat. An infant

Deaths from gunshot wounds are almost as great in number as deaths from automobile accidents and will be greater by the year 2003 if the current trend continues, according to a January 1994 report by the United States Department of Health and Human Services.

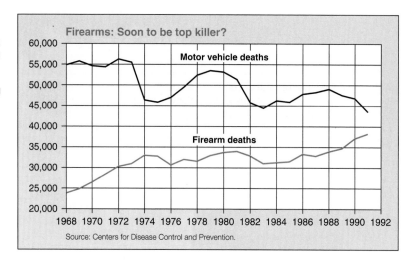

Firearms: Soon to be top killer?

Source: Centers for Disease Control and Prevention.

in the seat faces the rear of the car. The impact could be great enough to break the infant's neck or cause brain injury.

The NHTSA said the passenger-side airbag poses no danger for older children who have outgrown their infant seat and are large enough to face forward. But the agency recommended that both infants and older children be placed in the rear seat, which is the safest place in the car for a child.

Antilock brakes. Many motorists do not use antilock brakes properly, reducing the brakes' effectiveness in preventing accidents, a study by the Highway Loss Data Institute (HLDI) reported on January 27. Antilock brakes are designed to stop a car in a shorter distance, especially on wet or slippery pavement, without causing the car's wheels to lock. Locked wheels can result in uncontrollable skids.

The HLDI, an insurance industry group based in Detroit, compared accidents among cars with antilock brakes to those among cars with conventional brakes. Researchers found no reduction in the number of accidents or in the average amount of damage to cars with antilock brakes. They said that many motorists making a sudden stop with antilock brakes pump the brakes, as they were taught to do with conventional brakes to prevent skids. But pumping decreases the effectiveness of antilock brakes. The HLDI advised motorists to apply steady pressure to antilock brakes,

and never pump the brake pedal in emergency stops.

Alcohol-related fatalities. On Dec. 3, 1993, the CDC reported that the number of alcohol-related traffic fatalities in the United States declined by 30 percent from 1982 to 1992, dropping from 25,165 to 17,699. The decrease occurred despite a 40 percent increase in the number of miles that Americans drove during this period.

CDC officials said the decrease resulted from a number of measures taken to discourage drunken driving. These include prompt suspension of driving licenses for people who drive while intoxicated; reductions in the legally permissible blood-alcohol concentration; wider use of sobriety checkpoints by police; and greater public awareness of the dangers of drinking and driving.

But the CDC recommended adoption of additional measures to further reduce the number of deaths and injuries caused by people who drink and drive. It cited a need for new restrictions on the use of alcohol by underaged youth, more alcohol-abuse treatment programs, and intensified efforts to make people aware of the risk of being arrested for drunken driving.

Guns in the home. Despite the widespread belief that gun ownership can protect people from crime, keeping a gun at home increases the risk that a family member will be killed, according to a study of homicides in three states reported in October 1993.

Researchers in Tennessee, Washington, and Ohio studied the circumstances surrounding 1,860 homicides that occurred in the late 1980's and early 1990's in three large counties that included the cities of Memphis, Seattle, and Cleveland. Their report, published in *The New England Journal of Medicine,* compared 388 of the victims with control subjects who lived in the same neighborhood and were similar to the victims in age, income, race, and other characteristics.

The study found that homicide victims were more likely to live alone, to rent rather than own their residence, and to live in a household with an illicit drug abuser or with someone who had been hit or hurt in a family fight. Researchers said physicians and law enforcement officials should make a greater effort to protect victims of battering and family violence, because they face a high risk of being murder victims.

But the major difference setting homicide victims apart was availability of a gun in the home. The risk of a homicide was 2.7 times greater in households with a gun than in those without a gun. Most of the killings occurred when a family member or close acquaintance shot someone else in the household. There was no evidence that keeping a gun increased personal safety even among the small number of homicides that involved forced entry.

The American Academy of Pediatrics (AAP) in May 1994 began a nationwide public education program to warn parents that a gun in the home is more likely to be used to kill a family member or an acquaintance than an intruder. The AAP is sponsoring the program with the Center to Prevent Handgun Violence, a nonprofit organization based in Washington, D.C., that tries to reduce gun-related injuries and deaths.

The AAP said that 14 children and adolescents are killed each day in gun-related murders, suicides, and accidents. Guns account for about 11 percent of all deaths annually among children and adolescents. The program includes distribution of patient education brochures and efforts to encourage pediatricians to counsel parents about the risks of keeping a gun at home.

Parents who do decide to keep a gun at home should keep the weapon unloaded in a locked drawer or cabinet, with the ammunition stored in a separate locked place, AAP said.

□ Michael Woods

In the Special Reports section, see HOME, SAFE HOME. In the Health Matters section, see TREATING BURNS. See also ENVIRONMENTAL HEALTH. In WORLD BOOK, see SAFETY.

Sexually Transmitted Diseases

In January 1994, the Centers for Disease Control and Prevention (CDC), in Atlanta, Ga., announced a new program designed to prevent the spread of sexually transmitted diseases, including AIDS, among young people. Various national, state, and local groups that work to prevent AIDS helped develop the program, called the Prevention Marketing Initiative, in consultation with marketing experts.

The initiative included a series of 12 radio and television public service announcements targeting sexually active people aged 18 to 25. The announcements encourage young people to refrain from sexual activity or to use condoms if they do engage in sexual intercourse. "Young people need to know that the surest way to prevent AIDS is to refrain from having sex, but we also need to be realistic," said Donna Shalala, secretary of the Department of Health and Human Services, which oversees the CDC.

The CDC was responding to concerns generated by the growing number of sexually active young people and their inconsistent use of condoms. Abundant evidence has shown that consistent and correct condom use is effective for preventing STD's.

The CDC also produced a step-by-step brochure to help people use condoms correctly. Single copies of the brochure are available free of charge by phoning the CDC National AIDS Hot Line at 800-342-AIDS.

Teens and gonorrhea. The highest rates of gonorrhea in the United States occur among teen-agers, according to an August 1993 CDC report. Adolescents accounted for 24 to 30 percent of all cases of gonorrhea from 1981 through 1991. Although gonorrhea rates among older age groups declined during these years, rates among teen-agers rose or remained unchanged. Higher levels of sexual activity and inconsistent use of condoms may account for some of the increase.

In 1991, female adolescents aged 15 to 19 had the highest gonorrhea rates of any group, with more than 1 percent of all girls in that age group

infected. The total number of cases among this group was about 84,000. Among boys aged 15 to 19, slightly less than 1 percent had gonorrhea in 1991, a total of about 76,000 cases. Gonorrhea is caused by bacteria and is treated with antibiotics. Symptoms may be mild and go unnoticed. The infection is most serious when left untreated in women because it can spread through the uterus to the fallopian tubes and lead to sterility.

Sex education. The CDC commissioned a review of 23 studies of school-based sex education programs and reported the findings in the spring of 1994. The review found that some programs succeeded in reducing risky adolescent sexual activity but that other programs had no such impact. Reductions in risky activity included later age at first intercourse, less frequent intercourse, fewer sexual partners, and use of condoms or other contraceptives.

The effective programs all focused on these risky behaviors. In addition, they included activities to personalize the information, addressed social or media influences on sexual behaviors, and were designed to strengthen individual and group values against unprotected sex.

Currently, 46 states either strongly recommend or require sex education in schools, and all 50 states either recommend or require AIDS education programs. By the late 1980's, about 85 percent of all U.S. schools offered sex education. Of these, at least 85 percent included information on abstinence, contraception, pregnancy, and STD's, including AIDS.

The authors of the report pointed out that the United States has one of the highest teen-age pregnancy rates of any industrialized nation. More than 40 percent of American women become pregnant before age 20, and more than 1 million teen-agers become pregnant each year.

New chlamydia guidelines issued by the CDC in August 1993 advise health care providers to screen women routinely for chlamydia, an infection that is widespread among young people. Because the infection usually produces no symptoms, testing is crucial

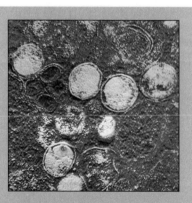

Chlamydia trachomatis, the bacteria that cause chlamydia.

Facts about chlamydia

- Chlamydia (pronounced *kluh MIHD ee uh*) is a sexually transmitted disease that strikes an estimated 4 million men and women in the United States each year.

- It's possible to have a chlamydia infection for years without symptoms.

- When symptoms do appear, women may notice a vaginal discharge, burning during urination, lower abdominal pain, pain during intercourse, or bleeding between menstrual periods.

- Men with a chlamydia infection may notice a discharge from the penis, burning during urination, burning and itching around the opening of the penis, or pain and swelling in the testicles.

- If left untreated, chlamydia can cause reproductive problems, including sterility, and it can infect newborns.

- Testing is the only sure way to detect a chlamydia infection, even in the absence of symptoms. Anyone whose partner develops chlamydia should be tested.

- Chlamydia is a bacterial infection and can be treated with antibiotics.

Source: American Social Health Association.

to identify and treat the disease before complications develop. Complications include *pelvic inflammatory disease* (infection of the fallopian tubes), infertility, and tubal pregnancy. Most chlamydia tests involve using a swab to collect cells from the mucous membranes of the genitals and then testing the cell sample for the presence of the bacteria that cause chlamydia.

The new guidelines encourage screening for two groups of women: all sexually active women under age 20, and women aged 20 and over who have not used barrier contraception—condoms or diaphragms—consistently or who have had a new partner or more than one partner in the previous three months. Women under age 20 should be screened at each pelvic examination, and older women who meet the screening criteria should be tested annually.

The CDC guidelines encourage health care providers to screen men for chlamydia when possible. A new chlamydia test for men reported in November 1993 involves testing a urine sample from the patient for signs of the bacteria that cause chlamydia. This method offers a noninvasive alternative to the painful method of inserting a swab into the urethra for a tissue sample.   □ Katherine Stone

See also AIDS. In WORLD BOOK, see AIDS; SEXUALLY TRANSMITTED DISEASE.

Public fears were aroused by a study reporting that sunscreen use failed to protect mice against a deadly form of skin cancer called melanoma. In the study, reported in May 1994 by researchers in Houston, the mice were exposed to ultraviolet (UV) light—a form of electromagnetic radiation released by the sun. The researchers conducted the study to see if sunscreen alone could prevent the development of melanoma.

Sunscreens were applied to the ears and tails of the mice 20 minutes prior to their exposure to UV radiation, which occurred two times a week for three weeks. After the last exposure, researchers injected melanoma cells into the ears of the mice, which they checked for a week. They found that the sunscreen failed to protect the mice from developing melanoma.

After reading newspaper accounts of the study, many people erroneously concluded that sunscreens did not protect against skin cancer. However, the Houston study looked at cancerous growth in the skin after cancer cells had been artificially introduced. It did not investigate the start of tumor growth in the skin, which is what can happen to people after prolonged sunlight exposure. Researchers concluded that factors besides exposure to ultraviolet light must contribute to the development of melanoma.

On the basis of the study, dermatologists are recommending that people with fair complexions use sunscreen, wear hats with wide brims and protective clothing of a tightly woven fabric, and seek out shaded spots. Dermatologists also point out that sunscreens do protect against the two most common forms of skin cancer: basal cell and squamous cell.

Sunscreen protection. Medical researchers reported in October 1993 that regular use of sunscreens prevents the development of actinic keratoses, the most common premalignant skin tumors caused by the sun. Such growths are forerunners of squamous cell carcinoma.

The study was conducted in Australia on 588 people 40 years of age or older who had already developed actinic keratoses. Some participants used sunscreen with a sun-protection factor of 17. Others used a cream that lacked the active ingredients of the sunscreen. The participants applied sunscreen or cream daily to the head, neck, forearms, and hands. They also received instructions to avoid the midday sun and to wear protective clothing in strong sunlight. People in the group using sunscreen lost about one growth, on average, whereas those using the base cream gained one. Researchers concluded that sunscreen use prevents the development of actinic keratoses and thus may reduce the risk of skin cancer.

New medication for psoriasis. The U.S. Food and Drug Administration in

December 1993 approved the marketing of a medicated ointment called calcipotriene for treating mild to moderate psoriasis, a skin disease characterized by scaly, red patches. Researchers believe psoriasis results when cells in the outer layer of skin divide more rapidly than normal, producing large amounts of flaky skin.

Calcipotriene became available as a prescription drug in March 1994 under the name Dovonex. It is a synthetic form of vitamin D_3, which is called the sunshine vitamin because it forms in the skin when the body is exposed to sunlight.

Most patients with psoriasis improve with exposure to sunlight. Re-

searchers have theorized that vitamin D stimulates this improvement. In FDA tests, about 70 percent of the people treated with calcipotriene showed improvement after about two weeks. Side effects among some of those treated included burning, itching, and other skin irritation.

Calcipotriene has generally proven to be as effective as other ointments applied to the skin, such as topical steroids. However, the medication can irritate the sensitive skin of the face and other areas. Physicians believe calcipotriene is most effective in skin folds, such as under the breasts and in the groin, areas where topical steroids can thin the skin.

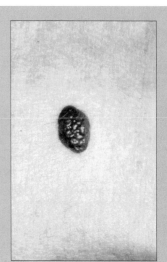
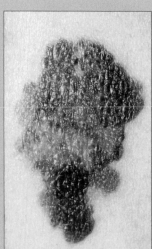

Melanoma:
A deadly cancer of the skin
Melanoma is the least common but most dangerous form of skin cancer. A melanoma can be surgically removed if detected early but can be fatal if allowed to spread to other parts of the body. To recognize a melanoma tumor, look for an abnormally shaped mole or discoloration on the skin, especially one that seems to change rapidly. A normal mole, *far left,* usually appears round or oval and has smooth edges. A melanoma, *left,* typically has an irregular shape and rough edges. Also, most normal moles are brown. Melanomas may be black, red, blue, white, or a combination of colors.

A steady rise
Melanoma cases have risen steadily in the United States since the early 1970's, with newly diagnosed cases increasing at the rate of about 4 percent a year, *below left.* The American Cancer Society estimates that about 32,000 Americans will be diagnosed with melanoma in 1994. Scientists believe that exposure to ultraviolet radiation from the sun plays a role in the development of melanoma. And a study reported in 1994 found that sunscreens may not protect against melanoma.

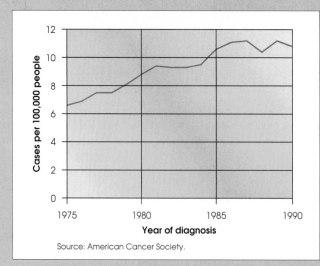

Source: American Cancer Society.

Low-fat diet and skin cancer. Researchers at Baylor College of Medicine in Houston reported in May 1994 that a low-fat diet can decrease the development of actinic keratoses. Researchers believe up to 25 percent of these tumors have the potential to develop into squamous cell carcinoma. In some cases, this type of skin cancer can invade surrounding tissues or spread to distant parts of the body through the bloodstream.

In the Baylor study, 76 individuals who had already been diagnosed with skin cancer other than melanoma were divided into two groups. One group followed their normal diet and the other group restricted fat intake to 20 percent of their total calorie intake.

After two years, the total number of actinic keratoses had decreased in the individuals who ate a low-fat diet during the study period. Study participants on the unrestricted diet, who took in an average of 36 percent of their daily calories as fat, developed new skin cancers four times as often as the participants in the low-fat group. Dietary fat has also been linked to the development of a number of other cancers, including those of the breast, colon, ovaries, and prostate gland. □ Kathryn E. Bowers

In the Health Matters section, see A GUIDE TO DRY SKIN AND MOISTURIZERS. In WORLD BOOK, see SKIN.

Despite 30 years of public health warnings, large numbers of adolescents continue to use tobacco in some form, according to a report released in March 1994 by U.S. Surgeon General M. Joycelyn Elders. The report stated that more than 3 million young people under the age of 18 smoked cigarettes and more than 1 million male adolescents used smokeless tobacco in early 1994.

The rate of smoking increased from 7 percent to 8 percent among 8th-graders, from 12 to 14 percent among 10th-graders, and from 17 to 19 percent among 12th-graders in 1993, according to a University of Michigan survey released in January 1994. Most adolescent smokers also reportedly want to quit but say they are unable to do so.

The surgeon general called for renewed efforts to examine the nature and scope of adolescent tobacco use in order to prevent young nonsmokers from becoming smokers. About half of the nation's 46 million smokers started smoking regularly before the age of 18, according to the American Cancer Society. Thus, if adolescents can be kept from using tobacco, researchers believe that most will never start using it.

Smoking and breast cancer risk. A woman's risk of dying from breast cancer increases by 25 percent if she is a smoker, according to a study released in May 1994 by the American Cancer Society. The study found that the risk of fatal breast cancer rose as the number of cigarettes smoked daily increased and as the number of years spent smoking increased. Among women who smoke two packs or more per day, the risk of developing fatal breast cancer goes up by 75 percent, compared with nonsmokers.

The researchers studied more than 600,000 women who were cancer-free at the start of the study in 1982. After six years, researchers observed 880 cases of fatal breast cancer.

The study did not propose that smoking is a direct cause of breast cancer or that smokers are more likely to get the disease than nonsmokers. Instead, researchers speculate that smokers are at an increased risk of fatal breast cancer because of overall poor health or delayed diagnosis. For example, smokers may be at increased risk of fatal breast cancer because many of them have respiratory and cardiovascular problems that threaten their survival. In addition, data from previous research suggest that smokers are less likely to receive mammograms than nonsmokers or former smokers. Thus, cancerous tumors are less likely to be detected at an early stage.

Smoking linked to bone loss. Medical researchers from the University of California at San Diego reported in September 1993 that smoking is associated with a loss of bone mass in

Smoking

A Commissioner's Crusade: Regulating Cigarettes

The burning issue for American smokers in 1994 was whether the United States Food and Drug Administration (FDA) would regulate cigarettes as drugs. In February, FDA Commissioner David A. Kessler expressed his willingness to do so.

In a letter to an antismoking coalition on February 25, Kessler stated, "Evidence brought to our attention is accumulating that suggests that cigarette manufacturers may intend that their products contain nicotine to satisfy an addiction on the part of some of their customers." The American Cancer Society and other health groups had formed the coalition.

Under U.S. law, the FDA can regulate a substance as a drug only if it can show that the maker intends the substance to be used as a drug. Therefore, Kessler needed to demonstrate that the tobacco industry manipulates nicotine in cigarettes with the intention of enhancing the addictive effects.

Kessler compiled tobacco industry memos, patents, and manufacturing practices that he said supported his contention that manufacturers do indeed regard tobacco as an addictive drug. He then asked Congress for guidelines on how to proceed in bringing tobacco under FDA control. He stated he would take action on his own if Congress did not act.

In response, the House Subcommittee on Health and the Environment, headed by Henry A. Waxman (D., Calif.), opened hearings in March 1994 on the effects of smoking on health. Kessler, representatives from various health groups and the American Medical Association, and the heads of America's seven largest tobacco companies testified.

In his testimony, Kessler cited a 1983 study by a Philip Morris researcher that had found nicotine to be addictive in rats. In the study, the rats had pressed a bar to receive bursts of nicotine into their veins in doses equivalent to those provided to a human smoker in a cigarette.

Philip Morris executives had had the paper withdrawn after it had been accepted for publication in a scientific journal and afterward closed down the research group. Kessler pointed out that this study had preceded by five years a 1988 declaration by the surgeon general that nicotine was an addictive substance.

One aspect of the tobacco debate focused on the reason cigarettes contain nicotine. The tobacco industry claims that nicotine is an important flavoring agent. Kessler disputed the claim, countering that the industry often tries to mask nicotine's harsh, unpleasant flavor. Furthermore, cigarette companies have the technology to remove nicotine and other harmful chemicals from their products, according to Vedpal S. Malik, a biochemist who worked for Philip Morris for 11 years. Malik said the companies have not encouraged the development of this process for large-scale manufacturing.

Quite the contrary, according to Kessler and others who accuse tobacco companies of manipulating nicotine levels in their products. On April 14, Waxman produced a study by tobacco company researcher Alexander W. Spears that indicated companies have engaged in such practices since 1981. Waxman said that the study's existence meant that the tobacco executives had lied to his subcommittee when they denied manipulating nicotine levels.

Waxman's revelation was

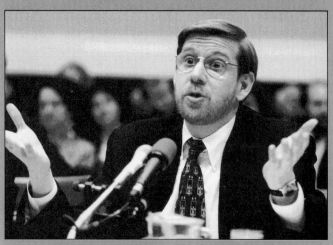

Food and Drug Commissioner David A. Kessler testifies on smoking.

supported by another 1981 report, which had been presented to a tobacco chemists' conference that year. The report stated that "current research is directed toward increasing the nicotine levels while maintaining or marginally reducing the tar deliveries." (Tar refers to tiny particles in cigarette smoke that have been linked to cancer and other diseases.)

The tobacco industry controls nicotine content in various ways, according to Kessler. Among these are growing and using varieties of tobacco that are naturally high in nicotine, blending varieties of tobacco with different concentrations of nicotine, and chemically transferring nicotine from one type of tobacco to another during processing. Nicotine content also is boosted by treating filters or paper wrappers with the substance and spraying tobacco with a nicotine compound that tempers the harsh natural flavor of nicotine.

In August, an FDA advisory panel on drug abuse supported Kessler's efforts. It concluded that nicotine fits the description of an addictive drug and that current nicotine levels in cigarettes can lead to addiction.

Most observers felt it was unlikely, however, that Congress would ban cigarettes in 1994. For one thing, Congress was not certain how to stop people from smoking. Second, a ban would likely lead to illegal trafficking, according to Kessler. Instead, new regulations might restrict advertising or force manufacturers to gradually lower nicotine levels until cigarettes became nonaddictive.   □ Gayle R. Hamilton

the hip and that this loss tends to be greatest among the heaviest smokers. The study evaluated the smoking patterns of 544 men and 822 women from 1972 to 1974 and again 16 years later, when bone density measurements were taken. Researchers believe that the loss of bone mass increases the risk of hip fracture among people over 60. However, the rate at which bone density is lost appears to slow if a person stops smoking, even in later life.

According to a study published in February 1994 by researchers at the University of Melbourne in Australia, women who smoke one pack of cigarettes each day throughout adulthood will lose an average of 5 to 10 percent of their bone mass by the time they reach menopause, the time of life when menstruation stops. Such bone loss may lead to an increased risk of fractures in women who are heavy smokers.

The study included 41 pairs of female identical twins who ranged in age from 27 to 73. The researchers sought a comparison between identical twins of the same sex so that they would not have to account for differences in bone density due to age, gender, and genetic composition, all of which are major factors affecting bone density.

Lifetime tobacco use of each twin was calculated in terms of pack-years. One pack-year means one pack of cigarettes smoked daily for one year. The twins chosen for the study had to be at least 5 pack-years apart in their smoking habits. So, for example, if one twin smoked one pack of cigarettes each day for 5 years (a 5-pack-year habit), and the other smoked one pack each day for 11 years (an 11-pack-year habit), the difference between the twins would be 6 pack-years.

Bone density was measured in the spine and *femur* (thighbone) in each of the twins. Researchers found that among twins whose habit differed by more than 20 pack-years, the woman who smoked more had an average of 5 to 10 percent less bone mass than her twin.

Leukemia risk. Cigarette smoking may increase an adult's risk of contracting leukemia, according to a study published in December 1993 by the National Cancer Institute. Leukemia is a cancer of white blood cells.

The study evaluated 1,200 people over the age of 60, half of whom had leukemia. It found that the risk of two types of leukemia—acute myeloid and acute lymphocytic—was at least twice as great for smokers as for nonsmokers. The researchers concluded that as many as 37 percent of leukemia cases among people 60 years of age and older may be attributable to regular cigarette use.

Earlier studies had failed to find such a strong link between smoking and leukemia, the researchers sug-

gested, because the studies had looked at all types of leukemia rather than the two acute forms, which are most common among older people. Although the mechanism by which smoking might contribute to leukemia is not yet known, the researchers pointed out that cigarette smoke contains benzene and other chemicals that have been associated with the development of leukemia.

Danger to a fetus. Researchers in Toronto, Canada, have found the first physical evidence that secondhand smoke can reach a pregnant woman's unborn child, according to a study published in February 1994. The study

---

Smoking and medication: A poor mix

Smoking can not only cause health problems, it also can make certain medications less able to do their job. Tobacco smoke speeds the breakdown of certain drugs so they exit the body too soon to reach their targets. For this reason, doctors may need to prescribe larger or more frequent doses of a drug for patients who smoke.

Medicines affected by smoking

Generic name (common brand names)	Commonly used for
Theophylline (Bronkodyl, Quibron, Slo-Phyllin, Theo-Dur)	Treating bronchial asthma, bronchitis, and emphysema
Chlordiazepoxide (Librium) Diazepam (Valium)	Relieving the symptoms of anxiety
Amitriptyline (Elavil), Desipramine (Norpramin) Imipramine (Tofranil) Nortriptyline (Aventyl, Pamelor)	Treating depression
Pentazocine (Talwin) Propoxyphene (Darvon)	Relieving pain
Heparin	Preventing blood clotting
Insulin	Controlling diabetes
Propranolol (Inderal)	Reducing high blood pressure, relieving angina, preventing heart attacks

Critically reviewed by Daniel A. Hussar, Philadelphia College of Pharmacy and Science.

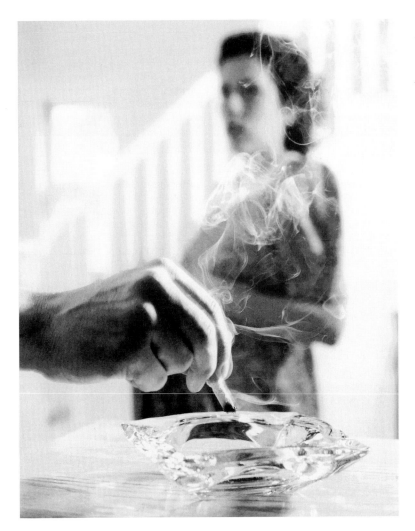

Exposing the unborn
Secondhand smoke can reach a pregnant woman's unborn child. Evidence of nicotine has been found in the hair samples of newborns whose mothers were exposed to secondhand smoke during pregnancy, indicating that passive smoke can reach a child in the womb.

measured levels of cotinine, the metabolized form of nicotine, in hair samples of newborns. It included the infants of 36 women who smoked, 23 nonsmokers who were regularly exposed to secondhand smoke, and 35 nonsmokers who were not exposed to secondhand smoke.

Among infants of women exposed to secondhand smoke, the amount of cotinine discovered was about twice as great as that found in infants of nonexposed women. It was also about one-fourth that found in the hair of smokers' children.

The study did not investigate the effects of secondhand smoke on newborns. However, previous research has indicated that children whose mothers were exposed to second-hand smoke while pregnant face an increased risk of problems with attention span and communication skills.

Kicking the habit for life. Quitting smoking at any age can help improve a person's health. A study published in November 1993 by researchers in Boston, reported that a smoker's risk of developing heart disease or having a stroke could decrease by as much as 24 percent within two years of quitting the habit. Within 10 to 14 years, the risk of heart disease and stroke could become comparable to that of nonsmokers. Smokers have nearly five times the risk of dying of heart disease as nonsmokers do.

☐ Gayle R. Hamilton
In WORLD BOOK, see SMOKING.

Stroke

Stroke patients taking aspirin to prevent recurrent strokes may develop a resistance to aspirin's anticlotting effects. That finding was reported in February 1994 by researchers at the University of Illinois at Chicago.

Many strokes and heart attacks are caused by blood clots that form or become wedged in clogged arteries, shutting off blood flow. Aspirin inhibits clotting and thus reduces the risk of strokes and heart attacks.

Two hundred stroke patients took part in the study. Each patient was given one standard 325-milligram (mg) aspirin tablet daily. The patients were also given a blood test to measure the tendency of their blood to clot. If the initial aspirin dose did not adequately inhibit clotting, the dosage was increased in 325-mg increments until the desired anticlotting effect was achieved. No one was given more than 1,300 mg per day.

After 3½ years, the investigators found that about 20 percent of the patients in the ongoing study required increased aspirin dosages. Some patients regained the anticlotting effect with higher doses of aspirin, but in others higher doses were only partially effective. A few patients had become totally resistant to aspirin's anticlotting effect, even at the highest dose.

Extreme neck motions may cause stroke
Activities in which the head is bent or turned to an extreme position may restrict blood flow to the brain and cause a stroke, according to a study at New York Medical College at Valhalla, reported in May 1994. Such activities can include having one's hair washed at a beauty salon or painting a ceiling. The risk was found to be greatest for the elderly and for people who have already suffered a stroke or who have had *transient ischemic attacks* (temporary obstructions of blood flow to the brain).

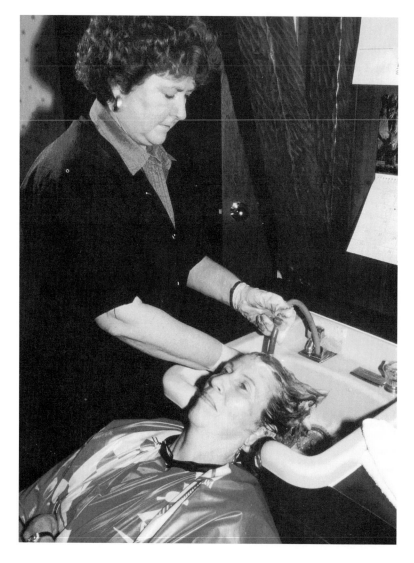

The researchers said these findings mean that physicians may no longer be able to use a standard approach in treating stroke and heart attack patients. Different patients may need different aspirin doses, and patients may need periodic blood tests to determine if their dose is still sufficient.

Fish in diet reduces stroke risk.

Eating fish reduces the risk of stroke, researchers at the National Institute of Public Health in Bilthoven, the Netherlands, reported in February 1994. They made that finding in a long-term study of 552 Dutch men.

The men were signed up for the study in 1960 and questioned about their eating habits. In 1970, and for 15 years thereafter, the investigators continued to study the men. During the follow-up period, 42 first-time strokes occurred among the group.

The researchers found that fish consumption was much lower among the men who had strokes. They determined that eating ⅔ ounce (19 grams) or more of fish a day can cut the risk of stroke by about half. An average serving of fish weighs about 3 ounces (85 grams).

The scientists explained that the consumption of certain fats found in fish, called omega-3 fatty acids, may help prevent the formation of blockages in arteries in the brain and in those leading to the brain. They said that eating at least one portion of fish each week might help protect people against strokes.

A blood clue for clogged arteries.

A high level of lipoprotein (a), a fatty substance in the blood, is a strong predictor of diseased arteries in the brain. That finding was reported in February 1994 by researchers at the Biotechnology Research Institute in Rockville, Md.

The scientists studied health data collected from 265 men and women who had suffered strokes or who had other symptoms, such as episodes of temporary paralysis in parts of the body, indicating diseased brain arteries. The data included information on other blood fats as well as lipoprotein (a). The data was correlated with ultrasound images of the patients' neck arteries, which are usually blocked when arteries in the brain are.

Ninety-one of the people studied had a lipoprotein (a) blood level of 18 mg per deciliter (0.1 liter) or higher. The investigators found that those individuals were more than 20 times as likely to have clogged arteries in their brain as people in a control group with low lipoprotein (a) levels. Elevated amounts of lipoprotein (a) in the blood had previously been shown to be a strong risk factor for heart attacks. But a high level of lipoprotein (a) appears to be an even more potent predictor of stroke. ☐ Julie Foreman

In WORLD BOOK, see STROKE.

Angela Lakeberg, one of two conjoined twins surgically separated in a widely publicized operation in August 1993, died on June 9, 1994. Her twin sister had died during the operation, when surgeons reconstructed the twins' shared heart and gave it to Angela, who was judged to have the best chance of survival.

The operation created a furor among medical ethicists, physicians, and surgeons, many of whom believed that the surgery had little hope of success, given the twins' anatomy. Although Angela Lakeberg lived months longer than many experts had predicted, the infant never grew strong enough to leave the hospital or be removed from a respirator.

Options for breast cancer surgery.

A partial mastectomy is just as effective as more extensive surgery for the treatment of breast cancer in its earliest stages, according to a September 1993 report by researchers at the Cleveland Clinic Foundation in Ohio. A partial mastectomy, also called *lumpectomy*, is an operation in which a cancerous tumor and a margin of healthy tissue around it are removed from the breast.

Since the 1970's, the standard treatment for early-stage breast cancer has changed from the radical mastectomy—removal of the entire breast, the muscles beneath it, and all the lymph nodes in the area—to less disfiguring operations such as the par-

Surgery

343

tial mastectomy and the modified radical mastectomy. In the latter operation, surgeons remove the entire breast but leave the underlying muscle.

The Ohio researchers compared the effectiveness of various types of breast cancer surgery by surveying statistics on survival and cancer recurrence among patients who had surgery during the period from 1975 to 1988. The scientists found that the rates of long-term survival were equivalent among the patients who had modified radical mastectomies, partial mastectomies, and radical mastectomies.

Physicians sometimes prescribe radiation therapy after partial mastectomy to destroy any remaining cancer cells in the breast. The 1993 study examined the health of women with early stage breast cancer who had partial mastectomies without follow-up radiation therapy. At 5 and 10 years after surgery, these patients and women who had undergone radiation therapy had similar rates of cancer recurrence. (See also CANCER.)

Hysterectomy complications in African Americans. African-American women who have a *hysterectomy* (surgical removal of the uterus) may run a greater risk of long hospitalizations and dying in the hospital than white women undergoing the same operation. That was the November

"Virtual" eye surgery
A medical researcher practices eye surgery using a virtual reality computer system under development in 1994 at the Georgia Institute of Technology in Atlanta and the Medical College of Georgia in Augusta. The new system consists of a computer, a surgical tool, and a microscope that displays pictures of a human eyeball. As a user manipulates the surgical tool, the computer analyzes the motion and sends updated images of the eyeball to the microscope. Researchers say the simulator could help train eye specialists and allow surgeons to rehearse difficult operations.

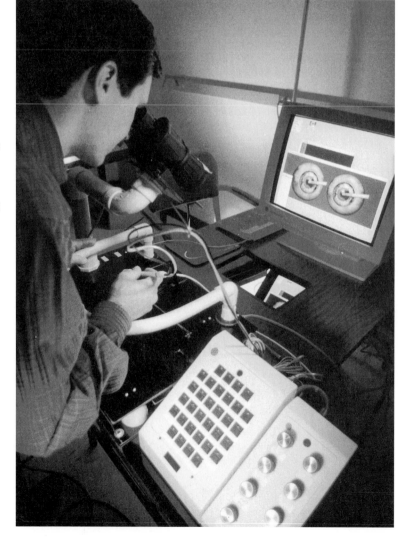

1993 report of researchers with the University of Maryland in Baltimore. Hysterectomy is most often performed to treat noncancerous fibroid tumors of the uterus.

The researchers studied hospital discharge records for all women receiving hysterectomies at nonmilitary hospitals in Maryland from 1986 to 1991. More than 53,000 women were treated, 70 percent of them white and 26 percent African American. After analyzing the data, scientists found that African-American women as a group showed a 40 percent greater risk of complications from infection than did white women. The African-American women were almost three times more likely to be hospitalized for longer than 10 days and three times more likely to die in the hospital. The authors of the study said that further research is needed to find explanations for the different rates of complications.

Limiting repeat organ transplants.
The procedures for allocating organs to people with heart or liver failure should be changed to favor those who have not had a previous, unsuccessful transplant. That was the November 1993 recommendation of physicians at the University of Pittsburgh in Pennsylvania and the University of Minnesota in Minneapolis. The selection process for organ recipients is a matter of life or death because donated livers and hearts are very scarce. Some 10 to 17 percent of the people on the waiting lists for those organs die before transplantation.

Currently, to get on the U.S. waiting lists for a donated liver or heart, a patient must have terminal heart or liver failure and must be considered medically suitable for a transplant. Patients may be ruled out for lack of insurance, as well as lack of family support, emotional stability, and other factors that could affect their ability to live with the transplant.

Organs are matched with people on the waiting list according to such criteria as the recipient's blood type, body size, and medical urgency. Because people whose previous transplants have failed are critically ill and in dire need of an organ, these patients often come out at the top of the waiting list.

A better way to fix a broken jaw
Breaking a jaw typically has meant having the jaws wired shut and living for six weeks or more on liquids sucked through a straw. But surgeons have a new technique called rigid fixation in which they use tiny screws, either alone or with a metal plate, to hold the fractured bone securely together, leaving the jaws mobile. Surgeons find that a patient can eat soft foods immediately after surgery and resume a normal diet in about a week. Surgeons also say that the chance of postoperative infection is reduced with the new technique because the patient can easily open his or her mouth for cleaning. In most cases, the screws and plates are permanent.

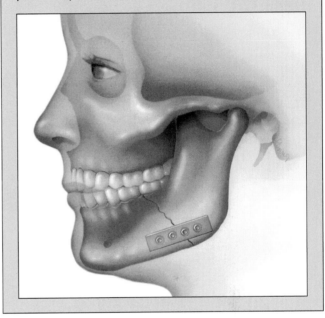

The Minnesota and Pennsylvania physicians surveyed research on the outcome of approximately 10,000 liver transplants and 5,000 heart transplants. According to that research, 77 percent of patients receiving first liver transplants survived at least one year. Of those receiving a second liver transplant, 54 percent survived one year. For patients getting a third liver, the figure dropped to 44 percent. First-time heart transplant recipients had a one-year survival rate of 82 percent, compared with 57 percent for repeat transplant recipients.

The physicians argued that scarce organs should be given to patients who have the best chance of long-term survival. To ensure that, the doctors suggested the U.S. organ-match-

Teeth
See Dentistry

Transplants
See Surgery

ing registry be altered so that first-time transplant candidates are given preference over retransplant candidates. Because survival rates for successive transplants are low, the scientists further recommended that people who have received two failed transplants be removed from the waiting list.

Rethinking a test for colon cancer. A blood test commonly used to detect new malignancies after colon cancer surgery is largely ineffective, a team of U.S. researchers reported in August 1993. The test measures blood levels of a molecule some colon cancer cells produce called carcinoembryonic antigen (CEA). An estimated 500,000 Americans who have had colon cancer surgery have taken a CEA test at least once to help determine whether another operation was necessary to remove a regrowth of cancer.

The research team, led by cancer specialist Charles G. Moertel of the Mayo Clinic in Rochester, Minn., monitored the health of 1,216 colon cancer patients. The scientists found that the CEA test missed many recurrences of cancer and sometimes suggested the presence of cancerous growths when none existed. In addition, using the test did not appear to significantly increase patients' survival odds.

◻ Julie Foreman

In WORLD BOOK, see SURGERY.

Urology

Men who consume large amounts of animal fat—particularly fat from red meat—have an 80 percent greater chance of developing advanced prostate cancer on average than do men who eat a low-fat diet. That was the conclusion of a study reported in October 1993 by cancer researcher Edward Giovannucci and his colleagues at Harvard Medical School and the Harvard School of Public Health in Boston.

The prostate is a walnut-sized gland that lies at the base of the bladder and surrounds the urethra. The gland produces a substance that helps nourish sperm.

In the United States, prostate cancer is the second most deadly cancer among men, following lung cancer. About 35,000 American men die each year from prostate cancer, according to the American Cancer Society, and an estimated 200,000 men will be diagnosed with the disease in the United States in 1994.

The Harvard study tracked the dietary habits of approximately 48,000 male health professionals from 1986 to 1990. During that time, 300 men in the study were diagnosed with prostate cancer, and in 126 of those cases, the cancer had spread beyond the prostate gland and was no longer curable.

The study did not find a link between the initial risk of developing prostate cancer and a high-fat diet. But the study reported that diets high in alpha-linolenic acid, a fat found in red meat, increased the risk that the cancer would progress more quickly to an advanced stage. Other sources of alpha-linolenic acid are chicken with the skin on, and butter. Men with the highest intake of these foods were nearly 3½ times more likely to develop advanced prostate cancer than men with the lowest intake, according to the study. Diets rich in such fat were also associated with an increased risk of dying of prostate cancer.

The Harvard study supports a long-held suspicion among medical researchers that environmental factors rather than genetic flaws account for the high rate of death from prostate cancer among American men. American men are 4½ times more likely to die of prostate cancer than are Japanese men, for instance. Among Japanese men who immigrate to the United States, however, the risk of developing prostate cancer increases until it is nearly equal that of native-born Americans.

Cranberry juice can help prevent urinary tract infections (UTI's) in women, according to a study reported in March 1994 by urologists from Harvard Medical School. Physicians have long sought a simple and inexpensive way of preventing UTI's, which are a major health problem for older women. Such infections can produce sudden chills, high fever, and other symptoms that may require hospital treat-

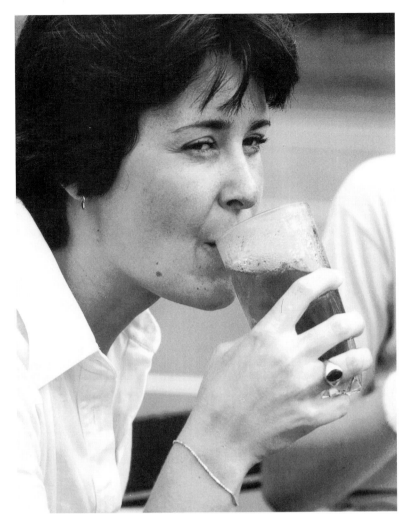

A cup a day
Drinking cranberry juice may help older women prevent urinary tract infections, researchers at Harvard University reported in March 1994. In the study, women who drank a cup of cranberry juice a day experienced nearly half as many urinary tract infections as the women who drank no cranberry juice.

ment. Many women over age 65 experience at least one UTI per year, and about 12 percent of older women have more than one UTI a year.

The Harvard researchers gave 153 older women who suffered from frequent UTI's a daily cup of cranberry juice or a beverage that looked and tasted like the juice but had no cranberry content.

After six months, the researchers found that 28 percent of the women who had not received cranberry juice developed a UTI, compared with 15 percent of the women in the group that drank cranberry juice. Researchers believe that cranberry juice may work by keeping bacteria from attaching to the bladder lining and causing infection.

Prostate cancer prevention trial.
The National Cancer Institute began a study in autumn 1993 to find out whether the drug finasteride (sold as Proscar) can decrease the incidence of prostate cancer. Finasteride blocks the conversion of the male hormone testosterone into a form that physicians believe helps prostate tumors grow. Physicians now prescribe Proscar to help shrink enlarged noncancerous prostate glands. The study was enrolling men over age 55 who were in good health and had no sign of prostate cancer. During the study, the men will be examined for signs of prostate cancer.　　□ Glenn S. Gerber

See also CANCER (CLOSE-UP). In WORLD BOOK, see CANCER, PROSTATE GLAND.

Venereal Diseases
See Sexually Transmitted Diseases

Veterinary Medicine

Veterinarians should vaccinate dogs against Lyme disease in any geographic area with a high incidence of the disease in human beings. The Lyme Disease Committee of the National Association of State Public Health Veterinarians announced this recommendation in December 1993.

Lyme disease is named for the town of Lyme, Conn., where in the mid-1970's local physicians first noticed its symptoms. The physicians observed an unusual pattern of recurrent joint disease that appeared mainly in children during the summer and early fall. Researchers eventually discovered that the disease was caused by *Borrelia burgdorferi,* a bacterium living in certain ticks of the Northeast and upper Midwest and along the West Coast. People can become infected through tick bites on walks in tick-infested woods or from ticks carried home by their pets. The ticks are also carried by deer and other animals.

The symptoms of *B. burgdorferi* infection in a dog usually include fever, recurrent lameness, lethargy, and loss of appetite. Studies have found, however, that in areas with a high incidence of Lyme disease, from 25 to 50 percent or more of free-roaming dogs have been infected without showing any symptoms. The same can be true of infected cats, livestock, and wildlife.

Veterinarians have had a Lyme disease vaccine for dogs since June 1992. The vaccine reportedly protects the dog for at least six months. But because a vaccinated dog may still carry infected ticks home, the Lyme Disease Committee warned dog owners against complacency. Owners should promptly inspect a dog or cat for any attached ticks and remove them immediately. Studies have shown that the transmission of *B. burgdorferi* is minimal during the first 48 hours after the tick attaches itself.

Disease from cats. Evidence was mounting in 1993 and 1994 that the domestic cat carries a type of bacteria responsible for two diseases in human beings. The bacteria appear to cause no harm to the cat. *Rochalimaea henselae* has been implicated in cat scratch disease (CSD) and bacterial angiomatosis (BA), an infection that is particularly dangerous to people with weakened immune systems, such as people with AIDS or organ transplant patients.

Researchers at the University of California at San Francisco found that four patients with BA had among them seven cats. Blood samples from the cats showed the presence of *R. henselae.* Fleas feeding on one of the infected cats harbored the organism as well. The researchers also tested 61 additional pet or stray cats in the area and found the infection in 25 of them, a 41 percent rate of infection.

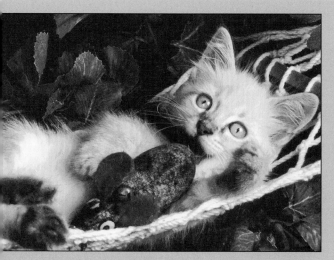

**Love it, or leave it—
it's all in a "catnip gene"**
Many cats love playing and rolling in catnip. They frolic in delighted frenzy after sniffing catnip leaves. What attracts cats is actually an oil on the leaves. But not all cats react to the weed in this way. Some pay no attention to it at all. The explanation, researchers say, lies in the cat's genes. A cat without the "catnip gene" is immune to the weed's allure. And even a cat with the gene may not always react so joyfully when given a catnip toy. The response depends upon the cat's emotional state, age, and environment. And then there are the highly sensitive cats that can detect the presence of catnip when its oil constitutes only one part per billion parts of air.

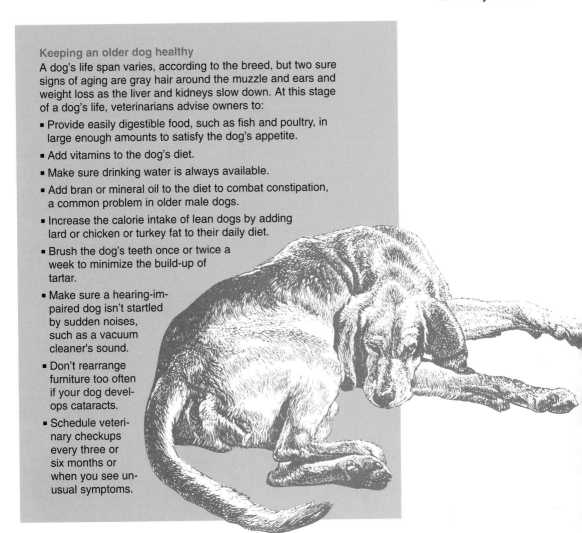

Keeping an older dog healthy

A dog's life span varies, according to the breed, but two sure signs of aging are gray hair around the muzzle and ears and weight loss as the liver and kidneys slow down. At this stage of a dog's life, veterinarians advise owners to:

- Provide easily digestible food, such as fish and poultry, in large enough amounts to satisfy the dog's appetite.

- Add vitamins to the dog's diet.

- Make sure drinking water is always available.

- Add bran or mineral oil to the diet to combat constipation, a common problem in older male dogs.

- Increase the calorie intake of lean dogs by adding lard or chicken or turkey fat to their daily diet.

- Brush the dog's teeth once or twice a week to minimize the build-up of tartar.

- Make sure a hearing-impaired dog isn't startled by sudden noises, such as a vacuum cleaner's sound.

- Don't rearrange furniture too often if your dog develops cataracts.

- Schedule veterinary checkups every three or six months or when you see unusual symptoms.

In another 1993 study, researchers in Connecticut determined that exposure to kittens, rather than older cats, put people at significant risk for developing CSD. Moreover, a person who had been scratched by a kitten with fleas was 29 times more likely to develop CSD than someone who had a kitten free of fleas.

Researchers say that people need not give up their pets on the basis of such findings. Instead, they advise owners to wash their hands after handling a cat and to clean a scratch or bite with soap and warm water.

A new diagnostic test, which became available in January 1994, will help breeders detect a defective gene in English springer spaniels, according to researchers at the University of Pennsylvania in Philadelphia who developed the test. The defective gene causes a deficiency of a protein needed for normal cell functioning. The deficiency can be life-threatening.

A dog must inherit a copy of the defective gene from each parent to develop the deficiency. A dog with one normal copy and one defective copy is healthy but can transmit the defective copy to offspring. Using only a few drops of blood, the new test can determine whether a dog has the deficiency, carries the defective gene, or is healthy.   □ Jeffrey E. Barlough

In the Health Matters section, see FRIENDS INDEED: PETS AND YOUR HEALTH. In WORLD BOOK, see VETERINARY MEDICINE.

Weight Control

A natural craving for fat
Increased levels of a chemical produced in the brain stimulate a craving for fatty foods in adolescent girls, according to a study reported in October 1993. Scientists speculate that this appetite for fat, which begins at puberty, serves as preparation for pregnancy, when the body requires additional energy.

Even though most people in the United States realize that lowering fat intake can help maintain good health, American diets still consist of 34 percent fat on average, according to the Third National Health and Nutrition Examination Survey conducted by the Centers for Disease Control and Prevention (CDC) in Atlanta, Ga. The CDC reported the results in February 1994, noting that the survey is conducted to find out if Americans are lowering their fat consumption to reach the CDC's goal for the year 2000. That goal is a diet in which less than 30 percent of daily calories come from fat.

Another CDC goal for the year 2000 is to lower the number of overweight American adults to no more than 20 percent of the population. The percentage of overweight adults is increasing, however, according to a July 1994 study that compared the results of the third survey with those of the first two surveys. From 1960 to 1980, about 25 percent of U.S. adults were overweight (defined as weighing at least 20 percent more than their ideal body weight). From 1980 to 1991, the figure rose to 33 percent.

Is even less fat better? Some diet regimens publicized in 1993 and 1994

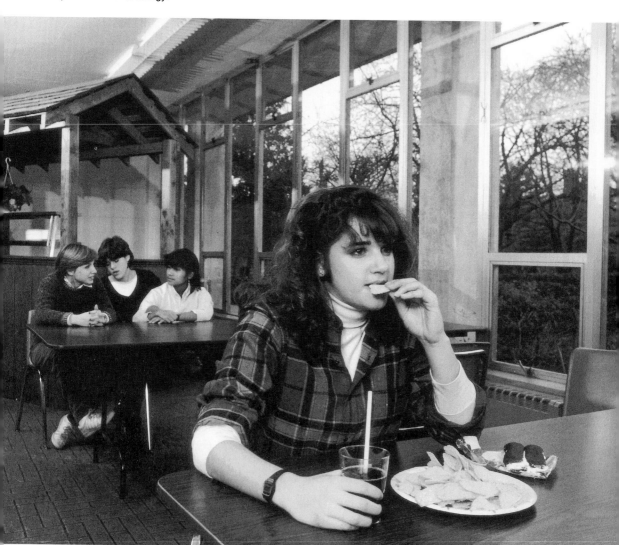

suggested that people eat far less fat than the CDC goal—obtaining as few as 10 percent of their total calories from fat. But not only is this advice difficult to follow, it may be dangerous, nutrition experts warn.

A diet at 10 percent fat may be dangerous on two counts, according to Wayne Calloway, an obesity specialist at George Washington University in Washington, D.C. First, too little fat can slow growth in young people, who continue to grow until age 20 but tend to be very weight-conscious. And second, the substitution of *carbohydrates* (starches and sugars) for fats can hamper the body's ability to get rid of fluids, thereby increasing a person's weight.

According to the books that tout a very-low-fat diet, calories that would otherwise come from fat should come from complex carbohydrates, such as beans, grains, pasta, and potatoes. Ounce for ounce, carbohydrates contain half the calories of fats. One problem with such a substitution, however, is that it can overload the digestive system with bulky starch and fiber. Another problem is that many people substitute cookies and cake for the vegetables and other complex carbohydrates that the books recommend.

Jeanne Goldberg, a nutritionist at Tufts University in Boston, points to a related problem with very-low-fat diets: a generally poor understanding of good nutrition among Americans. She adds that people who rely on readily available prepared foods simply cannot build a healthful diet from products labeled "low fat" and "no fat."

Getting the fat out. One way to cut down on fat would be to digest less of it, so that more of it passed out of the body. A two-year clinical trial was underway in the United States and Europe in 1994 to test a drug that helps the body do just that. The drug, called orlistat, interferes with enzymes that normally break down fats until they are small enough to pass through the cells lining the small intestine. The drug's interference enables some fat to leave the body undigested.

In earlier tests, orlistat had blocked the absorption of about 30 percent of the fat that people consumed, no matter how much of the drug they took. A large amount of fat was still absorbed because the stomach and small intestine produce so much of the fat-digesting enzyme.

The new trials were scheduled to end in 1995, and scientists may then be able to determine how long people can take the drug safely, how quickly they gain weight after discontinuing the drug, and what diet and exercise plans should accompany the drug. Side effects have included greasy bowel movements and diarrhea.

Testing fat substitutes. The U.S. Food and Drug Administration (FDA) is revamping its methods of analyzing replacement substances that have the taste and consistency of fats, according to an April 1994 report. The FDA currently calls for studies that feed laboratory animals 100 times the amount of the substance that a person would consume. Feeding animals such huge amounts could produce symptoms that might never arise in humans, according to George Pauli, director of FDA's division of product policy in the Center for Food Safety and Applied Nutrition.

Nutritionists are concerned that the consumption of fat substitutes might lead to a deficiency in fat-soluble vitamins, such as A and E. These vitamins must be dissolved in fat before the body can use them.

Obesity as a disability. People who are obese in adolescence and young adulthood are more likely to have lower incomes and less education and to remain single than people who are not obese. This was the finding of a study reported in September 1993 by nutrition researcher William H. Dietz and colleagues at the Harvard School of Public Health, the New England Medical Center, and Harvard Medical School, all in Boston. Furthermore, they found that being very overweight has greater social and economic consequences than do many other chronic health conditions.

The researchers reviewed data from a national survey of 10,039 people who were between the ages of 16 and 24 in 1981 and who had answered questionnaires annually until 1988. The researchers classified 370 of the survey participants as obese.

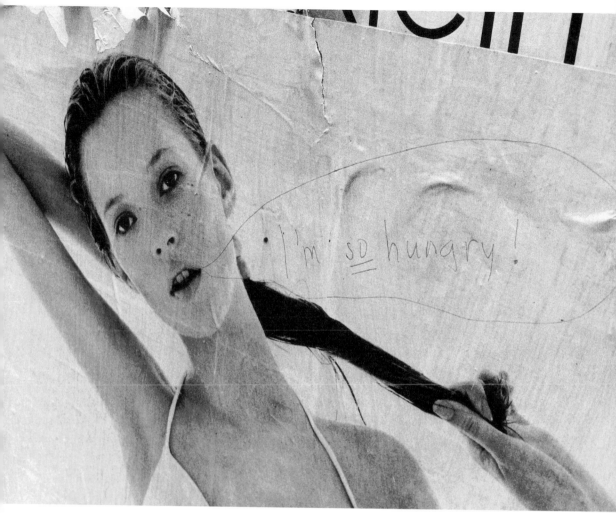

An impossible dream
A billboard featuring ultra-thin model Kate Moss bears an anonymous scrawl that reflects the position of Boycott Anorexic Marketing. The group, which is based in Boston, claims that such advertising encourages starvation diets and eating disorders among American women who strive to look like reed-slim models.

The researchers compared the responses of this group with those of a nonobese group who had chronic health conditions, such as asthma, skeletal abnormalities, and diabetes.

During the period between 1981 and 1988, the obese young women had completed a third of a year less schooling, were 20 percent less likely to have married, and had earned an average of $6,710 less per year than the women in the comparison group. The obese young men had completed only slightly less schooling, but were 11 percent less likely to have married and had earned $2,876 less per year than the comparison group. Psychological tests, however, showed that obese men and women did not lack self-esteem.

The researchers concluded that obese people have a "social disability" that can be attributed to their obesity. They found no evidence of social disability among the comparison group, whose chronic conditions for the most part were not physically apparent.

The researchers suggested that the stigma attached to being very overweight caused the social disability. In addition, people often perceive obesity as preventable and blame obese individuals for their condition. To help remedy this situation, Dietz and his colleagues suggested that obese people be included in the Americans with Disabilities Act, which prohibits discrimination in employment practices against people with disabilities. □ Ricki Lewis

In WORLD BOOK, see WEIGHT CONTROL.

Index

How to use the index
This index covers the contents of the 1993, 1994, and 1995 editions of *The World Book Health & Medical Annual*.

Caffeine, 95: 324, **94:** 322, **93:** 49, 280-281, 358 (il.)
Calcipotriene (drug), 95: 336
Calcium
  bone health, **95:** 240, 258, **94:** 128, 240-241, 259 (il.), 301-302, 322
  food sources, **94:** 35, **93:** 291
  hypertension, **93:** 360-361
  kidney stones, **94:** 300, 316
  lead poisoning, **95:** 331
Calories, 94: 32-35, 66, 351-352
Camel cigarettes, 93: 375-377
CANCER, 95: 265-271, **94:** 266-270, **93:** 298-304
  aging, **93:** 171, 174
  books, **94:** 259-260, **93:** 292-293
  cellular phones, **94:** 333
  diet, **95:** 19, 61-73, 337, 346, **94:** 35, 64-66, **93:** 125, 303, 341, 354-355
  drugs, **94:** 270, **93:** 298-301
  electromagnetic fields, **94:** 289
  gene therapy, **95:** 230, 265-267, 299, **93:** 223, 301-302
  genetic basis, **95:** 212-215, 224-225, 228, 297-299, **94:** 256-257, 267 (il.), 296-297, **93:** 214-215, 299-301, 335
  heart disease link, **95:** 306
  phone information, **95:** 40, **94:** 38
  smoking, **95:** 337, **93:** 111-112, 124-125
  surgery, **95:** 343-344, **93:** 123-124, 213
  vitamins, **95:** 309, 324-325
  see also **Chemotherapy; Radiation therapy;** and specific cancer types
CAPD. See **Ambulatory dialysis**
Captopril (drug), 95: 277
Carbamepazine (drug), 95: 185
Carbohydrates, 95: 105, 162, 170
  see also **Fruits; Vegetables**
Carbon monoxide poisoning, 95: 152, **94:** 289
Carcinogens. See **Cancer**
Cardiac arrest, 94: 312, **93:** 322
Cardiac emergency units, 94: 287
Cardiopulmonary resuscitation, 95: 159, 240-241, **94:** 312, **93:** 321, 345 (il.)
Cardiovascular disease. See **Heart disease**
Carotenoids, 94: 71
Carotid arteries, 95: 307, **94:** 89, 93, 96-97
Carotid endarterectomy, 94: 96-99
Carpal tunnel syndrome, 95: 253 (il.)
Carrots, 95: 293 (il.)
Cartilage, 95: 254, **94:** 252
CAS. See **Computer-assisted surgery**
CAT scan. See **Computerized tomography**
Cataracts, 95: 32-35, 294-295, **94:** 242, 293-295, **93:** 324
Catheters, 94: 92, 96
Catnip, 95: 348 (il.)

Each index entry gives the last two digits of the edition year and the page number or numbers. For example, this entry means that information on caffeine may be found on page 324 of the 1995 edition.

When there are many references to a topic, they are grouped alphabetically by clue words under the main topic. For example, the clue words under the general reference for calcium group the other references under several subtopics.

An entry in all capital letters indicates that there is a Health & Medical News Update with that name in at least one of the three volumes covered by this index. References to the topic in other articles may also appear after the topic name.

An entry that only begins with a capital letter indicates that there are no Health & Medical News Update articles with that title but that information on this topic may be found in the edition and on the pages listed.

The "see" and "see also" cross-references indicate that references to the topic are listed under another entry in the index.

The indication (il.) after a page number means that the reference is to an illustration only.

A

Abortion, 94: 235, 308, **93:** 340-342
Accidents. See **Automobile safety; Emergency medicine; Safety**
ACE (drug), 95: 308
Acer, David J., 94: 244, **93:** 276
Acetaminophen (drug), 95: 281, **93:** 46, 50
Acetylsalicylic acid. See **Aspirin**
Acne, 93: 244
Acquired immune deficiency syndrome. See **AIDS**
Actinex (drug). See **Masoprocol**
Actinic keratoses, 95: 335, 337
Acupressure, 94: 182, 325 (il.)
Acupuncture, 94: 175 (il.), 178 (il.), 181-182
Acute stress disorder, 95: 320
Acyclovir (drug), 93: 347
ADA deficiency. See **Adenosine deaminase deficiency**
ADAM (program), 94: 148, 156 (il.)
Addiction. See **Alcohol and drug abuse**
Addison's disease, 94: 301
Adenocarcinoma, 93: 115-119
Adenosine deaminase deficiency, 95: 221, 228-229
Adenosine triphosphate. See **ATP**
Adjuvant treatment, 93: 299
Adolescents
  alcohol/drug abuse, **95:** 246, **94:** 73-85, 245-246, **93:** 279
  birth control use, **95:** 254
  delinquent girls, **94:** 273-274
  firearm deaths, **95:** 333
  gonorrhea, **95:** 334
  smokeless tobacco, **94:** 339-341
  smoking, **95:** 337, **94:** 290-291, **93:** 120, 307
  weight control, **94:** 350-351, **93:** 383-384
  see also **Puberty**
Adrenal glands, 94: 301, **93:** 248
Adult respiratory distress syndrome, 94: 327
Advance directives, 94: 223
Aerobic exercise, 95: 106-107, 111-114, 117, 285 (il.)
Africa, and AIDS, 95: 53
African Americans. See **Blacks**
AGING, 95: 240-242, **94:** 240-242, **93:** 274-275
  AIDS, **95:** 245
  alcoholism, **94:** 248
  book, **95:** 259
  cataracts, **95:** 32
  child rearing, **95:** 81-82
  dizziness, **95:** 193-195
  dry skin, **95:** 29
  exercise/fitness, **95:** 117, 241, 292-293, **94:** 241-242, **93:** 174-176, 292 (il.)
  genes, **93:** 176-177, 334-335
  health plans, **94:** 236-237, **93:** 260, 331
  home safety, **95:** 157
  longevity research, **93:** 168-181
  pets and health, **95:** 13-15
  psychiatric drugs, **95:** 185
  sleep needs/problems, **95:** 121, 129
  tuberculosis, **93:** 65
  see also **Alzheimer's disease; Bone disorders; Menopause; Senility**

Agoraphobia, 95: 178
Agriculture, 95: 57, **93:** 135-138
  see also **Nutrition and food; Pesticides**
Agriculture, U.S. Department of, 94: 57-71
  see also **Nutrition and food**
AIDS, 95: 242-245, **94:** 242-245, **93:** 276-278
  books, **95:** 259, **94:** 259, **93:** 292
  condoms, **95:** 245, **94:** 334-335
  drug approval, **95:** 245, **94:** 281-282, **93:** 315-316
  drug-resistant virus, **94:** 315
  emergence, **95:** 46, 48, 53
  ethical issues, **94:** 226-228, 234
  health care workers, **93:** 341
  health plan benefits, **94:** 305-306
  other sexually transmitted diseases, link with, **93:** 372
  phone information, **95:** 40, **94:** 38
  pregnancy, **95:** 243 (il.), 325
  testing, **94:** 243, **93:** 276, 289 (il.)
  tuberculosis, **93:** 56, 62-63
  vaccine, **95:** 245, **94:** 245, **93:** 278
  see also **AZT**
AIDS-like illness, 94: 245
Air pollution, 95: 286 (il.), 290, **93:** 324
Air travel, 93: 21, 369
Airbags, Automobile, 95: 331-332, **93:** 365
ALCOHOL AND DRUG ABUSE, 95: 246-249, **94:** 245-248, **93:** 279-282
  artery disease, **94:** 100
  children/adolescents, **95:** 246, **94:** 73-85, 245-246, **93:** 279
  phone information, **95:** 40, **94:** 38
  social environment, **93:** 350-351
  traffic deaths, **95:** 332
  treatments, **94:** 317-319
  tuberculosis, **93:** 63-64
  violence, **94:** 50-51
Alcohol consumption, 94: 294, **93:** 361, 383 (il.)
Alcoholism. See **Alcohol and drug abuse**
Aleve (drug), 95: 281
Alexander technique, 94: 182-183
Allergic rhinitis, 93: 70
ALLERGIES AND ASTHMA, 95: 249-252, **94:** 248-251, **93:** 282-284
  arthritis and diet, **93:** 285
  aspirin, **93:** 42-43
  book, **93:** 293
  drugs, **95:** 249-250, **94:** 250-251, 328, **93:** 363
  insect bites, **94:** 30-31
  near-fatal asthma, **95:** 329
  phone information, **95:** 40, **94:** 38
  pregnancy, **94:** 323
  seasonal allergies, **93:** 69-81
  see also **Antihistamines; Immune system; Immunotherapy**
Alpha interferon (protein), 93: 107
Alprazolam (drug), 95: 284-285
ALS. See **Amyotrophic lateral sclerosis**
Alternative medicine, 94: 173-185
Altitude sickness, 93: 21-22
Alzheimer's disease, 95: 202-215
  beta-amyloid, **94:** 265 (il.), **93:** 296
  dementia, **94:** 240
  drug, **95:** 282
  estrogen, **95:** 242, 262 (il.)
  gene, **95:** 211-212, 261-262
  phone information, **95:** 40, **94:** 38

women, **94:** 131
AMA. See **American Medical Association**
Amantadine (drug), 93: 146, 153
Ambulatory dialysis, 94: 315-316
American Medical Association, 94: 19, 218, 312, **93:** 258, 259, 269
Americans with Disabilities Act, 93: 340
Amino acids, 95: 218
Amniocentesis, 93: 360
Amoxicillin (drug), 93: 319-320
Amphetamines, 94: 79
Amygdala, 94: 320
Amyl nitrite (drug), 94: 79
Amylin (protein), 95: 173
Amyotrophic lateral sclerosis, 94: 262-264, 297-299
Anabolic steroids, 93: 249
Anaerobic exercise, 95: 106
Anafranil (drug). See **Clomipramine**
Analgesics, 93: 41-42
Anaphylactic shock, 94: 31, **93:** 81
Androgen, 93: 248
Anemia, 93: 137-138
  see also **Iron-deficiency anemia; Sickle cell anemia**
Anencephaly, 94: 221, 324, **93:** 322
Aneurysms, 94: 89, 90, 93, 101, 248
Angel dust. See **PCP (drug)**
Angelman syndrome, 93: 332-333
Anger, and heart attack, 95: 308 (il.)
Angina pectoris, 94: 89, 344-345, **93:** 48, 345
Angiography. See **Coronary angiography; Digital subtraction angiography**
Angioplasty. See **Coronary angioplasty**
Animals. See **Veterinary medicine**
Anopheles mosquito, 93: 198-209
Anorexia nervosa, 93: 243, 244
Antacids, 94: 280
Antianxiety drugs, 95: 181, 186
Antibiotics, 95: 57, 95-101, 328, **94:** 280, **93:** 231-235, 317-318
Antibodies
  allergic reactions, **93:** 72
  diabetes, **95:** 278
  hepatitis, **93:** 100-101, 105-106
  immunization, **93:** 29
  influenza virus, **93:** 150
  rabies, **94:** 166, 169
  transplant rejection, **93:** 283
  ulcers, **95:** 99
Anticoagulants, 94: 311
Antidepressant drugs, 95: 175-176, 180, 182-183, 316-317, **94:** 318
Antigens, 93: 105, 335
Antihistamines, 95: 251, 309, **94:** 282, **93:** 78-79, 319
Anti-inflammatory drugs, 94: 250-251, **93:** 41-42, 192-194
  see also **Nonsteroidal anti-inflammatory drugs**
Antioxidants
  aging, **94:** 70-71, **93:** 170-174, 176 (il.)
  cancer prevention, **95:** 63-73, 324-325, 329
  muscle health, **94:** 292
Antipsychotic drugs, 95: 181, 187
Antipyretics, 93: 41-42
Anxiety disorders, 95: 178, 186, **94:** 104

Aortic aneurysm, **94:** 90, 93, 101
APACHE (program), 94: 150-151
Apnea. See **Sleep apnea**
ApoE4 gene, 95: 211, 261-262
Appetite. See **Eating disorders; Weight control**
Arrythmia. See **Heartbeat**
Arsenic, 93: 113
Arteries, 94: 88
   hardening, **95:** 241, 292-293
   see also **Atherosclerosis; Heart disease**
ARTHRITIS AND CONNECTIVE TISSUE DISORDERS, 95: 252-254, **94:** 252-254, **93:** 285-287
   ancient skeletons, **93:** 134-135
   aspirin, **93:** 41-42, 49
   books, **95:** 259, **94:** 259
   phone information, **95:** 40, **94:** 38
   see also **Osteoarthritis; Rheumatoid arthritis**
Artificial eyes, 95: 294
Artificial insemination, 95: 314
Asbestos, 93: 113, 114 (il.), 124-125
Ashe, Arthur, 94: 242-243, **93:** 276
Aspartame (sweetener), 95: 273
Aspirin, 93: 38-53
   colon cancer, **94:** 266-267, **93:** 304
   heart attacks, **94:** 134-135, 278, **93:** 46-51
   influenza, **93:** 148
   side effects, **95:** 281
   stroke, **95:** 342-343, **94:** 134, **93:** 49-51, 318-319
   ulcers, **95:** 91, 100, **93:** 42
Assisted-living facilities, 95: 214-215
Asthma. See **Allergies and asthma**
Astigmatism, 93: 16-17, 328-329
Atherectomy, 94: 96, 99 (il.)
Atherosclerosis, 94: 87-101
   diabetes, **95:** 167
   drugs, **95:** 306-307, **94:** 309
   hypothyroidism, **93:** 164
   lipoprotein, **95:** 343
   mental health, **93:** 350
   weight control, **94:** 350, 351
   see also **Heart disease**
Athletics, 94: 290-291, **93:** 295 (il.)
   see also **Exercise and fitness**
Atovaquone (drug), 94: 281
ATP, 95: 105-106, 111, 114
Atrial fibrillation, 94: 343, **93:** 50
Audiologists, 94: 24-25, 285 (il.)
Aural rehabilitation, 94: 27
Autism, 93: 353-354
Autoimmune diseases, 93: 159
Automobile safety, 95: 242, 248, 331-332, **94:** 329, 332-333, **93:** 365
Autonomic nervous system, 95: 167
Autonomy, Principle of, 94: 218, 225
Ayala, Anissa, 94: 211
Azacitidine (drug), 95: 257
Azithromycin (drug), 93: 317-318, 370-371
AZT (drug), 95: 243 (il.), 245, 325, **94:** 244, 315, **93:** 278

B

Babies. See **Infants**
Baboon liver transplants, 94: 232, 346, **93:** 312
Baby and Child Care (Spock), **95:** 75-87

Baby Fae, 94: 232
Back pain, 95: 257, **94:** 180, 253, 258
Bacteria
   food, **94:** 331-332, 332 (il.), **93:** 369
   genetic engineering, **95:** 219
   infectious diseases, **95:** 45-50, 56-59, 310 (il.)
   Loofah sponges, **94:** 338
   pet health, **95:** 348
   tuberculosis, **95:** 328, **94:** 314-315, **93:** 56-59
   ulcers, **95:** 89-101, **94:** 280, **93:** 314
Bacterial meningitis, 95: 286
Balance, Sense of, 95: 189-201, **94:** 241-242
Baldness, 94: 309 (il.)
Balloon angioplasty, 95: 306, **94:** 95-96, 311, 345
Barbiturates, 94: 79
Basal ganglia, 94: 110-112, 298
Base pairs, 95: 221, 232
Basic Four food groups, 94: 57, 58
BCG (vaccine), 93: 62
Bed-wetting, 95: 125
Bee stings, 94: 28-31
Behavior therapy, 94: 113-115
Bellybutton surgery. See **Laparoscopy**
Beneficence, 94: 218, 225
Benign positional vertigo, 95: 194, 199, 201
Benign tumors. See **Tumors, Benign**
Benzodiazepines (drugs), 95: 186, **93:** 316-317
Bergalis, Kimberly, 94: 228, **93:** 276
Beta-amyloid, 94: 265 (il.), **93:** 296
Beta-blockers (drugs), 94: 95, **93:** 160-161
Beta carotene
   aging, **93:** 174, 176 (il.)
   artery/heart disease, **95:** 309, **94:** 70-71
   cancer, **95:** 63-66, 69-72, 309, 324-325, 329
   sources, **95:** 64
Beta interferon (drug), 94: 264-265
Beta 2 agonists (drugs), 95: 249, **94:** 251, 328
Betaseron (drug), 95: 281-282
BGH. See **Bovine growth hormone**
Bicycle safety, 94: 334, **93:** 367-368
Bile, 95: 280
Bioenergetics, 94: 185
Bioequivalence of drugs, 94: 18-19
Biofeedback, 94: 129, 173 (il.), 184, 275 (il.)
Biologic response modifiers, 93: 213-215
Biological clock, 94: 21-23
Biopsy, 95: 99-100, **94:** 208 (il.), **93:** 117 (il.), 302 (il.)
Biotechnology. See **Genetic engineering**
Bipolar disorder, 95: 178, 183
BIRTH CONTROL, 95: 254-255, **94:** 254-255, **93:** 287-288
   Healy interview, **94:** 142
   warning labels, **94:** 335 (il.)
   see also **Condoms; Intrauterine devices; Norplant contraceptive**
Birth defects, 94: 324, 339 (il.), **93:** 359-360
   see also **Anencephaly; Down syndrome; Pregnancy and childbirth; Spina bifida**
Bismuth (drug), 95: 95

Bites
   insect, **94:** 28-31
   pet, **95:** 15
   rabid animal, **94:** 159-171
Blacks
   asthma in children, **94:** 249
   drug use, **95:** 246-247
   hysterectomies, **95:** 344-345
   life expectancy, **93:** 341
   salt intake, **93:** 349 (il.)
   sickle cell anemia, **93:** 30, 290
   stroke, **93:** 378
   syphilis study in 1930's, **94:** 233
   violence, **94:** 44, 45, 48, 50, 53
   vitiligo, **94:** 336
   see also **Sickle cell anemia**
Blastomycosis, 94: 281
Bleeding, 93: 312-314
   see also **Hemophilia**
Blepharoptosis, 93: 327-328
Blindness. See **Eye and vision**
BLOOD, 95: 256-257, **94:** 256-257, **93:** 289-290
   fetal abnormalities, **93:** 360
   kidney dialysis, **93:** 349-350
   lead levels, **93:** 324
   malaria infection, **93:** 200-203
   see also **Anemia; Bleeding; Leukemia; Red blood cells; White blood cells**
Blood clots, 94: 89, 91 (il.), **93:** 42, 44-45, 48-51
Blood donation, 94: 257
Blood pressure, 95: 12-13, 194, 200, 312-313, **93:** 174
   see also **Hypertension**
Blood sugar. See **Diabetes; Hypoglycemia**
Blood testing
   diabetes, **95:** 166, 172
   hepatitis, **93:** 101, 105-106, 108
   leukemia, **94:** 206-207, 208 (il.)
   prostate cancer, **95:** 266
   see also **AIDS**
Blood transfusions, 93: 101
Blue-baby syndrome, 93: 91
Blue Cross and Blue Shield, 93: 259-261, 270, 331
Boating safety, 94: 333-334
Body dysmorphic disorder, 94: 317-318
"Bog people," 93: 128-129
Bone cancer, 93: 138 (il.)
BONE DISORDERS, 95: 257-258, **94:** 257-259, **93:** 290-292
   posture, **93:** 25-26
   puberty, **93:** 244
   smoking, **95:** 337-339
   see also **Arthritis and connective tissue disorders; Osteoporosis; Spine disorders; Women**
Bone marrow, 94: 202
   biopsy, **94:** 206-207, 208 (il.)
   transplants, **95:** 256, 257, **94:** 209-212, 214 (il.), 256, **93:** 289
BOOKS OF HEALTH AND MEDICINE, 95: 259-261, **94:** 259-261, **93:** 292-294
Botox, 93: 374
Bovine growth hormone, 95: 322-323
BPV. See **Benign positional vertigo**
BRAIN AND NERVOUS SYSTEM, 95: 261-265, **94:** 262-266, **93:** 295-298
   aging, **93:** 173, 175-176
   alcohol effects, **95:** 249

ancient human remains, **93:** 129-130
aneurysms and cocaine, **94:** 248
artery disease, **95:** 343
aspirin and strokes, **93:** 49-51
depression, **94:** 318 (il.), 320
diabetes, **95:** 167, 168
dizziness, **95:** 190-201
dyslexia, **94:** 188, 190-191
menstruation, **94:** 118
obsessive-compulsive disorder, **94:** 110-113
optic neuritis, **95:** 295-296
psychiatric drug effects, **95:** 176, 179-183
rabies, **94:** 161-162
sleep stages, **95:** 120-121
spinal cord injuries, **95:** 135-137
violence, **94:** 52-53
see also **Alzheimer's disease; Mental health; Multiple sclerosis; Nerve cells; Parkinson disease; Spine disorders; Stroke**
Brain cancer, 95: 301, **94:** 333, **93:** 302-304, 315 (il.)
Brain stem, 94: 161
Brain tissue transplants, 94: 345-346
Brakes, Antilock, 95: 330 (il.), 332
Breast cancer
aging, **94:** 270 (il.)
birth control drug, **94:** 254
books, **95:** 259, **93:** 292-293
breast-feeding, **95:** 269 (il.), 327
chemotherapy, **93:** 213, 215, 298-301
diet, **95:** 61, 65-68, 323, **94:** 64-66, 267-268, 321-322
Healy interview, **94:** 136-137, 139
hormone replacement therapy, **94:** 126, 136
menstruation onset, **95:** 292
pesticides, **95:** 288-289
screening, **95:** 267-268, **94:** 268-269
smoking, **95:** 337
surgery, **95:** 265, 343-344
Tamoxifen risk, **95:** 270-271
Breast-feeding, 95: 269 (il.), 327, **93:** 361
Breast implants, 93: 366-367
Broccoli, 95: 323, **94:** 59
Bronchi, 93: 112, 115
Bronchodilators, 95: 249, **94:** 250-251, 328, **93:** 283 (il.), 284
Bronchoscope, 93: 121
Bulimia, 93: 243, 244
Bungee jumping, 95: 295 (il.)
Burns, 95: 36-39
Bush, George and Barbara, 93: 155-156, 159-160, 313
Buspirone (drug), 94: 348
Butyl nitrite (drug), 94: 79
Butyrate (drug), 93: 290
Byrd, Dennis, 95: 134-135, 140-141, **94:** 263

C

Caffeine, 95: 258 (il.), 324, **94:** 322, **93:** 49, 280-281, 358 (il.)
Calcipotriene (drug), 95: 336
Calcium
bone health, **95:** 240, 258, **94:** 128, 240-241, 259 (il.), 301-302, 322
food sources, **94:** 35, **93:** 291
hypertension, **93:** 360-361
kidney stones, **94:** 300, 316

lead poisoning, **95:** 331
Calories, 94: 32-35, 66, 351-352
Camel cigarettes, 93: 375-377
CANCER, 95: 265-271, **94:** 266-270, **93:** 298-304
aging, **93:** 171, 174
AIDS, **95:** 243-244
antihistamines, **95:** 251
books, **95:** 259-260, **93:** 292-293
cellular phones, **94:** 333
chlorinated water, **94:** 288
diet, **95:** 19, 61-73, 337, 346, **94:** 35, 64-66, 89, **93:** 125, 303, 341, 354-355
dogs, **93:** 380
drugs, **94:** 270, **93:** 298-301
electromagnetic fields, **94:** 289
gene therapy, **95:** 230, 265-267, 299, **93:** 223, 301-302
genetic basis, **95:** 212-215, 224-225, 228, 297-299, **94:** 256-257, 267 (il.), 296-297, **93:** 214-215, 299-301, 335
heart disease link, **95:** 306
new treatments, **93:** 210-223
obesity, **93:** 384
octreotide scanning, **95:** 300-301
phone information, **95:** 40, **94:** 38
smokeless tobacco, **94:** 339
smoking, **95:** 337, **93:** 111-112, 124-125
stress, **95:** 317-319
surgery, **95:** 266, 343-344, **93:** 123-124, 213
vitamins, **95:** 61-73, 309, 324-325
women, **94:** 132, 136-137
see also **Chemotherapy; Radiation therapy;** and specific cancer types
CAPD. See Ambulatory dialysis
Captopril (drug), 95: 277
Carbamazepine (drug), 95: 185
Carbohydrates, 95: 105, 162, 170
see also **Fruits; Vegetables**
Carbon monoxide poisoning, 95: 152, **94:** 289
Carcinogens. See Cancer
Cardiac arrest, 94: 312, **93:** 322
Cardiac emergency units, 94: 287
Cardiopulmonary resuscitation, 95: 159, 240-241, **94:** 312, **93:** 321, 345 (il.)
Cardiovascular disease. See Heart disease
Carotenoids, 94: 71
Carotid arteries, 95: 307, **94:** 89, 93, 96-97
Carotid endarterectomy, 94: 96-99
Carpal tunnel syndrome, 95: 253 (il.)
Carrots, 95: 293 (il.)
Cartilage, 94: 252
CAS. See Computer-assisted surgery
CAT scan. See Computerized tomography
Cataracts, 95: 32-35, 294-295, **94:** 242, 293-295, **93:** 324
Catheters, 94: 92, 96
Catnip, 95: 348 (il.)
Cats
health, **95:** 348-349, **94:** 348-349
owner health, **95:** 12-15
rabies, **94:** 163, 169
Cauda equina, 95: 135, 137
CD-4 cells, 94: 242
CD-ROM, 94: 153
Cellular phone safety, 94: 333
Central nervous system, 95: 135-137, 142-143, **94:** 161-162, 207

Cerebrospinal fluid, 93: 192
Cervical cancer, 95: 66, **94:** 335-336, **93:** 219, 357-358
Cervical intraepithelial neoplasia, 94: 336
CF. See Cystic fibrosis
CFC's. See Chlorofluorocarbons
Change of life. See Menopause
Chemotherapy, 94: 207-209, 212, **93:** 212, 213, 216-217, 300
Chewing gum, 94: 275-276
Chickenpox, 94: 314, **93:** 347
CHILD DEVELOPMENT, 95: 271-274, **94:** 271-274, **93:** 304-307
AIDS, **93:** 277
alcohol/drug abuse, **94:** 73-85, **93:** 279-280
allergies and asthma, **95:** 249-250, **94:** 248-251, 328
Alzheimer's disease anxiety, **95:** 213
bone disorders, **94:** 257-258
books, **94:** 260
child abuse, **94:** 43-45, 48-49
depression, **95:** 317
dyslexia, **94:** 187-199, **93:** 304-305
ear and hearing, **95:** 286, **94:** 284-285, **93:** 225-235
eye disorders, **95:** 294, 296
firearm deaths, **95:** 333
hepatitis, **93:** 100
home safety, **95:** 151-152, 155, 156
immunization, **95:** 310, **94:** 313-314, **93:** 27-29
iron supplement dangers, **94:** 333
lead poisoning, **95:** 286-289, **93:** 86-87, 322-323
leukemia, **95:** 289-290, **94:** 203-204, 207-209, 212
over-the-counter drugs, **95:** 283
posture, **95:** 26
precocious puberty, **94:** 282
psychiatric drugs, **95:** 184
research on humans, **94:** 234
Reye's syndrome, **93:** 43
sleep problems, **95:** 125
smokeless tobacco, **94:** 339-341
smoking, **94:** 340-341, **93:** 307
Spock interview, **95:** 75-87
violence causes, **94:** 53-54
see also **Adolescents; Birth defects; Day care; Infants; Pregnancy and childbirth; Puberty; Rheumatoid arthritis; Safety**
Chiropractic, 94: 173, 176, 180-181
Chlamydia, 95: 334-335, **93:** 317-318, 370-371
Chlorine, 94: 288, **93:** 84-85, 92, 347-348
Chlorofluorocarbons, 94: 288
Chloroquine (drug), 93: 206, 208
Chlorpromazine (drug), 95: 179, 186
Chocolate, 95: 321 (il.)
Cholera, 95: 46, 48, **93:** 19, 83, 92
Cholesteatoma, 93: 230-231
Cholesterol
artery disease, **94:** 60-62, 100, 123
diabetes, **95:** 170
diet, **95:** 321 (il.), **94:** 32-35, 60-67, 70, **93:** 358 (il.)
drugs, **95:** 307-308, **94:** 309-310
exercise effects, **93:** 324-325
gene therapy, **93:** 333 (il.)
good and bad, **95:** 18-19
pet ownership, **95:** 12, **94:** 350
self-test, **94:** 311 (il.)
see also **Familial hypercholes-**

terolemia; Heart disease; High-
density lipoprotein; Low-density
lipoprotein; Plaque
Chorionic villus sampling, 93: 359-
360
Chromosomes
cancer, **94:** 215, 296
fetal abnormalities, **93:** 360
genetic code, **95:** 218-219, 223-224
genetic imprinting disorders, **93:** 332-
333
immune system disease, **94:** 300
mapping, **95:** 233-234
see also **DNA; Genes**
Cigarette smoking. See Smoking
Circadian rhythms, 95: 264-265, **94:**
22
Cirrhosis, 95: 280, **93:** 100, 104
Claudication, 94: 90
Claustrophobia, 95: 178
Cleaning products, 93: 368-369
Cleft palate, 93: 228
Climacteric, 94: 120, 121
Clinical bioethicists, 94: 219-220
Clinton, Bill, 95: 302-304, **94:** 302-305
Clinton, Hillary Rodham, 95: 302, **94:**
302, 305 (il.)
Clomipramine (drug), 94: 112-113,
318, **93:** 354
Cloning, 95: 219, 226, 314
Clostridium botulinum **(bacteria), 93:**
374
Clozapine (drug), 95: 316
CNS. See Central nervous system
Cocaethylene (drug), 93: 282
Cocaine
aneurysms, **94:** 248
child/adolescent use, **95:** 246, 247,
94: 76, 78, 85, 245, **93:** 279, 281-
282
gene for abuse, **95:** 248
violence, **94:** 50
Cochlear implants, 94: 285
Codons, 95: 218, 232
Coffee. See Caffeine
**Cognex (drug). See Tacrine hy-
drochloride**
Cognitive therapy, 95: 127
Colds, 95: 328 (il.), **94:** 183-184, **93:**
70, 145, 352
**Colitis, Ulcerative. See Ulcerative col-
itis**
Collagen, 95: 254
Collagenase (enzyme), 95: 297
Colon cancer
aspirin, **94:** 266-267, **93:** 51, 304
diet, **94:** 64-65
gene, **95:** 225, 297-298, **94:** 267 (il.),
279, 296-297, **93:** 299, 301
polyp removal, **95:** 269-270
screening, **95:** 270, 346, **94:** 280
stress, **95:** 317-319
Colon disorders, 95: 278-280, **94:** 278-
279, 344 (il.)
see also **Colon cancer; Ulcers**
**Colorectal cancer. See Colon cancer;
Rectal cancer**
Coma, 94: 161-162, **93:** 163
**Compulsions. See Obsessive-com-
pulsive disorder**
Computer-assisted surgery, 95: 344
(il.), **94:** 145-147, 151 (il.)
Computerized tomography, 94: 92-93,
147-148, **93:** 133 (il.), 192

Computers
child rearing, **95:** 86
health effects, **94:** 293 (il.)
medical assistance, **95:** 309 (il.), **94:**
145-157
Condoms
AIDS, **95:** 245
cost/effectiveness, **95:** 255
sexually transmitted diseases, **95:**
333, **94:** 334-335, **93:** 370, 371
vaginal, **94:** 254-255, **93:** 287-288
Confidentiality, 94: 225-229
Conjoined twins. See Siamese twins
**Connective tissue disorders. See
Arthritis and connective tissue dis-
orders**
Contact lenses, 95: 293-294, **94:** 295,
93: 16-18
Continuous passive motion, 94: 252-
253
Contraception. See Birth control
Cooperative centers, 94: 12-13
Cornea, 95: 293-294, **94:** 295, **93:** 16-
18
Coronary angiography, 94: 92, 97 (il.),
310 (il.)
Coronary angioplasty, 95: 306, **94:** 95-
96, 311, 312, 344-345, **93:** 345
**Coronary artery disease. See
Atherosclerosis; Heart disease**
Coronary bypass surgery, 95: 306,
308-309, **94:** 95, 344-345
Corticosteroids, 95: 249-250, 296-297,
94: 251, 328, **93:** 80, 194, 363-364
**Costs of health care. See Financing
medical care; Health care issues**
Cotinine (chemical), 95: 341
**CPR. See Cardiopulmonary resusci-
tation**
Crack. See Cocaine
Cramps, 95: 116
Cranberry juice, 95: 346-347
Crayons, Lead in, 95: 330-331
Crick, Francis H. C., 95: 218
Crime, Violent. See Violence
Crohn's disease, 95: 280
Cromolyn (drug), 93: 80
Cruzan, Nancy Beth, 94: 222-223, **93:**
26
Cryptosporidium, **94:** 329
Crystal healing, 94: 185
**CT scan. See Computerized tomogra-
phy**
Cushing's syndrome, 94: 302, **93:** 116
(il.)
CVS. See Chorionic villus sampling
Cyclosporine (drug), 95: 280, **94:** 278-
279
Cystic fibrosis
drug, **95:** 282
gene therapy, **95:** 230, **94:** 297
phone information, **95:** 40, **94:** 38
screening, **95:** 224 (il.), **93:** 362-363
Cystic kidney disease, 95: 313-314
Cytokines, 93: 349-350
Cytomegalovirus, 93: 317
Cytotoxic drugs, 94: 207, **93:** 213-215

D

Dairy products, 95: 258 (il.), 322-323,
94: 57-62
Dalla Corte, Rossana, 95: 315 (il.)
Day care, 95: 81, **94:** 12-16, 284-285,
93: 305 (il.), 307

DDC (drug). See Dideoxycytidine
DDE (chemical), 95: 288
DDI (drug). See Dideoxyinosine
DDT, 95: 288-289, **93:** 207-208
Deafness. See Ear and hearing
Death, Definition of, 93: 221-222
Deaths
antihistamines, **95:** 309
highway, **94:** 332
smoking, **93:** 280, 375
violence, **94:** 44, 50
see also **Right to die; Safety;** and
specific diseases
Decongestants, 93: 79-80
Deer mice, 95: 51-52, 328
Deer ticks, 95: 58-59
Defibrillation, 94: 345 (il.), **93:** 344-345
Delinquent behavior, 94: 273-274
Delta-wave sleep, 95: 120
Dementia, 95: 204, 244, **94:** 240
see also **Alzheimer's disease**
Dengue, 95: 56
DENTISTRY, 95: 275-276, **94:** 275-276,
93: 308-309
ancient humans, **93:** 129 (il.), 136 (il.)
fluoridated water, **93:** 92-94
pets, **94:** 348-349
Deoxyribonucleic acid. See DNA
Depo Provera (drug), 95: 255, **94:** 254,
93: 288
Depression
adolescence, **93:** 246-247
brain changes, **94:** 318 (il.), 320
childhood, **95:** 317
drugs, **95:** 175-176, 182-183, 316-317
heart disease, **93:** 350
memory, **93:** 352-353
rise in rates, **94:** 317
women, **94:** 123, 131-132
Dermatitis, 95: 29
Dermatology. See Skin
DIABETES, 95: 276-278, **94:** 276-278,
93: 309-311
cataracts, **95:** 33
dizziness, **95:** 194
drug, **95:** 300
exercise, **95:** 170, 172, **93:** 175, 326
eye surgery risk, **95:** 294-295
kidney disease, **93:** 349
phone information, **95:** 40, **94:** 38
tight blood sugar control, **95:** 262-263,
276-277, 314
Type II complications, **95:** 161-173
Diabetic retinopathy, 95: 166-167, 277,
294-295, **94:** 276, **93:** 309 (il.)
*Diagnostic and Statistical Manual of
Mental Disorders,* **95:** 319-320
Dialysis, 95: 313, **94:** 315-316, **93:** 349-
350
Diaphragms (birth control), 95: 255
Diarrhea, 95: 279, **93:** 20-21, 313
Diazepam (drug). See Valium
**Didanosine (drug). See Dideoxyino-
sine**
Dideoxycytidine (drug), 93: 278, 315
Dideoxyinosine (drug), 95: 245, **93:**
278, 315
Diet. See Nutrition and food
DIGESTIVE SYSTEM, 95: 278-280, **94:**
278-280, **93:** 312-314
diabetes, **95:** 167
see also **Colon disorders; Stomach;
Ulcers**
Digital rectal examination, 95: 266, **94:**
269

Digital subtraction angiography, **94:** 93

Diphtheria, 94: 314

Disabled, 93: 340 (il.)

spinal cord injuries, **95:** 132-145, **94:** 263

Disequilibrium, 95: 193, 198

Dissociation, 95: 195

Dissociative identity disorder, 95: 320

Dizziness, 95: 189-200

DNA

ancient human remains, **93:** 129-131

cancer, **95:** 297, **94:** 296, **93:** 217-218

discovery, **93:** 218

free radical damage, **95:** 62, 65, **94:** 70

genetic disease, **95:** 221-222

genetic engineering, **95:** 219, 229

Huntington's disease gene, **94:** 298-299

mapping, **95:** 232-234

see also **Chromosomes; Genes**

DNase (drug), 95: 282

Dogs

health, **95:** 348, 349, **94:** 348, 349 (il.), **93:** 380

owner health, **95:** 12-15

rabies, **94:** 162-163, 169

Dominant genes, 95: 220 (il.), 223

Donor organs. See Transplants

Dopamine, 95: 186-187, **94:** 345, **93:** 281-282

Doppler ultrasound, 94: 93

Dornase alfa (drug). See DNase

Dovonex (drug). See Calcipotriene

Down syndrome, 95: 40-41, 326-327, **94:** 39, 213

Doxycycline (drug), 93: 370-371

Dreaming, 95: 120-121, 125, 131

Drinking water. See Water

Drug abuse. See Alcohol and drug abuse

DRUGS, 95: 281-283, **94:** 281-284, **93:** 315-319

bacterial resistance, **95:** 57, 328

birth control, **93:** 288

books, **95:** 259

computer medicine, **94:** 153-154

generic, **94:** 17-20

genetic engineering, **95:** 226

health care costs, **93:** 254

herbal medicine, **94:** 178-179

home safety, **95:** 149, 151-152

psychiatric, **95:** 175-187

sleeping pills, **95:** 129

smoking interaction, **95:** 340

tobacco regulation, **95:** 338-339

see also **Alcohol and drug abuse; Chemotherapy; and specific drugs and disorders**

Duodenal ulcers. See Ulcers

Duodenum, 95: 90

Durable power of attorney, 94: 223

Dyslexia, 94: 187-199, **93:** 304-305

E

EAR AND HEARING, 95: 284-286, **94:** 284-285, **93:** 319-320

auditory dyslexia, **94:** 195, **93:** 189

book, **95:** 260

dizziness, **95:** 190-201

hearing aids, **94:** 24-27

otitis media, **94:** 284-285, **93:** 225-235

otosclerosis, **94:** 147

phone information, **95:** 41, **94:** 39

Earthquake, Los Angeles, 95: 318

Eating disorders, 93: 244

Ebola hemorrhagic fever, 95: 46, 48, 59

ECG. See Electrocardiography

Echocardiography, 94: 92

Ectopic pregnancy, 93: 359

Education, 95: 351-352, **94:** 271-272

Effexor (drug). See Venlafaxine hydrochloride

Effusion, 94: 254

EKG. See Electrocardiography

Elderly. See Aging

Electrical wiring safety, 95: 158

Electrocardiogram. See Electrocardiography

Electrocardiography, 94: 92, 97 (il.)

Electroencephalograph, 95: 120

Electromagnetic fields, 94: 289

Embryos, 93: 314

EMERGENCY MEDICINE, 94: 286-287, **93:** 321-322

emergency room visits, **93:** 12-15

observation units, **93:** 321

stroke, **93:** 378

see also **Cardiopulmonary resuscitation; First aid**

EMF's. See Electromagnetic fields

Emotions. See Mental health

Endometrial cancer, 95: 271, **93:** 180, 301

Endoscopy, 95: 100

Endothelium, 94: 88

Endurance, 95: 110-114

Enhancemate (computer system), 94: 155

ENVIRONMENTAL HEALTH, 95: 286-290, **94:** 287-289, **93:** 322-324

genetic mutation, **95:** 222, 224

infectious diseases, **95:** 52-55

see also **Air pollution; Water pollution**

Epidemics. See specific diseases

Epilepsy, 95: 41, 283, **94:** 39, 264, 349 (il.)

Epinephrine, 94: 251

Episiotomy, 93: 360

Erythromycin (drug), 93: 346

Escherichia coli **(bacteria), 95:** 45, **94:** 330

Esophagus, 94: 266-267

Essential fatty acids, 94: 65-66

Estrogen

aging, **93:** 335-336

Alzheimer's disease, **95:** 242, 262 (il.)

breast cancer, **94:** 66, **93:** 300

menstruation, **94:** 118-124, **93:** 248

pesticide mimics, **95:** 288-289

see also **Hormone replacement therapy**

Ethical issues. See Medical ethics

Euchromatin, 93: 335

Eugenics, 95: 237, **94:** 229

Eustachian tube, 93: 226-228

Evoked response studies, 93: 190-191

Exclusive-provider organizations, 95: 22

EXERCISE AND FITNESS, 95: 290-293, **94:** 290-292, **93:** 324-326

artery/heart disease, **95:** 103, 117, 290-291, **94:** 100, 101, 291

asthma, **95:** 250

benefits, **95:** 103-117

books, **93:** 293-294

diabetes, **95:** 170, 172, **93:** 175, 326

dizziness, **95:** 201

elderly, **95:** 117, 241, 292-293, **94:** 241-242, **93:** 174-176, 292 (il.)

joint diseases, **94:** 252, **93:** 285-287

posture, **95:** 26

spinal cord injuries, **95:** 140-141

women, **95:** 327, **94:** 128

Experimental autoimmune encephalomyelitis, 93: 295-296

Exposure (therapy), 94: 113

EYE AND VISION, 95: 293-297, **94:** 292-295, **93:** 327-329

AIDS, **93:** 317

diabetes, **95:** 161-162, 166-167

dizziness, **95:** 190-201

Graves' disease, **93:** 159, 162 (il.)

multiple sclerosis, **93:** 185, 190-191

phone information, **95:** 41, **94:** 39

sleep movements, **95:** 120

surgery, **95:** 32-35, 344 (il.), **94:** 293-295, **93:** 328-329

visual dyslexia, **94:** 188-189, 195

see also **Cataracts; Contact lenses; Cornea; Diabetic retinopathy**

Eyelid surgery, 93: 327-328

F

Factor VIII (protein), 94: 257, **93:** 289-290

Falling injuries, 95: 149-151

False memories, 95: 271-272

Familial adenomatous polyposis, 95: 270, **94:** 279-280

Familial hypercholesterolemia, 95: 221, 229, 230

Family

alcoholism, **93:** 279

Alzheimer's disease patients, **95:** 212-213

day care, **94:** 12-16

drug abuse, **94:** 73-85

health history, **93:** 30-33

Spock interview, **95:** 80

violence, **94:** 45, 48-49, 51

see also **Child development**

Family and Medical Leave Act, 94: 303

Family-care centers, 94: 12

Fat, Body. See Weight control

Fat, Dietary, 95: 16-19

aging, **93:** 171

cancer, **95:** 321-323, 337, 346, **94:** 267-268, 321-322

diabetes diet, **95:** 170

food labels, **94:** 32-35

guidelines, **95:** 350-351, **94:** 57-66, 309-310, 321

school lunches, **93:** 354 (il.)

Fat substitutes, 95: 351

Fatty acids, 95: 16-19, 343, **94:** 63, 65-66, 321

FDA. See Food and Drug Administration, U.S.

Feet, and diabetes, 95: 168

Felbamate (drug). See Felbatol

Felbatol (drug), 95: 283

Feline mouth diseases, 94: 349

Ferrets, Rabies in, 94: 169-170

Fertility, 94: 253

Fetal alcohol syndrome, 93: 281

Fetal tissue transplants, 95: 143-144, **94:** 235, **93:** 340-341

Fetus. See Pregnancy and childbirth

Fever, 93: 41-42
Fialuridine (drug), 95: 315
Fiber, Dietary, 94: 35, 66-67
Fibrillation, 94: 343, 93: 50, 344-345
Fibroblasts, 93: 335
Fibromyalgia, 93: 286-287
Fillings, Dental, 95: 275-276
Filters, and allergies, 95: 251-252
FINANCING MEDICAL CARE, 93: 330-
332
see also **Health care issues; Health
policy; Medicaid; Medicare**
Finasteride (drug). See **Proscar**
Fire prevention, 95: 153-158
Firearms, 95: 79-80, 158, 332-333, 94:
50-52, 55
First aid, 95: 37, 38, 159, 93: 20, 294
Fish oils, 95: 19, 343
Fitness. See **Exercise and fitness**
Five-a-Day For Better Health Pro-
gram, 95: 73
FK506 (drug), 93: 312
Fleas, 95: 348-349, 94: 28-30
Flexibility, Body, 95: 107-110, 114-115
Flu. See **Gastroenteritis; Influenza**
Fluoridated water, 93: 92-94
Fluoxetine (drug). See **Prozac**
Fly bites, 94: 29, 30
Folate, 95: 64, 66
Folic acid, 94: 324, 93: 357-358
Follicle-stimulating hormone, 93: 247-
248
Food. See **Nutrition and food**
Food and Drug Administration, U.S.,
95: 338-339, 94: 18-19, 32-35, 179,
235 (il.), 93: 151-152
see also **Drugs; Nutrition and food**
Food Guide Pyramid, 94: 57-71
Foscarnet, 93: 317
Four Corners disease, 95: 45, 47 (il.),
48, 51-52, 312, 94: 287-288, 313 (il.),
314
Foxes, Rabies in, 94: 170-171, 93: 382
Framingham Heart Study, 94: 60
Fraud. See **Medical ethics**
Free radicals, 95: 62-65, 94: 70-71,
292, 323, 93: 174 (il.), 178
Fruits
cancer, 95: 62-73
Food Guide Pyramid, 94: 57-61, 66-
67
vision, 95: 293
see also **Pesticides**

G

GABA (neurotransmitter), 95: 185
Gabapentin (drug), 95: 283
Gametocytes, 93: 199, 201-202
Gammalinolenic acid, 95: 254
Gancyclovir (drug), 95: 303-304, 317
Gangrene, 95: 167, 168
Garrod, Sir Archibald E., 95: 220
Gastric bypass surgery, 93: 310
Gastritis, 95: 92-94
Gastroenteritis, 93: 145, 313
Gene splicing. See **Genetic engineer-
ing**
Gene therapy
cancer, 95: 230, 265-267, 299, 93:
223, 301-302
cholesterol, 95: 229, 93: 333 (il.)
cystic fibrosis, 95: 230, 94: 297
development, 95: 228-230
hemophilia, 95: 257

severe combined immune deficiency
disease, 94: 300
General Motors Corp., 94: 332-333
Genes, 95: 218-237
aging, 93: 176-177
alcohol/drug abuse, 95: 248, 94: 247-
248, 93: 281
allergies, 93: 284
Alzheimer's disease, 95: 211-212,
261-262
amyotrophic lateral sclerosis, 94: 262-
264, 297-299
ancient human remains, 93: 129-130
bone disorders, 95: 240, 257-258
catnip, 95: 348 (il.)
circadian rhythms, 95: 264-265
diabetes, 95: 173, 94: 278, 93: 310-
311
dog disease, 95: 349
dyslexia, 94: 189-191
family health history, 93: 30-33
Huntington's disease, 94: 298-299
mapping, 95: 232-235, 299-300, 94:
139, 229
mental illness, 95: 176, 182
multiple sclerosis, 93: 187-188
obsessive-compulsive disorder, 94:
115
rheumatoid arthritis, 95: 252
stress disorder, 94: 319-320
stroke, 93: 377-378
see also **Cancer; Gene therapy; Genetic engineering; Genetic
medicine**
Genetic counseling, 95: 230, 94: 229
Genetic engineering, 95: 219, 226-231,
236-237, 277 (il.), 322-323, 93: 302
Genetic imprinting, 93: 333
GENETIC MEDICINE, 95: 297-300, 94:
296-300, 93: 332-335
cancer, 95: 297-299
development, 95: 226-231
see also **Gene therapy; Genes; Genetic engineering**
Genetic screening, 95: 230, 236-237
Genetics, 95: 218-237
see also **Genetic medicine**
Genistein (compound), 95: 65
Genital herpes, 93: 371
Genitals, and menopause, 94: 121,
127
Genome, 95: 232, 300
Gentamicin (drug), 93: 320
Gertz, Alison, 94: 243
Gestational diabetes, 94: 276-277
Gingivitis, 93: 308 (il.)
Ginseng, 94: 129
GLANDS AND HORMONES, 95: 300-
301, 94: 300-302, 93: 335-337
aging, 93: 173, 180-181
bovine growth hormone, 95: 322-323
cancer-fighting drugs, 93: 213-215
Graves' disease, 93: 159-160, 162
menopause, 94: 118-120
puberty, 93: 242 (il.), 247-249
see also **specific glands and hor-
mones**
Glaucoma, 95: 297
Glucokinase, 93: 310-311
Glucose, 95: 162
see also **Diabetes**
Glutamate decarboxylase (molecule),
95: 278
Glycogen, 95: 105-106, 111, 115, 93:
98

GM-1 ganglioside (drug), 95: 135,
139-140, 94: 263
Goiter, 93: 157, 162 (il.)
Gonadotropin-releasing hormone, 93:
247
Gonorrhea, 95: 334
Gout, 93: 42
Grains, in diet, 94: 57-61, 66-67
Graves' disease, 93: 159-160, 162
Ground water, 93: 83-84
Growth hormone, 93: 247-249
see also **Human growth hormone**
Guaiac (extract), 94: 280
Guar gum, 93: 382-383
Gulf War syndrome, 95: 305
see also **Persian Gulf War**
Gum disease, 95: 276, 94: 275, 93:
308-309
Guns. See **Firearms**

H

Haemophilus influenzae type b, 94:
314
Hair cells (ear), 94: 284
Hair loss. See **Baldness**
Haitian refugees, 94: 306-307
Halcion, 93: 316-317
Handguns. See **Firearms**
Hansen's disease. See **Leprosy**
Hantaviruses, 95: 45, 48, 51-52, 312,
328-329, 94: 314
Harvard Community Health Plan, 94:
155-156
Hashimoto's disease, 93: 163
Hashish, 94: 78
Hay fever, 93: 70
HDL. See **High-density lipoprotein**
Headache, 95: 41, 94: 39, 322, 93: 52
see also **Migraine**
Health and Human Services, Department of, 94: 233-234
Health care information, 95: 40-41,
94: 38-39, 93: 34-35
HEALTH CARE ISSUES, 95: 302-305,
94: 302-308
books, 95: 259-260
computers and costs, 94: 153-155
emergency room visits, 93: 14-15
generic drug costs, 94: 20
health care system reform, 95: 302-
305, 94: 236-237, 302-305, 93:
252-271, 339-340
managed-care plans, 95: 20-23
see also **Medical ethics**
HEALTH CARE ORGANIZATIONS, 93:
337-339
see also **Hospitals; Nursing homes**
Health care system. See **Health care
issues**
Health maintenance organizations,
95: 20-23, 93: 262, 269-270, 331
HEALTH POLICY, 93: 339-342
see also **Financing medical care;
Health care issues**
Healy, Bernadine, 94: 131-143
Hearing. See **Ear and hearing**
Hearing aids, 94: 24-27
HEART AND BLOOD VESSELS, 95:
306-309, 94: 308-312, 93: 342-346
cardiac arrest, 94: 312, 93: 322
defects, 93: 322
exercise benefits, 95: 105, 94: 111-
115
see also **Arteries**

359

Heart attacks, 94: 89, 94 (il.)
angioplasty, **94:** 311
aspirin, **94:** 134-135, 278, **93:** 46-51
bald men, **94:** 309 (il.)
computer diagnosis, **94:** 149
depression, **93:** 350
drug treatment, **95:** 308, **94:** 310-311
exercise, **95:** 290-291
nicotine patch, **93:** 374-375
social factors, **93:** 342-343
surgery choices, **95:** 306
Heart disease, 94: 87-101
books, **95:** 260, **94:** 261, **93:** 293, 294
cancer link, **95:** 306
cardiac emergency units, **94:** 287
causes, **95:** 307, 308 (il.)
computer model, **94:** 148-150
diabetes, **95:** 162, 167-168
diet, **95:** 19, **94:** 35, 60-64, 71
exercise, **95:** 103, 117, 290-291, **94:** 100, 101, 291
hormone replacement therapy, **94:** 126-127, **93:** 343-344
insulin resistance, **93:** 311
iron in blood, **94:** 322-323
pet ownership, **95:** 12, **94:** 350
phone information, **95:** 41
smoking, **95:** 341, **93:** 345-346, 377
social factors, **93:** 342-343
vitamins, **95:** 68, 309, **94:** 320-321, **93:** 358
weight control, **94:** 350, 351, **93:** 383, 384
see also **Atherosclerosis; Cholesterol; Coronary angioplasty; Coronary bypass surgery; Heart attacks; Women**
Heart rate, 95: 115, 116
Heart transplants, 95: 345
Heartbeat, 95: 309, **94:** 343, 345 (il.)
Heartburn, 94: 280
Heimlich maneuver, 95: 159
Helicobacter pylori **(bacteria), 95:** 89-101, **94:** 280, **93:** 314
Hellerwork, 94: 182
Hematologists, 94: 207
Hemodialysis, 94: 315-316
Hemoglobin, 95: 256-257, **94:** 256 (il.), **93:** 290
Hemolytic-uremic syndrome, 94: 330
Hemophilia, 95: 221 (il.), 243, 257, **94:** 257, **93:** 289-290
Hepatic vein, 93: 312-314
Hepatitis, 95: 315, **94:** 346, **93:** 97-109, 347-348
Herbal medicine, 94: 128-129, 173, 177 (il.), 178-179
Hereditary disorders. See Genes
Hereditary nonpolyposis colorectal cancer, 94: 296
Heredity. See Genes
Heroin, 95: 247
Herpes, 95: 244-245
Heterochromatin, 93: 335
High blood pressure. See Hypertension
High-density lipoprotein, 95: 18-19, 291, **94:** 63-64, 310
Hip disorders, 95: 339, **94:** 145-147, 253-254, 301-302
Hip pads, 94: 241
Hippocratic Oath, 94: 218, 220
Hismanal (drug), 93: 79, 319
Histamine, 93: 72
Histoplasmosis, 94: 281

Histrelin acetate, 94: 282
HIV. See AIDS
Hives, 95: 250-251
HMO's. See Health maintenance organizations
Hodgkin's disease, 94: 210
Home safety, 95: 147-159
Homelessness, 93: 58 (il.), 63-64
Homeopathy, 94: 177 (il.), 179-180
Homework, 95: 272
Homicide, 94: 44, 50
Homosexuality, 95: 53, 243, **93:** 297
Hormone replacement therapy, 95: 301, **94:** 101, 124-128, 135-136, **93:** 179-180, 343-344
Hormones. See Glands and hormones
Hornet stings, 94: 29, 30
Horses, 94: 350
Hospices, 94: 261
Hospitals, 94: 286-287, **93:** 12-15, 252 (il.), 337-339
Hosts, 95: 50
Hot flashes, 94: 120-121, 124, 125, 129
HRT. See Hormone replacement therapy
H_2-blockers (drugs), 95: 94
Hughes, Howard, 94: 109-110
Human diploid cell vaccine, 94: 166-169
Human Genome Project, 95: 233, 299-300, **94:** 139, 229
Human growth hormone, 95: 226, **93:** 180-181, 254
Human immunodeficiency virus. See AIDS
Human leukocyte antigens, 95: 252, 253, **94:** 211, 316
Human papillomavirus, 94: 335-336, **93:** 357-358
Huntington's disease, 95: 230, 232, **94:** 298-299, **93:** 30
Hydrogenation, 95: 18, 19, **94:** 62-63, 321
Hydrophobia, 94: 161
Hydroxyurea, 93: 290
Hyperactivity, 95: 272-273
Hypercholesterolemia. See Familial hypercholesterolemia
Hyperkalemic periodic paralysis, 94: 350
Hypertension
artery disease, **94:** 100
diet, **94:** 66, **93:** 345
exercise, **93:** 325-326
eye disorders, **94:** 294
mind-body techniques, **94:** 184, 185
pregnancy, **93:** 360-361
stress, **95:** 317
Hyperthyroidism, 93: 157-162
Hypnosis, 95: 319, **94:** 184-185
Hypoglycemia, 95: 171-172, 277
Hypotension, 95: 194
Hypothalamus, 93: 45, 247, 297
Hypothyroidism, 93: 162-165, 336
Hysterectomy, 95: 344-345

I

Ibuprofen (drug), 95: 281, **93:** 46, 50
Imitrex (drug). See Sumatriptan succinate
Immune globulin, 93: 108
Immune system

alternative medicine, **94:** 183-184
aspirin, **93:** 53
drug resistance, **95:** 57
genetic medicine, **95:** 221, 228-229
influenza virus, **93:** 143-144, 150
inherited deficiency, **94:** 299-300
pathogen defenses, **95:** 50
sexually transmitted diseases, **93:** 372
sleep needs, **95:** 123-124
stress, **94:** 265
tissue rejection, **93:** 282-283
tuberculosis, **93:** 57
viral disease vaccines, **95:** 312
vitamins, **94:** 240 (il.)
see also **AIDS; Allergies and asthma; Antibodies; Rheumatoid arthritis; Vaccines**
Immunization. See Vaccines
Immunoglobulin E, 93: 72-76
Immunology. See Allergies and asthma; Antibodies; Vaccines
Immunotherapy, 95: 251, **93:** 80-81
Impaired glucose tolerance, 95: 166
In vitro fertilization, 95: 314
Income, and obesity, 95: 351-352
Indemnity insurance, 95: 20-22, **93:** 259-261
Indians, American. See Native Americans
Individual practice associations, 95: 23
Infants
blindness, **93:** 327
diet, **95:** 273 (il.)
hearing, **95:** 285-286, **94:** 24, 285
inborn knowledge, **94:** 274
lung disease, **93:** 362
premature, **94:** 323-324
safety, **95:** 331-332, 365-367
secondhand smoke, **94:** 341
water contamination, **93:** 91
see also **Birth defects; Child development; Day care; Pregnancy and childbirth**
Infection
contact lenses, **93:** 18
diabetes risk, **95:** 168
ear, **93:** 225-235
eye, **94:** 295
INFECTIOUS DISEASES, 95: 310-312, **94:** 313-315, **93:** 346-348
origin of new, **95:** 45-59
Inflammation, 93: 38, 41-42, 46
Influenza, 94: 314, **93:** 141-153
Inhalants (drugs), 94: 75, 76, 79, 245-246
Injuries. See Safety and specific injuries
Insect bites and stings, 94: 28-31
Insomnia, 95: 124-128, 242, **93:** 316-317
Insulin, and diabetes. See Diabetes
Insurance. See Financing medical care; Health care issues
Intelligence, 95: 273-274, **94:** 188, 193-194, 197
Interferon, 95: 281-282, **93:** 215
Interleukin (protein), 94: 275, **93:** 146, 215, 335-336
Intestinal parasite, 94: 279 (il.), 288, 329-331
Intrauterine devices, 95: 255
Intron A. See Alpha interferon
Iodine, 93: 156-157, 161-162, 166
Iron, 94: 322-323, 333, **93:** 42
Iron-deficiency anemia, 93: 42
Islet cell transplantation, 93: 309-310

Isoniazid (drug), **93**: 61-62, 66 (il.)
Itraconazole (drug), **94**: 281-282
IUD's. See **Intrauterine devices**

J

Jack-in-the-Box restaurants, **94**: 330
Jackson, Michael, **94**: 336, 337
Jaundice, **93**: 99, 104 (il.)
Jaw, **95**: 345 (il.), **94**: 275 (il.)
Jet lag, **94**: 21-23
Job-related injuries, **95**: 330
Jogging, **95**: 114. See **Running**
Johnson, Earvin (Magic), **93**: 276
Johnson, Sherry, **94**: 244
Joints. See **Arthritis and connective tissue disorders; Bone disorders**
JRA. See **Juvenile rheumatoid arthritis**
Justice, Principle of, **94**: 218
Juvenile rheumatoid arthritis, **95**: 56, **93**: 287

K

Kennedy, John F., **94**: 301
Keratoses, **95**: 335, 337, **93**: 282
Keratotomy, Trapezoidal, **93**: 328-329
Kessler, David A., **95**: 338-339
Kevorkian, Jack, **95**: 316, **94**: 224, 307-308
KIDNEY, **95**: 312-314, **94**: 315-316, **93**: 349-350
  aspirin, **93**: 42
  diabetes, **95**: 162, 167, 277, 314
  food poisoning, **94**: 330
  kidney stones, **95**: 313 (il.), **94**: 300, 316
  transplants, **95**: 313
  see also **Urinary disorders**
Knees, **94**: 253 (il.), 259, **93**: 285-286
Kruk, John, **95**: 268 (il.)
Kudzu, **95**: 246 (il.)
Kyphosis, **95**: 26

L

L-dopa (drug), **94**: 346
L-glutamate (protein), **93**: 298
Labor. See **Pregnancy and childbirth**
Labyrinth (ear), **95**: 190-201
Lactic acid, **95**: 115
Lakeberg twins, **95**: 305, 343
Langerhans cells, **94**: 265
Language, **95**: 202, 206, **93**: 306
  see also **Dyslexia**
Laparoscopy, **94**: 286, **93**: 378-379
Laser surgery, **94**: 96, 295
Latex allergy, **95**: 251
Laughing gas. See **Nitrous oxide**
LDL. See **Low-density lipoprotein**
Lead poisoning, **95**: 286-289, 330-331, **94**: 287, 331-332, **93**: 86-90, 322-323
Learning. See **Child development; Education**
Leg disorders, **95**: 124-127, 168
Legionnaire's disease, **95**: 46, 48
Lemieux, Mario, **94**: 210
Leprosy, **93**: 138-139
Leukemia, **94**: 201-215
  drugs, **93**: 214, 215
  electromagnetic fields, **94**: 289

gene, **94**: 212-215, 256-257
  radiation link, **95**: 289-290
  smoking, **95**: 339-340, **94**: 215, 341
  umbilical cord blood, **95**: 256
Leuprolide acetate (drug), **94**: 282
Levodopa (drug). See **L-dopa**
Levonorgestrel (drug). See **Norplant contraceptive**
Life expectancy, **94**: 118, 291, **93**: 168-170, 341 (il.)
"Light" foods, **94**: 35
Lightheadedness, **95**: 194
  see also **Dizziness**
Limbic system, **94**: 185
Lipoprotein (a), **95**: 343
  see also **High-density lipoprotein; Low-density lipoprotein**
Liposomes, **95**: 267
Listeriosis, **93**: 369
Lithium (drug), **95**: 183-185
Liver disorders. See **Cirrhosis; Familial hypercholesterolemia; Hepatitis; Liver transplants**
Liver spots, **93**: 275
Liver transplants, **95**: 345, **94**: 232, 346, **93**: 312
Living wills, **94**: 223, **93**: 23-26
Loofah sponges, **94**: 338
Lordosis, **95**: 25
Lou Gehrig's disease. See **Amyotrophic lateral sclerosis**
Lovastatin (drug), **95**: 307-308, **93**: 318 (il.)
Low-density lipoprotein
  artery/heart disease, **95**: 68, **94**: 88, 123, 309-310
  diabetes, **95**: 170
  exercise, **95**: 291
  food sources, **95**: 18-19, **94**: 66, 70, 320
LSD, **94**: 76, 78
Lumpectomy, **95**: 265, 343
Lung cancer, **95**: 111-125
  radon in water, **93**: 90
  smoking, **93**: 346
  vitamins, **95**: 66, 71-72, 324-325, 329
Lungs, **95**: 40, 111-114, **94**: 38
  see also **Allergies and asthma; Lung cancer; Pneumonia; Respiratory system; Tuberculosis**
Lupron (drug). See **Leuprolide acetate**
Lupus, **93**: 287
Luteinizing hormone, **93**: 247-248
Lyme disease, **95**: 46, 48, 56-59, 348, **93**: 348
Lymph nodes. See **Lymphatic system**
Lymphatic system, **94**: 202, 210, **93**: 113
Lymphocytes. See **White blood cells**
Lymphoma, **94**: 210, **93**: 380

M

Macular degeneration, **95**: 293
"Magic bullets." See **Monoclonal antibodies**
Magnetic resonance imaging, **94**: 92-93, 97 (il.), 147-148, 264, **93**: 187 (il.), 192, 254
Major histocompatibility complex (genes), **94**: 129-130, 284
Malaria, **93**: 196-209
Malignancy. See **Cancer**
Malpractice suits, **93**: 255-256, 271

Mammary cancer. See **Breast cancer**
Mammography, **95**: 267-268, **94**: 268-269
Managed-care plans, **95**: 20-23
Managed competition, **94**: 304
Mania, **95**: 178, 183
Manic-depressive illness. See **Bipolar disorder**
Mantoux test. See **Tuberculin skin test**
MAO inhibitors. See **Monoamine oxidase inhibitors**
Margarine, **95**: 19, **94**: 63, 321
Marijuana, **95**: 246, 247, **94**: 75-76, 78, 85, 245, **93**: 279
Masoprocol (drug), **94**: 282
Mastectomy, **95**: 265, 343-344
Mastoid cavity, **93**: 230-231
Mastoidectomy, **93**: 235
Maternal serum screening, **95**: 326-327
Mathematics, **94**: 271-272, 274
Measles, **95**: 310, **93**: 27-29
Meat, **95**: 321-323, 346, **94**: 57-62, 330-331, 332 (il.)
Medicaid
  health care costs, **93**: 252, 257, 331
  health care reform plans, **95**: 302, 305, **94**: 304, **93**: 268, 340
  provisions, **93**: 264
MEDICAL ETHICS, **95**: 314-316, **94**: 218-227
  AIDS, **94**: 234
  books, **94**: 261, **93**: 293
  genetic medicine, **95**: 236-237
  medical fraud, **95**: 265, **93**: 257, 271
  see also **Right to die**
Medicare
  health care costs, **93**: 253, 260, 271, 330-331
  health care reform plans, **95**: 303, **93**: 268
  provisions, **93**: 263
"Medigap" policies, **93**: 263-264
Meditation, **94**: 182 (il.), 185
Mefloquine (drug), **93**: 209
Meister, Joseph, **94**: 170
Melanoma, **95**: 299, 335, 336
Melatonin, **94**: 22, 302, **93**: 247
Memory, **95**: 202-208, 271-272, **94**: 241 (il.), **93**: 175, 305, 352-353
Menarche. See **Menstruation**
Mendel, Gregor Johann, **95**: 218
Ménière's disease, **95**: 193, 199, 201, **93**: 320
Meningitis, **95**: 286, **93**: 231
Menopause, **94**: 117-129
  bone health, **95**: 240
  book, **93**: 294
  exercise, **95**: 291
  Healy interview, **94**: 135-136
  osteoporosis, **94**: 322, **93**: 326
  pregnancy after, **95**: 314
  see also **Hormone replacement therapy**
Menstruation, **95**: 291-292, **94**: 118-120, 274, **93**: 238, 240-241, 248
MENTAL HEALTH, **95**: 316-320, **94**: 317-320, **93**: 350-354
  books, **93**: 294
  cancer patients, **93**: 222
  dizziness, **95**: 195
  insomnia, **95**: 124
  menopause, **94**: 122-123
  pet ownership, **95**: 14
  phone information, **95**: 41, **94**: 39

psychiatric drugs, **95:** 175-187
unfair tests, **95:** 315-316
violence, **94:** 52-53
see also **Brain and nervous system; Child development; Psychotherapy;** and specific disorders
Mepron (drug). See Atovaquone
Mercury, in dental fillings, 95: 275
Merozoites, 93: 199-202
Metabolism, 93: 156
Metastasis (cancer), 93: 113, 116, 212
Methamphetamine (drug), 94: 79
Methylprednisolone (drug), 95: 135, 139-140, **94:** 263, **93:** 329
Microbes, and disease, 95: 50
Microtubules, 93: 298-299
Midazolam (drug), 94: 286
Middle ear infection. See Otitis media
Mifepristone (drug). See RU-486
Migraine, 95: 193, **94:** 282-283
see also **Headache**
Miliary tuberculosis, 93: 59-60
Milk. See Dairy products
Milwaukee water contamination, 94: 279 (il.), 288, 329-331
Mind and body, 94: 183-185, 261
see also **Brain and nervous system**
Miscarriage, 95: 324
Mitral valve prolapse, 94: 308-309
Modified Burch colposuspension, 94: 346
Moisturizers, 95: 28-31
Monoamine oxidase (chemical), 95: 300
Monoamine oxidase inhibitors (drugs), 95: 180, 182, 183
Monoclonal antibodies, 93: 222-223, 283
Monounsaturated fat, 95: 18, 19, 170, **94:** 62-64
Mood disorders, 95: 177-178, 183-185
Mood stabilizers (drugs), 95: 181, 183-185
Moral center of brain, 95: 263-264
Morning sickness, 94: 325 (il.)
Mosquitoes, 95: 56, **94:** 28-30, **93:** 198-209
Moss, Kate, 95: 352 (il.)
Motion sickness, 95: 191-193
Motrin (drug). See Ibuprofen
Mount Pinatubo eruption, 94: 288
Moving, and child behavior, 95: 274
Mozart, Wolfgang Amadeus, 95: 273-274
MRI. See Magnetic resonance imaging
Multiple personality disorder, 95: 320
Multiple sclerosis, 95: 195, 281-282, 295-297, **94:** 264-265, **93:** 183-195, 295-296
Mummies, 93: 128-134
Mumps, 93: 27-28
Murder, 94: 49
see also **Violence**
Muscles
atherosclerosis, **94:** 90-91, 94 (il.)
balance, sense of, **95:** 191
bone replacement, **93:** 291-292
exercise benefits, **95:** 104-116
fibromyalgia, **93:** 286
posture, **95:** 24-27
vitamin E, **94:** 292
see also **Multiple sclerosis**
Music, and intelligence, 95: 273-274

Mutations, 95: 50-51, 57, 221-225
Mycobacterium avium complex, 94: 245, 281
Mycobacterium tuberculosis **(bacteria), 94:** 314-315, **93:** 56-60
Mycobutin (drug). See Rifabutin
Myelin, 94: 264, **93:** 184-185, 190-195
Myopia, 95: 294
Myotonic dystrophy, 93: 334
Myxedema. See Hypothyroidism

N

Nafarelin acetate (drug), 94: 282
Naltrexone (drug), 94: 246-247, 319
Napping, 95: 124, 128
Naproxen sodium (drug). See Aleve
National Institutes of Health, 94: 131-143
National Marrow Donor Program, 94: 256
Native Americans, 95: 45, 51, **94:** 313 (il.), **93:** 137-138, 281
Natural killer cells, 94: 183
Nausea, 95: 190, 198, **94:** 325 (il.)
Navajo Indians, 95: 45, 51, **94:** 313 (il.)
NDP (enzyme), 93: 298
Nearsightedness, 95: 294
Nerve cells, 95: 142-145, 179-185, **94:** 112-113, 262, **93:** 184, 296
Nervous system. See Brain and nervous system
Neural tube defects, 94: 324
Neurological disorders. See Brain and nervous system
Neurons. See Nerve cells
Neurontin (drug). See Gabapentin
Neuropathy, 95: 167, 262-263
Neurotransmitters, 95: 179-185, **94:** 52, 112, 265, 345
see also **Dopamine; Serotonin**
Neurotrophic growth factors, 93: 181
"New Age" medicine, 94: 178, 185
Nicotine, 95: 338-339, 341
see also **Smoking**
Nicotine inhalers, 94: 338-339
Nicotine nasal spray, 94: 339
Nicotine patches, 95: 278-280, **93:** 317, 374-375
Night sweats, 94: 121, 125
Night terrors, 95: 125
Nightmares, 95: 125, **93:** 351-352
Nitrates, 93: 88 (il.), 91-92
Nitric oxide, 94: 327, **93:** 297-298
Nitroglycerin, 94: 93-95
Nitrosamines, 93: 91
Nitrous oxide, 94: 73, 78
Nodules (thyroid), 93: 160, 165
Non-Hodgkin's lymphoma, 94: 210
Nonmalificence, 94: 218, 225
Non-REM sleep, 95: 120-121
Nonsteroidal anti-inflammatory drugs, 95: 91, 96, 100, **93:** 45-46
Norepinephrine, 95: 182, 183
Norplant contraceptive, 95: 254-255, **94:** 255 (il.)
Nuclear radiation. See Radiation
Nureyev, Rudolf, 94: 243
Nurses, 94: 155
Nursing homes, 95: 214-215, **93:** 65, 339
NUTRITION AND FOOD, 95: 321-325, **94:** 320-323, **93:** 354-358
aging, **93:** 170-171, 170-174, 178-179, 275

allergies, **94:** 251, **93:** 285
behavior, **93:** 383
birth defects, **94:** 324
books, **93:** 294
cancer prevention, **95:** 19, 61-73, 337, 346, **94:** 35, 64-66, **93:** 125, 303, 341, 354-355
Cushing's syndrome, **94:** 302
diabetes, **95:** 168-170, 276-277
drug side effects, **94:** 283
early humans, **93:** 135-138
exercise benefits, **93:** 324-325
Food Guide Pyramid, **94:** 57-71
food poisoning, **94:** 330-331, **93:** 369
labeling, **95:** 16, **94:** 32-35
phone information, **95:** 41, **94:** 39
stroke, **95:** 343, **94:** 71, 343 (il.)
sugar and hyperactivity, **95:** 272-273
see also **Calcium; Cholesterol; Fat, Dietary; Heart disease; Pesticides; Weight control**
Nystagmus, 95: 194, 199-200

O

"Oat cell" cancer, 93: 116-119
Obesity. See Weight control
Obsessive-compulsive disorder, 95: 178, **94:** 103-115, **93:** 354
Obstetrics. See Pregnancy and childbirth
OCD. See Obsessive-compulsive disorder
Octreotide (hormone), 95: 300-301
Oils, in diet, 95: 13-19, 343, **94:** 58-64
see also **Fat, Dietary**
OKY-046 (drug), 95: 249
Olive oil, 95: 19
Omega-3 fatty acids, 95: 19, 343
Omeprazole (drug), 95: 95
Oncogenes, 94: 296
Operations. See Surgery
Opiates, 94: 319
Optic neuritis, 95: 295-296, **93:** 329
Orbital cortex, 94: 111
Oregon health plan, 94: 237, 304
Organ donation, 94: 221, 230-232
Organ transplants. See Transplants
Oriental sore (disease), 93: 373-374
Orlistat (drug), 95: 351
Orthostatic hypotension, 95: 194, 200
Ossicles, 93: 226
Osteoarthritis, 94: 252, **93:** 41, 134, 285-286
Osteoclasts, 93: 335-336
Osteoporosis
ancient humans, **93:** 135, 137 (il.)
calcium in diet, **94:** 322
delayed puberty, **93:** 290-291
estrogen research, **93:** 335-336
exercise, **95:** 291, **94:** 291-292, **93:** 170, 326
genetic basis, **95:** 257-258
Healy interview, **94:** 132, 133
hyperthyroidism, **93:** 164-165
menopause, **94:** 123-125
phone information, **95:** 41, **94:** 39
Otitis media, 94: 284-285, **93:** 225-235
Otologists, 94: 24
Otorhinolaryngologists, 94: 24
Otosclerosis, 94: 147
Otoscope, 93: 230 (il.)
Ovarian cancer, 94: 137, 270, 283-284, **93:** 215

Ovaries, 94: 118-119, 93: 247-248, 335-336
Ovulation, 93: 240-241
Oxidation, in cells, 95: 62
Oxygen radicals. See Free radicals
Ozonation (water treatment), 93: 92
Ozone depletion, 94: 288-289

P

Pacific yew tree, 94: 281 (il.), 283, 93: 298-299
Pain, 95: 268-269, 94: 181-182, 93: 41, 44-45
Pain relievers, 95: 281
Paleopathology, 93: 127-139
Palmtop computers, 94: 155
Pancreas, 95: 162, 163, 173, 277 (il.)
Paralysis, 95: 132-145, 94: 263, 350
Paraplegia, 95: 137
Parathyroid hormone, 94: 301
Parkinson disease, 95: 41, 187, 94: 39, 345-346
Passive-aggressive personality disorder, 95: 320
Pasteur, Louis, 94: 170
Pathogens, 95: 50-51
Patient rights. See Medical ethics
Patient Self-Determination Act, 94: 223-224, 93: 26
Pauling, Linus, 95: 221
PCP (drug), 94: 76
Peanuts, 94: 251
Penis, 93: 241-243
Peptic ulcers. See Ulcers
Perimenopause, 94: 118
Periodontal disease, 95: 276, 94: 275, 93: 308-309
PerioGlas (dental material), 95: 276
Peripheral nervous system, 95: 135, 94: 161
Persian Gulf War, 95: 305, 93: 373
Persistent vegetative state, 94: 222
Pertussis, 94: 314, 93: 27, 347
Pesticides, 95: 287, 288-289, 94: 334
PET scans. See Positron emission tomography
Pets. See Veterinary medicine
p53 (gene), 95: 228
Phencyclidine (drug). See PCP
Phobia, 95: 178
Phonics, 93: 306-307
Phonoangiography, 94: 93
Photodynamic therapy, 93: 123-124
Physical examinations, 94: 36
Physical fitness. See Exercise and fitness
Physical therapy, 95: 27, 140-141, 201, 210 (il.)
Physicians
    AIDS transmission, 93: 276-277
    fees, 94: 306
    health care history, 93: 258
    managed-care plans, 95: 22-23
    medical ethics, 94: 218-219, 224
    minority groups, 95: 305
    primary care, 94: 307, 93: 271
    training costs, 93: 254-255
    women, 94: 143
Pituitary gland, 93: 156, 158 (il.), 163, 247
Placebos, 94: 175
Plagues. See Infectious diseases

Plaque
    arterial, 95: 306-307, 94: 88-91, 345, 93: 171, 318 (il.)
    brain, 95: 211, 93: 184
    dental, 93: 308-309
Plasmodia, 93: 199-203
Plastic surgery, 94: 346
Platelets, 94: 202, 206, 93: 48-49
Play-or-pay health plans, 93: 268-269
Pneumonia, 94: 281, 93: 133, 142, 148-149, 346-347
PNS. See Peripheral nervous system
Point-of-service plans, 95: 22
Poisoning, 95: 151-152
    see also Asbestos; Carbon monoxide poisoning; Lead poisoning; Nutrition and food; Pesticides
Polio, 95: 310
Pollen. See Hay fever
Pollution. See Air pollution; Environmental health; Water pollution
Polyglycolic acid, 93: 292
Polymerase chain reaction, 95: 219, 93: 130-131
Polyps
    colon, 95: 269-270
    nasal, 93: 76
Polysomnography, 94: 328
Polyunsaturated fat, 95: 18-19, 94: 62-63
Popcorn, 95: 324
Portal vein, 93: 312, 314
Positron emission tomography, 94: 111, 147, 320, 93: 296 (il.)
Post-traumatic stress disorder, 95: 318-320, 94: 319-320
Posture, 95: 24-27
Poverty, and violence, 93: 48
Power of attorney, 93: 24-26
PPO's. See Preferred provider organizations
Prader-Willi syndrome, 93: 332-333
Prednisone (drug), 93: 329
Preeclampsia, 93: 52-53
Preferred provider organizations, 95: 20, 22, 93: 261-262
PREGNANCY AND CHILDBIRTH, 95: 325-327, 94: 323-326, 93: 359-362
    AIDS, 95: 243 (il.), 325
    aspirin, 93: 52-53
    caffeine and miscarriage, 95: 324
    diabetes, 95: 164
    ethical issues, 95: 314
    gestational diabetes, 94: 276-277
    hormones, 93: 336-337
    menstruation, 94: 118
    psychiatric drugs, 95: 185
    rheumatoid arthritis, 95: 252-253
    smoking risk, 95: 340-341
    substance abuse, 93: 280-281
    sudden infant death, 93: 365
    see also Birth defects; Child development; Genetic screening; Infants; Premature infants
Prehistoric people. See Paleopathology
Premature infants, 94: 323-324, 93: 327
Prevention Marketing Initiative, 95: 333
Privacy, 94: 225-229
Pro-MED (program), 95: 59
Progesterone (hormone), 94: 118, 125, 126, 254, 93: 180, 248
Progressive relaxation, 94: 185

Proscar (drug), 95: 347, 93: 319, 379 (il.)
Prostaglandins, 93: 44-46, 48
Prostate cancer
    diet, 95: 65, 321-323, 346, 94: 64-65
    drug, 95: 347
    screening, 95: 266-267, 94: 269-270, 93: 378-379
    vasectomy risk, 94: 347-348
Prostate gland, 95: 261, 94: 347 (il.), 348, 93: 319
    see also Prostate cancer
Prostate-specific antigen, 95: 266, 94: 269-270, 348
Protein
    aging, 93: 177-178
    diet, 95: 312-313
    synthesis by genes, 95: 218-222, 226, 232
Protozoa, 93: 200-202
Prozac (drug), 95: 175, 183, 317, 94: 318
Psoriasis, 95: 335-336
PSTD. See Post-traumatic stress disorder
Psychiatry. See Mental health
Psychogenic vertigo, 95: 195
Psychological disorders. See Mental health; Psychotherapy; Stress
Psychoneuroimmunology, 94: 183
Psychosis, 95: 179
Psychotherapy, 95: 127-128, 319, 94: 113-115
Puberty, 93: 237-249
    bone disorders, 93: 290-291
    delayed, 94: 302
    delinquent girls, 94: 273-274
    precocious, 94: 282
Public health. See Health care issues; Health policy
Pushups, 95: 111, 112

Q

Quadriplegia, 95: 137
Quick Medical Reference (program), 94: 150
Quill, Timothy, 94: 224
Quinine, 93: 205-206
Quinlan, Karen Ann, 94: 222
Quinolones, 93: 66

R

RA. See Rheumatoid arthritis
Rabies, 94: 159-171, 93: 381
Raccoons, Rabies in, 94: 163, 171, 93: 381
Radar guns, and cancer, 93: 302 (il.)
Radiation, 95: 289-290, 314-315, 93: 113, 177
    see also Radon; Ultraviolet radiation; X rays
Radiation therapy, 95: 344, 94: 209-211, 93: 123, 212, 213, 217-221
Radon, 93: 89 (il.), 90-91, 113, 122 (il.), 124-125
Ranitidine (drug), 93: 314
Rape, 94: 45, 228-229
Ras (gene), 93: 299-301
Ray, Ricky, 94: 243
RDA's. See Recommended Dietary Allowances

RDS. See **Respiratory distress syndrome**
Reading, 93: 306-307
  see also **Dyslexia**, **94:** 254-255
Reality (condom), 95: 254-255
Receptors, Cell, 95: 179-182, 248
Recessive genes, 95: 220 (il.), 223, 230
Recombinant DNA technology. See **Genetic engineering**
Recommended Dietary Allowances, 95: 70, 73, **93:** 355
Rectal cancer, 95: 317-319, **94:** 266-267
Red blood cells, 94: 202, **93:** 200 (il.), 202-203, 206
Reflexology, 94: 182
Regeneration, of spinal cord, 95: 141-145
Relaxation therapy, 95: 127, **94:** 185
REM sleep, 95: 120-121, 129-131
Remission, of leukemia, 94: 207, 209
Reno, Janet, 95: 302 (il.)
Research, on human beings, 95: 314-315, **94:** 233-235
Respiratory distress syndrome, 94: 327, **93:** 362
RESPIRATORY SYSTEM, 95: 328-329, **94:** 327-328, **93:** 362-364
  exercise benefits, **95:** 111-114
  see also **Allergies and asthma; Influenza; Legionnaire's disease; Lungs; Pneumonia; Sleep apnea; Smoking; Tuberculosis**
Response prevention, 94: 113
Restriction enzymes, 95: 219, 226, 233
Retina, 95: 166-167, **94:** 292, 295, **93:** 328 (il.)
  see also **Cataracts**
Retinitis pigmentosa, 94: 292
Retinopathy, Diabetic. See **Diabetic retinopathy**
Retinopathy of prematurity, 93: 327
Reye's syndrome, 93: 43, 148
Rheumatic fever, 93: 40
Rheumatoid arthritis, 95: 252-254, **94:** 253, **93:** 41, 134-135, 285
  juvenile, **93:** 287
RICE guideline, 95: 116
Rifabutin (drug), 94: 245, 281
Rifampin (drug), 93: 62
Right to die, 94: 221-224, **93:** 342
  see also **Suicide**
Risperidone (drug), 95: 316
Rituals. See **Obsessive-compulsive disorder**
Robbery, 94: 45
Robots, 94: 145-147, 150 (il.), **93:** 274 (il.)
Rodents, and disease, 95: 51-52, **94:** 314
Romanov family, 95: 221 (il.)
RU-486 (drug), 95: 255, **94:** 255
Running, 94: 252, 291

S

Safe Drinking Water Act, 93: 85-86
SAFETY, 95: 330-333, **94:** 329-334, **93:** 365-370
  drinking water, **93:** 83-95
  elderly drivers, **93:** 274

  exercise, **95:** 114-116
  home, **95:** 147-159
  phone information, **95:** 41, **94:** 39
  psychiatric drugs, **95:** 183
  sleep deprivation, **95:** 123
Saliva, and rabies, 94: 160-161, 164
Salmeterol (drug), 95: 249
Salt. See **Sodium**
Sand fly, 93: 373-374
Sanitariums, 93: 60, 62
Saturated fat, 95: 17-19, 324, **94:** 32-35, 62-63, 321
Scalds, 95: 36, 39
Scheuermann kyphosis, 94: 257-258
Schizophrenia, 95: 179, 186-187, 316
Schwann cells, 95: 144
Scleroderma, 93: 372-373
Sclerotherapy, 93: 312
Scoliosis, 95: 26, 258, **93:** 244
Screening tests, 94: 36-37
Scrotum, 93: 243
Seafood, 95: 251 (il.), **93:** 356-357
Sealant, Dental, 93: 308
Seismocardiogram, 93: 342 (il.)
Seizure, Epileptic. See **Epilepsy**
Seldane (drug), 95: 309, **93:** 79, 319
Selenium (mineral), 95: 65-66
Self-esteem, 94: 77, 272-273, **93:** 245-246
Semen, 93: 243
Senescence, 93: 335
Senility, 93: 53
Serotonin, 95: 182-183, **94:** 52, 53, 112-113
Serotonin re-uptake inhibitors (drugs), 95: 180, 182-183, **94:** 112-113
Set point theory, 94: 351-352
Severe combined immune deficiency disease, 94: 299-300
Sex cells, 95: 218-219, 222
Sex education, 95: 334
Sex hormones, 95: 297
  see also **Estrogen; Testosterone**
Sex-linked disorders, 95: 220 (il.), 223-224, **94:** 189, 300, **93:** 30
Sexual maturation. See **Puberty**
SEXUALLY TRANSMITTED DISEASES, 95: 333-335, **94:** 334-336, **93:** 370-372
  antibiotics, **93:** 317-318
  condoms, **94:** 254, 334-335
  phone information, **95:** 41, **94:** 39
  women, **94:** 132
  see also **AIDS**
Shellfish allergies, 95: 251 (il.)
Shiatsu, 95: 180 (il.), 182
Shoes, for runners, 94: 291
Shootings. See **Firearms**
Shoulder, Dislocated, 94: 258-259
Shyness, 93: 245
Siamese twins, 95: 305, 343, **94:** 344
Sickle cell anemia, 95: 221, 224 (il.), **94:** 256 (il.), **93:** 30, 290
"Sickness funds," 93: 266-267
SIDS. See **Sudden infant death syndrome**
Silicone-gel breast implants, 93: 366-367
Silver amalgam dental fillings, 95: 275
Simian immunodeficiency virus, 95: 53, **93:** 278
Sinuses, 95: 328 (il.)
SIV. See **Simian immunodeficiency virus**

Skeletal muscles, 95: 104-105
SKIN, 95: 335-337, **94:** 336-338, **93:** 372-374
  burns, **95:** 36-39
  computer diagnosis, **94:** 152
  menopause, **94:** 121
  moisturizers, **95:** 28-31
  sun damage, **94:** 282, 337 (il.)
Skin cancer
  diet, **95:** 337
  gene therapy, **95:** 265-267
  sun exposure, **95:** 335, **94:** 338, **93:** 324, 334 (il.), 372 (il.)
  see also **Lymphoma; Melanoma**
Sleep, 95: 119-131
  elderly, **95:** 242
  infant safety, **93:** 365-366
  jet lag, **94:** 21
  menopause, **94:** 121
  see also **Insomnia; Nightmares**
Sleep apnea, 95: 125, 128-129, **94:** 265-266, 327-328
Sleep restriction therapy, 95: 128
Sleeping pills, 95: 129
Sleepwalking, 95: 125
Smallpox, 95: 310-312
Smoke detectors, 95: 155-158
Smokeless tobacco, 94: 339-341
SMOKING, 95: 337-341, **94:** 338-342, **93:** 374-377
  advertising, **93:** 364, 375-377
  artery/heart disease, **95:** 341, **94:** 100, 101, **93:** 345-346, 377
  asthma, **94:** 250
  back pain, **95:** 253
  cancer, **95:** 337, **93:** 111-112, 124-125
  canine lung cancer, **93:** 380 (il.)
  deaths, **93:** 280, 375
  eye disorders, **95:** 242, 293, 294
  home safety, **95:** 154
  leukemia, **94:** 215, 341
  nicotine patch, **93:** 317, 374-375
  secondhand smoke, **95:** 340-341, **94:** 340-341, **93:** 114 (il.), 345-346, 377
  stroke, **95:** 341, **94:** 341-343
  students, **95:** 247, 337, **94:** 290-291, **93:** 120, 307
  ulcerative colitis, **95:** 279
  ulcers, **95:** 97, 101
Snare, Surgical, 94: 344 (il.)
Snoring, 95: 128-129
Snuff, 94: 339
Soap, 95: 30
Social learning theory, 94: 49-50
Sodium, 94: 32-35, **93:** 345
Sonograms. See **Ultrasound**
Spanish flu, 93: 147
Specific acceptance, 93: 350
Spectacle blur, 93: 17
Sperm, 94: 326
Spider bites, 94: 28-31
Spina bifida, 94: 324, **93:** 322
Spinal column, 95: 135-137
Spinal tap, 93: 192
Spine disorders
  back pain, **95:** 257
  chiropractic, **94:** 180-181
  posture, **95:** 24-27
  scoliosis, **95:** 26, 258, **93:** 244
  spinal cord injuries, **95:** 132-145, **94:** 263
Spirochete (bacteria), 95: 58
Spleen, 94: 202
Spock, Benjamin, 95: 75-87
Sporanox (drug). See **Itraconazole**

Sporozoites, **93:** 199, 201-202
Sports. See **Athletics**
Sprains, 95: 116
Squamous cell cancer, 95: 335, **93:** 116-119
Stab wounds, 94: 286
STD's. See **Sexually transmitted diseases**
Stem cells, 95: 229, **94:** 202, **93:** 289
Stents, 94: 99-101, **93:** 379-380
Stepparenting, 95: 83-85
Steroids. See **Corticosteroids**
Stillbirth, 94: 323-324
Still's disease. See **Juvenile rheumatoid arthritis**
Stimulants, 94: 79
Stimulus control therapy, 95: 127-128
Stomach, 93: 42, 45, 145, 310, 313
   see also **Ulcers**
Stomach cancer, 95: 98, **94:** 266-267, **93:** 314
Strains, Muscle, 95: 116
Strains, Viral, 93: 143-144
Strength, Body, 95: 110, 117
Streptococcus (bacteria), 95: 57, 310 (il.), **94:** 326, **93:** 346
Streptomycin (drug), 93: 61-62
Stress
   alternative medicine, **94:** 177-178, 182-185
   artery disease, **94:** 100, 101
   cancer, **95:** 317-319
   colds, **93:** 352
   Graves' disease, **93:** 160
   hypertension, **95:** 317
   immunity, **94:** 265
   insomnia, **95:** 124-127
   pets and health, **95:** 14
   trauma, **95:** 318-320
   ulcers, **95:** 89, 90, 92, 97
   violence causes, **94:** 52
Stretching, 95: 106-110, 114-115
STROKE, 95: 342-343, **94:** 342-344, **93:** 377-378
   aspirin, **95:** 342-343, **94:** 134, **93:** 49-51, 318-319
   atherosclerosis, **94:** 89, 94 (il.)
   book, **95:** 261
   dementia, **94:** 240
   depression, **93:** 350
   diabetes, **95:** 162, 167
   diet, **95:** 343, **94:** 71, 343 (il.)
   dizziness, **95:** 195
   drug prevention, **94:** 343, **93:** 318-319
   smoking risk, **95:** 341, **94:** 341-343
Substance abuse. See **Alcohol and drug abuse**
Sudden infant death syndrome, 95: 331, **93:** 365
Sugar, 95: 272-273, **94:** 57-58
Sugar, Blood. See **Diabetes**
Suicide, 95: 316, **94:** 224, 307-308, **93:** 246, 368
   see also **Right to die**
Sulfonylureas (proteins), 95: 171
Sulforaphane (chemical), 95: 65, 323, **93:** 354-355
Sumatriptan succinate (drug), 94: 282-283
Sunburn, 95: 37
Sunscreens, 95: 30, 335
Superoxide dismutase, 94: 262-264, 299
Support groups, 95: 320
Supprelin (drug). See **Histrelin acetate**

Surfactant, 93: 327, 362
SURGERY, 95: 343-346, **94:** 344-346
   atherosclerosis, **94:** 95-101
   bone disorders, **94:** 257-260
   cancer, **95:** 266, 343-346, **93:** 123-124, 213
   chest, **93:** 364 (il.)
   computer assistance, **95:** 344 (il.), **94:** 145-147, 151 (il.)
   ear, **93:** 320
   eye, **95:** 32-35, 294-295, 344 (il.), **94:** 293-295
   eyelid, **93:** 327-328
   plastic, **94:** 346
   see also **Coronary angiography; Coronary bypass surgery; Laser surgery; Transplants**
Surgical menopause, 94: 120
Sygen (drug). See **GM-1 ganglioside**
Synarel (drug). See **Nafarelin acetate**
Syphilis, 94: 233, **93:** 138-139, 308-309
Systemic lupus erythematosus, 93: 287

T

T cells, 94: 300, **93:** 191 (il.), 194-195, 284
Tacrine hydrochloride (drug), 95: 282
Tamoxifen (drug), 95: 270-271, **94:** 136-137, **93:** 300-301
Tanning (skin), 94: 337-338
Tardive dyskinesia, 95: 187
Taxol (drug), 95: 313-314, **94:** 137, 270, 281 (il.), 283-284, **93:** 298-299
Tay-Sachs disease, 95: 230, **93:** 30
TB. See **Tuberculosis**
Teen-agers. See **Adolescents**
Tele-Nurse (software), 94: 157
Teleconferencing, 94: 151-152
Telephone
   cellular phone safety, **94:** 333
   health information, **95:** 40-41, **94:** 38-39
Television, 95: 79-80, **94:** 50, 54-55, 271 (il.)
Telomeres, 93: 335
Tendinitis, 95: 116
Tendons, 95: 104, 116
Terfenadine (drug). See **Seldane**
Terminal illness. See **Hospices**
Testicular cancer, 95: 268 (il.)
Testosterone, 94: 52, **93:** 170, 248-249
Tetanus, 94: 314
Tetramune (vaccine), 94: 314
Tetraplegia, 95: 137
Thalassemia, 95: 256-257
Thalidomide, 94: 133
Thallium scan, 94: 92
Theophylline (drug), 94: 328
Therapeutic touch, 94: 182
Thorazine (drug). See **Chlorpromazine**
Thromboembolic disease, 94: 127
Thrombopoietin (protein), 95: 256
Thyroid cancer, 95: 301, **93:** 165
Thyroid gland, 95: 261, **93:** 155-167
Thyroid-stimulating hormone, 95: 301, **93:** 156
Thyroiditis, 93: 167
Thyrotropin (hormone), 93: 336
Thyroxine (hormone), 93: 156
TIA's. See **Transient ischemic attacks**
Tick bites, 95: 15, 58-59, 348, **94:** 29-31

Ticlopidine (drug), 94: 343, **93:** 318-319
Tics, 94: 110
Tinnitus, 95: 284-285, **93:** 42
Tissue transplants. See **Transplants**
Tobacco. See **Smokeless tobacco; Smoking**
Toothbrushes, 94: 275
Tourette syndrome, 94: 110
Toxic shock syndrome, 95: 46, 48, 57
Toys, 95: 79-80, **94:** 249 (il.)
Traffic lights, and elderly, 95: 242
Trans fatty acids, 95: 18, 19, **94:** 63, 321
Transforming growth factor beta, 94: 252, 316
Transient ischemic attacks, 95: 195, **94:** 89, 93, **93:** 49-50, 318-319
Transplants, 94: 230-232
   bone marrow, **95:** 256, 257, **94:** 209-212, 214 (il.), 256, **93:** 289
   heart, **95:** 345
   islet cell, **93:** 309-310
   kidney, **95:** 313
   liver, **95:** 345, **94:** 232, 346, **93:** 312
   repeat, **95:** 345-346
   tissue rejection, **93:** 282-283, 350
   umbilical tissue, **95:** 256
Trapezoidal keratotomy, 93: 328-329
Trauma, and stress. See **Post-traumatic stress disorder**
Traveling, 93: 19-22
Treadmill test, 94: 92, 97 (il.)
Treponema, 93: 139
Tretinoin (drug), 93: 275
Trichotillomania, 94: 108
Triglycerides, 95: 12
Trihalomethanes (chemicals), 94: 288, **93:** 92
Tsongas, Paul E., 94: 210
Tubal ligation, 95: 255
Tubercles (scar tissue), 93: 57
Tuberculin skin test, 93: 61, 63
Tuberculosis, 95: 57, 328, **94:** 314-315, **93:** 55-67, 133-134
Tumor necrosis factor, 95: 230, **93:** 302
Tumor suppressor genes, 95: 225, 228, 299, **94:** 296
Tumors, Benign, 94: 347 (il.), 348, **93:** 112-113, 138 (il.), 212, 275
Tumors, Cancerous. See **Cancer**
Tuskegee Study, 94: 233
Tylenol, 93: 46
Tympanic membrane, 93: 226, 231
Tympanometry, 93: 231, 234 (il.)
Tympanostomy tube, 93: 233-235
Typhoid, 93: 19-20

U

Ulcerative colitis, 95: 278-280, **94:** 278-279
Ulcerative keratitis, 95: 293-294, **94:** 295
Ulcers
   duodenal, **95:** 89-101, **94:** 280, **93:** 314
   gastric, **95:** 89-101, **93:** 42, 314
Ultrafast computerized tomography, 94: 92-93
Ultrasonography. See **Ultrasound**
Ultrasound, 95: 325-326, 327 (il.), **94:** 93, **93:** 218

Ultraviolet radiation, 93: 324, 334 (il.), 372-373
Umbilical cord tissue transplant, 95: 256
Unemployment, and violence, 94: 48
Uniform Anatomical Gift Act, 94: 230
Uniform Determination of Death Act, 94: 221
Unsaturated fat, 95: 17-19
Urethra, 94: 121
Urinary disorders, 95: 137, 346-347, **94:** 121, 346, **93:** 379-380
Urine spraying, by cats, 94: 348
UROLOGY, 95: 346-347, **94:** 347-348, **93:** 378-380
  see also **Prostate gland; Urinary disorders**
Ursodeoxycholic acid, 95: 280
Urticaria. See Hives
Uterine cancer, 94: 125, 136, **93:** 219, 384
  see also **Cervical cancer; Endometrial cancer**
Uterus, 95: 344-345, **93:** 44-45
Utricle, 94: 284
UV. See Ultraviolet radiation

V

Vaccines
  AIDS, **95:** 245, **94:** 245, **93:** 278
  child immunizations, **95:** 310, **94:** 313-314, **93:** 27-29
  genetic engineering, **95:** 226-228
  hepatitis, **93:** 108-109
  influenza, **93:** 149-153
  Lyme disease in dogs, **95:** 348
  malaria, **93:** 209
  pneumonia, **93:** 346-347
  rabies, **94:** 166-171, **93:** 381-382
  travel immunization, **93:** 19
  tuberculosis, **93:** 62
  viral diseases, **95:** 312
  see also **Allergies and asthma**
Valium (drug), 95: 186, **94:** 18
Vasectomy, 95: 255, **94:** 347-348, **93:** 288
Vectors, 95: 50
Vegetables
  cancer prevention, **95:** 61-73, 323
  Food Guide Pyramid, **94:** 57-61, 66-67
  infant diet, **95:** 273 (il.)
  vision, **95:** 293 (il.)
  see also **Pesticides**
Veins, 93: 312, 314
Venereal disease. See AIDS; Sexually transmitted diseases
Venlafaxine hydrochloride (drug), 95: 316-317
Venom, Insect, 94: 29-31
Ventricular fibrillation, 93: 344-345
Vertigo, 95: 190-201
Vestibular system, 95: 190-201
VETERINARY MEDICINE, 95: 348-349, **94:** 348-350, **93:** 380-382
  pets and health, **95:** 12-15, **94:** 350
  rabies, **94:** 159-171
  see also **Cats; Dogs**
Violence, 94: 43-55
  genetic basis, **95:** 299 (il.), 300
  hospital, **94:** 286-287

media, **95:** 79-80, 302 (il.), **94:** 50, 54-55
Virtual reality, 95: 344 (il.), **94:** 156 (il.)
Viruses
  feline calicivirus, **94:** 349
  Four Corners illness, **95:** 312, 328-329, **94:** 314
  gene therapy, **95:** 229, 267
  hepatitis, **93:** 99-105
  herpes, **95:** 244-245
  infectious diseases, **95:** 45-53
  influenza, **93:** 142-146
  rabies, **94:** 160-161, 166-169
  smallpox, **95:** 310-312
  vaccine technology, **95:** 226, 312
  see also **AIDS; Hantaviruses**
Vision. See Eye and vision
Vitamin A
  cancer, **95:** 63, 73, **94:** 135
  heart disease, **94:** 135
  vision, **94:** 292-293
Vitamin B, 95: 66
Vitamin C
  aging, **93:** 176
  cancer, **95:** 63-65, 69-73, **94:** 135
  heart disease, **95:** 69, **93:** 358
  sources, **95:** 64, **94:** 71
Vitamin D
  aging, **93:** 176
  bone health, **95:** 240, 257-258, **94:** 301
  cancer, **95:** 67-71
  sources, **95:** 64
Vitamin E
  aging, **93:** 176
  cancer, **95:** 63-66, 69-72, 309, 324, 329, **94:** 135
  exercise, **94:** 292
  heart disease, **95:** 68, 72, **94:** 135, 320-321
  menopause, **94:** 128
  sources, **95:** 64, **94:** 71
  vision, **94:** 292
Vitamins
  birth defects, **94:** 324
  cancer, **95:** 61-73
  dietary guidelines, **94:** 70-71
  elderly, **95:** 240, 241, **94:** 240 (il.)
  Healy interview, **94:** 135
  see also specific vitamins
Vitiligo, 94: 336-337
Volatile organic chemicals, 93: 88 (il.), 91-92
Vomiting, 95: 191, 198

W

Waist-to-hip ratio, 94: 350
Walking, 95: 27, 114, 115, 247, **93:** 174
Wanzer, Sydney H., 94: 224
Warfarin (drug), 95: 307, **94:** 343
Wasp stings, 94: 28-31
Water
  chlorinated, **94:** 288, **93:** 84-85, 92, 347-348
  fluoridated, **93:** 92, 94
  safety, **94:** 331, **93:** 83-95, 347-348
Water pollution, 93: 83-95
  intestinal parasite, **94:** 279 (il.), 288, 329-331
  lead, **94:** 287, 331-332, **93:** 86-90
  travel tips, **93:** 21
Watson, James D., 95: 218

WEIGHT CONTROL, 95: 350-352, **94:** 350-352, **93:** 382-384
  arthritis, **93:** 285
  diabetes, **95:** 164, 168-172, **94:** 278, **93:** 310
  heart/artery disease, **94:** 100
  low calorie diets, **93:** 355-357
  see also **Eating disorders**
Weightlifting, 95: 110
Whiplash, 95: 193
White blood cells, 95: 228-229, **94:** 183, 202, **93:** 70, 72, 284, 295-296, 303-304
  see also **Leukemia; T cells**
Whooping cough. See Pertussis
Wofford, Harris, 93: 268
Womb. See Uterus
Women
  AIDS, **94:** 243-244, **93:** 277
  alcoholism, **94:** 247-248
  Alzheimer's disease and estrogen, **95:** 242
  aspirin, **93:** 44-45
  bone disorders, **95:** 240, **94:** 123-126, 240-241, 259 (il.), 301-302, **93:** 135, 290-291
  books, **93:** 294
  breast implants, **93:** 366-367
  exercise, **95:** 291-292
  Healy interview, **94:** 131-143
  heart disease, **95:** 308-309, **94:** 122, 132-136, 312, **93:** 377
  research on humans, **94:** 234
  sexually transmitted diseases, **95:** 334-335
  stroke and smoking, **94:** 342-343
  thyroid disorders, **93:** 163, 167
  urological disorders, **95:** 346-347, **94:** 346, **93:** 380
  vaginal condom, **94:** 254-255, **93:** 287-288
  violence, **94:** 43, 45, 49, 51
  see also **Birth control; Breast cancer; Estrogen; Hormone replacement therapy; Menopause; Menstruation; Pregnancy and childbirth; Sex-linked disorders**
Women's Health Initiative, 94: 137-142

X

X rays, 94: 93, 97 (il.), **93:** 61, 65 (il.)
  see also **Radiation therapy**
Xenografts, 94: 232
Xerosis, 95: 28-31
XSCID (disorder), 94: 300
Xylitol (drug), 94: 275-276

Y

YAG laser capsulotomy, 94: 295
Yellow fever, 93: 19
Yew tree. See Pacific yew tree

Z

Zalcitabine (drug). See Dideoxycytidine
Zidovudine (drug). See AZT
Zollinger-Ellison syndrome, 95: 91-92
Zonalon (drug), 95: 250-251

Acknowledgments

The publishers of *The World Book Health & Medical Annual* gratefully acknowledge the courtesy of the following artists, photographers, publishers, institutions, agencies, and corporations for the illustrations in this volume. Credits should read from top to bottom, left to right on their respective pages. All entries marked with an asterisk (*) denote illustrations created exclusively for *The World Book Health & Medical Annual*. All maps, charts, and diagrams were prepared by *The World Book Health & Medical Annual* staff unless otherwise noted.

12 Blair Seitz, Photo Researchers
16 Yoav Levy, Phototake
21 Will and Deni McIntyre, Photo Researchers
28 Chris Harvey, Tony Stone Images
32 Biophoto Associates/Science Source from Photo Researchers
33 Richard Megna, Fundamental Photographs
34 Hank Morgan, Rainbow
44 John Lambert*
47 Centers for Disease Control and Prevention; UPI/Bettmann; AP/Wide World; Yoav Levy, Phototake
49 Centers for Disease Control and Prevention; CNRI/SPL from Photo Researchers
51 Centers for Disease Control and Prevention; Russell C. Johnson, University of Minnesota
54 M. Courtney-Clark, Photo Researchers; Jacques Jangoux, Tony Stone Images; Goddard Space Flight Center
55 Richard H. Smith, F.P.G.
57 CNRI/SPL from Photo Researchers
58 Centers for Disease Control and Prevention
60-61 Ralph Brunke*
63 Rose Zgodzinski
64 Ralph Brunke*
67 Ralph Brunke*; Rose Zgodzinski
68-71 Ralph Brunke*
73 Ralph Brunke*
74 Herb Swanson
75-77 © Marshall Williams
78 Wayne Miller, Magnum
80 © Marshall Williams
83 © Cartier-Bressen, Magnum
84 Herb Swanson
85-86 © Marshall Williams
88 P. Hawlin/CNRI/SPL from Photo Researchers; Mark Swindle*
91 Mark Swindle*
93-94 Mark Swindle*
96 Barry Slaven, M.D., Medical Images; Custom Medical
97 Mark Swindle*
99 Mark Swindle*
100 Dan Stultz*
102 Detail of drawing: *The Analysis of the Shoulder*

Girdle by Leonardo da Vinci (1510). Permission of Her Majesty Queen Elizabeth II (Royal Library, Windsor Castle, Windsor, England); Lew Long, The Stock Market
104-105 Charles Wellek*
106 OTIDRA Enterprises, Inc. (Ralph Brunke*)
107 Joe Rogers*
108-109 OTIDRA Enterprises, Inc. (Ralph Brunke*)
111 Joe Rogers*
112-113 OTIDRA Enterprises, Inc. (Ralph Brunke*)
115 Joe Rogers*
118 J. A. Hobson, M.D.
121-122 J. A. Hobson, M.D.
126 David R. Frazier
129 Ralph Brunke*
132 Jacques M. Chenet, Gamma/Liaison
133 Michael Ponzini, Focus on Sports
136 Barbara Cousins*
138 Bud Freund, West Light; Didier Givois, Agence Vandystadt from Photo Researchers
141 Paul R. Meyer, Northwestern Memorial Hospital; Barbara Cousins*
142 Oscar Izquierdo, Rehabilitation Institute of Chicago
143 Barry Slaven, M.D., Medical Images; The Upjohn Company
146 G. Brian Karas*
150-154 G. Brian Karas*
156-157 G. Brian Karas*
160 Carlos Fernandez/SPL from Photo Researchers; David Wagner, Phototake; Michael Seigel, Phototake; Gower Medical Publications/Biophoto Associates from Photo Researchers
164 Barbara Cousins*
166 Julie Pace*
169 Julie Pace*
170 Life Scan Inc.; Julie Pace*
171 Julie Pace*; Medic Alert
175 Cary Henrie*
179 Cary Henrie*
180-181 Cary Henrie*
183-186 Cary Henrie*
188 Superstock
192 Barry King, Gamma/Liaison
193 Colin Bidgood*

196 Dizziness and Balance Center, Wilmette, Ill. (Ralph Brunke*)
197-199 Neurocom International, Inc.; Dizziness and Balance Center, Wilmette, Ill. (Ralph Brunke*)
203 Dan Reynolds, Medical Images
205 Kevin Beebe, Custom Medical
207 Ira Wyman, Sygma
208 SIU from Photo Researchers
210 Catherine Pouedras/SPL from Photo Researchers; Ira Wyman, Sygma
213 Will and Deni McIntyre, Photo Researchers
214 Dan Reynolds, Medical Images
240 Bernd Kappelmeyer, FPG
243 Frank Founier, Contact Press Images
244 Association of Science Technology Centers
248 FDA
249 Hanley & Savage, The Stock Market
251 Ralph Brunke*
256 Michael A. Keller, The Stock Market
260 Ralph Brunke*
262 C. Dominique Toran-Allerand, M.D.
263 Paul Merideth
268 AP/Wide World
269 A. Sieveking, Photo Researchers
272 Lawrence Migdale
273 Gerber Products
275 3M Corporation
277 Gary Meek, Georgia Tech Research Corporation
285 OTIDRA Enterprises, Inc. (Ralph Brunke*)
286 Johan Elzenga, Tony Stone Images
288 Chuck Keeler, Tony Stone Images
291 Mugshots from The Stock Market
292 Roy Morsch, The Stock Market
295 Mark A. Johnson, The Stock Market
298 Steve Murez, Rapho from Black Star
299 Robert Yager, Tony Stone Images
302 AP/Wide World

303 Diane Walker,
     Gamma/Liaison
304 Jim Borgman, *Cincinnati
     Enquirer* © 1994. Reprinted
     with special permission of
     King Features Syndicate.
307 Gay Bumgarner, Tony Stone
     Images
308 Superstock
309 Gary Meek, Georgia Tech
     Research Corporation
310 Yvonne Hemsey,
     Gamma/Liaison
311 © 1994 Roz Chast
313 Terrence McCarthy, NYT
     Pictures; Mary Beth Saffo
315 Amendola, Imago 2000
318 Rick Rickman, Matrix
321 Archibald Candy
     Corporation
322 Stephen Crowley, NYT
     Pictures
326 Joe Feingersh, The Stock
     Market
327 Kevin Beebe, Custom
     Medical
328 Jack M. Gwaltney, Jr., M.D.,
     University of Virginia School
     of Medicine
330 Ralph Brunke*
334 CNRI/SPL from Photo
     Researchers
336 National Cancer Institute
338 AP/Wide World
341 Gary Buss, FPG
342 David R. Frazier
344 Stanley Leary, Georgia Tech
     Telephoto
345 Ellen Going Jacobs*
347 Ocean Spray Cranberries,
     Inc.
348 Norvia Behling
350 Yoav Levy, Phototake
352 Don Hogan Charles, NYT
     Pictures

World Book Encyclopedia, Inc., provides high-quality educational and reference products for the family and school. They include THE WORLD BOOK~RUSH-PRESBYTERIAN-ST. LUKE'S MEDICAL CENTER~MEDICAL ENCYCLOPEDIA, a 1,072-page fully illustrated family health reference; THE WORLD BOOK OF MATH POWER, a two-volume set that helps students and adults build math skills; THE WORLD BOOK OF WORD POWER, a two-volume set that is designed to help your entire family write and speak more successfully; and the HOW TO STUDY video, a presentation of key study skills with information students need to succeed in school. For further information, write World Book Encyclopedia, Inc.; 2515 E. 43rd St.; P.O. Box 182265; Chattanooga, TN 37422-7265.